Educational Audiology

IAN TUCKER and MICHAEL NOLAN

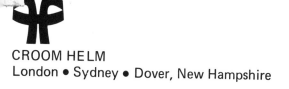

CROOM HELM
London • Sydney • Dover, New Hampshire

© 1984 Ivan Tucker and Michael Nolan
Croom Helm Ltd, Provident House, Burrell Row,
Beckenham, Kent BR3 1AT
Croom Helm Australia Pty Ltd, First Floor, 139 King Street,
Sydney, NSW 2001, Australia

British Library Cataloguing in Publication Data

Tucker, Ivan
  Educational audiology.
  1. Hearing disorders in children
  I. Title   II. Nolan, Michael
  618.92'0978   RF291.5.C45

ISBN 0-7099-2430-5
ISBN 0-7099-2464-X

Croom Helm, 51 Washington Street, Dover,
New Hampshire 03820, USA

Library of Congress Catalog Card Number: 84-45286
Cataloging in Publication Data applied for.

Printed and bound in Great Britain by
Biddles Ltd, Guildford and King's Lynn

CONTENTS

Foreword *Thomas J. Watson*   vii

Acknowledgements   xi

Introduction   1

1. The Ear   4
2. Diagnosis of Hearing-impairment in Children   9
3. Parent Guidance and Counselling   109
4. The Hearing Aid as a System   131
5. The Earmould   172
6. Technical Aspects Relating to the Efficient Use
    of Hearing Aids   202
7. Hearing Aids Not Entirely Worn on the Listener   236
8. Aid Fitting Procedures and Amplification
    Requirements of Children   288
9. The Developing Hearing-impaired Child   314
10. Educational Provision and Placement   352
11. The Child With Difficulties Additional to Deafness   381

Index   403

TO KATIE AND SHEILA

FOREWORD

Although several of the disciplines basic to the field of audiology had been developing over many years, the term itself only came into existence in the mid-1940s largely as a result of the aural rehabilitation services which were being provided for deafened veterans in the United States of America during the Second World War. The first textbook (*Hearing and Deafness*, edited by Hallowell Davis) appeared in 1947 and in 1950 the First International Course in Audiology took place in Stockholm. As one fortunate enough to participate in that course I can testify to the excitement that we felt at the possibilities which seemed likely to follow this synthesis of disciplines in the interests of deaf people and, even more specifically, deaf children. In 1951 David Kendall and I wrote a short paper in which we expressed our belief in the importance of this development for the educational treatment of deafness. Even then we discounted the idea of the 'Complete Audiologist' pointing out that no one could possibly be expected to be an expert in all the fields comprising this new discipline. That this is true has become more evident over the years with the increasing depth of knowledge that has been acquired by workers in the diverse fields which make up the totality of audiology. Increased knowledge of aetiology and preventive measures, new surgical techniques, acoustics, sound perception, linguistic development in children, the application of electronics to physiological measurement, and psychology, point only to some of the areas in which great advances have been made in the last 35 years and accentuate the fact that not only has the study of audiology been advancing on a broad front but that within each area of the front there has been a tremendous increase in the depth of that knowledge. Certainly no one person could claim to be an expert in all these areas and it has been the possibility of increased specialism that has made these developments possible.

One sector of this exciting and advancing field is educational audiology. Although I have called it a sector it is only so by virtue of its specific interest in children with impaired hearing. Like geriatric audiology, at the other end of the age-scale, it is dependent for its development upon information and expertise which come from other disciplines – psychology, communication engineering, electronics, neurophysiology, linguistics, education and others. Its particular significance as an essential area of further study and research was recognised as early as 1953 by the late Professor Henk Huizing of Groningen who, in that year, organised a course on what he called Paediatric Audiology. Since then, every new development that could contribute to our knowledge of deafness in childhood, its discovery, assessment and alleviation has widened this particular field. In 1958, the University of Manchester instituted the first Diploma in Audiology in the United Kingdom as a postgraduate course of study and practice. Although it did not relate solely to educational audiology, it was strongly oriented to that particular area and established a training ground for those who were to practise educational audiology in the field. Its early students, who came from all over Britain and from overseas, returned to posts in schools, in school health clinics, as organisers of services and as peripatetic teachers of the deaf where their newly-acquired knowledge and skills helped to change the pattern of assessment, guidance to parents and the educational treatment of deafness.

This book is a logical successor to these developments. My former colleagues at Manchester University, Ivan Tucker and Michael Nolan, from their different backgrounds, have put together the knowledge and expertise they have gained through their experience of teaching undergraduate and postgraduate students in clinics and in the lecture room and in counselling parents of countless hearing-impaired children. The result is not only a comprehensive and up-to-date account of the 'state of the art', but an equally valuable guide to practice. The scope of the work is in keeping with their exposition of the role of the educational audiologist. My own belief is that the function of the educational audiologist should be to enable a hearing-impaired child to obtain early and high quality listening experiences and to provide his parents with the support and knowledge that will enable them to ensure his optimal psychological, social and linguistic development. Such a description, in fact, corresponds fairly closely to the main areas which have been treated in the text below – early diagnosis and how it may be effected, the provision of hearing aids and how they may be used to best advantage, the importance of early and appropriate counselling of parents followed by ways in which they may contribute towards the child's linguistic development, and the problems that additional handicaps may bring to the management of a hearing-impaired child. This very brief summary of the contents of this book does less than justice to the authors who have, in fact, dealt with each of these major topics in several chapters which contain much detailed information essential to those already working in the field or wishing to become involved in it.

I believe that the range and depth of the information presented here contains a salutary and challenging message to those working in the field. The message is that educational audiology is a serious, wide-ranging and well-documented discipline with which practitioners need to be very familiar if they are to do the best that is possible for hearing-impaired children. This book charts a way, based on a long background of successful experience, by which that end may be achieved.

Thomas J. Watson

ACKNOWLEDGEMENTS

Our first thanks go to Dr Thomas Watson, now retired from the Department of Audiology at Manchester University, but an audiologist of international stature. Many areas of the world owe much to his influence and he would certainly be regarded as one of the first 'Educational Audiologists'. We owe him a lot for his kindness in agreeing to write the Foreword to this book and for his influence on our thinking about educational audiology.

We are also most grateful for the unstinting help of friends and colleagues, some of whom have read and commented on chapters of this book. We are particularly grateful to David Bond, Mary Hostler and Conrad Powell for help of this kind. We must acknowledge, however, our colleagues Wendy Lynas, Hilary Barratt, Elizabeth Midgeley and others from whom we have sought advice about various aspects of the book. Most of these people have, at some time or other, worked in the Department of Audiology and Education of the Deaf at Manchester University, under the Leadership of Professor Ian Taylor. Professor Taylor has provided us with the environment in which to develop our ideas and for this we are most grateful.

Many of our friends in the hearing aid industry have helped us with advice and some illustrations of equipment. Many thanks to David Griffiths (Photographer) and the University Department of Medical Illustration who have, between them, provided the bulk of our text illustrations.

INTRODUCTION

When we were planning this book we were hard pressed to find a suitable definition of an 'Educational Audiologist' since in this developing multi-disciplinary area the role of contributors to audiology is still being formed and shaped. In the United Kingdom the only provision for postgraduate educational audiology training is at the Manchester University Department of Audiology and Education of the Deaf. There are, however, many people in the field of education, who are doing some of the jobs we would regard as functions of the educational audiologist – but without the appropriate training. We hope that this book may help them, but at the same time stress the need for advanced training, and preferably, certification of all audiologists. Many visiting teachers of the deaf are doing largely educational audiology work rather than teaching support work and it is likely that only the keenest have read enough and attended a sufficient number of short courses and conferences really to do justice to the job. In the United States certification is conducted by the American Speech Language Hearing Association. It is only by advanced training and improvements in levels of skill that we feel there will be a move towards improvements in the services for hearing-impaired children. This also applies in audiological medicine and audiological science. The development, in the United Kingdom, of establishing a specialism in audiological medicine, with consultancy posts and a recognised training procedure has been a most important one. When the consultancy is well established it should mean that all children can be referred to an *audiological* specialist, not a specialist in another field with a 'smattering' of audiology. Similarly, we believe that schools and services for hearing-impaired children should be able to call upon the services of a specialist, qualified, educational audiologist.

We would be the first to admit that 'training' is not everything and would like to see an initial period after qualification being undertaken with a form of supervised 'practice'. This is already advocated for audiological scientists. The supervised practice in medical audiology could be at senior registrar level; in educational audiology it would not be so easy to manage, but early experience must be varied and *managed* if it is to be valuable.

The educational audiologist should be involved with other co-professionals in the initial assessment and be heavily responsible for the ongoing audiological management of the child, this bearing in mind the often limited information available from the initial assessments. We stress the need to work as a *team*; the medical person, the scientist and the educationalist each bringing something of their special skills to audiology. The hearing-impaired child will benefit from our co-operative approaches to assessment and problem solving. The initial fitting of amplification may well be a team responsibility with the educational audiologist taking on the follow-up amplification management. This would include 'educational' amplification such as FM systems. They should have detailed knowledge of earmould provision including the effects of texture and parameters relating to the acoustics of earmoulds.

Educational audiologists are frequently involved in training and assessing health visitors (who will have previous training as nurses) who carry out the initial screening procedures. In the United Kingdom there is a need for greater standardisation of training and monitoring of this screening service.

Work in guidance and counselling should be co-ordinated by educational audiologists and certainly there is a special component on this in the courses at Manchester. There is a great need for further training in the area for all teachers of the deaf who are involved.

The educational audiologist in the United Kingdom is highly likely to contribute to the team decision on educational placement and in the United States to be involved in the preparation of the Individualised Educational Programme (IEP). He will also provide support for children in ordinary schools in co-operation with visiting teachers of the deaf. In many education authorities the educational audiologist takes part in the progress monitoring of children so placed and they will certainly be involved in the detailed management and troubleshooting of hearing aid systems. There is also the growing role of fostering the links between audiological specialists and ordinary school teachers.

Finally, the educational audiologist has a major role to play in providing audiological management in schools for the deaf. It is his job, whatever the prevailing medium of instruction, to ensure that the children make the maximal use of their residual hearing. It is also his responsibility to ensure that if simultaneous methods of communication are used that he becomes proficient at the manual component. There is a growing, and we believe welcome, involvement of the educational audiologist in the management of the severely multiply handicapped child.

This book is primarily a book for practitioners. Indeed we think it is a book for anyone who sees the management of hearing-impaired children as going beyond the fitting of an aid — it goes into the efficiency of that fitting, into family relationships and interaction, into the school experience and social experience of the child — and when management takes this wide viewpoint we believe there is a real chance of better helping the hearing handicapped child to achieve his full potential.

1　THE EAR

The human ear basically comprises three distinct parts — outer, middle and inner ear (Figure 1.1).

The outer ear is made up of:

1. The pinna, which is a trumpet shaped flap of elastic cartilage attached to the head by ligaments and muscles.
2. The external auditory meatus, which is a bony canal lined with skin and cartilage continuous with that of the pinna. It has sebaceous glands (ceruminous glands) for secretion of cerumen (wax) which helps to keep the ear clean and clear of foreign bodies.
3. The tympanic membrane terminates the external auditory meatus. This is a thick semi-transparent partition of fibrous connective tissue. It has three layers — the outer layer being skin lined, the inner being covered with mucous membrane. The membrane not only acts as the receptor of vibrations, but also serves as a barrier to shelter the delicate contents of the middle ear. It provides an acoustic dead space so that air vibrations in the middle ear are broken up and dissipated and thus do not exert pressure against the round window in competition with vibrations coming through the cochlea in the other direction from the oval window.

The middle ear comprises a small air-filled cavity beyond the tympanic membrane which contains three tiny bones or ossicles. These bones are known as the malleus, incus and stapes. They are suspended across the middle ear cavity from eardrum to oval window, another smaller membrane situated in the bony wall between middle ear and inner ear. The malleus is in constant contact with the eardrum. The incus is connected to the malleus at one end and to the stapes at the other end. The footplate of the stapes fits snugly against the oval window.

The anterior wall of the middle ear provides an opening to the Eustachian tube, which is a narrow tube running from the nasopharynx to the middle ear. It is normally closed but opens to allow pressure equalisation in the middle ear upon swallowing or blowing of the nose.

The inner ear is a complicated arrangement of tubes filled with

4

Figure 1.1: The Ear

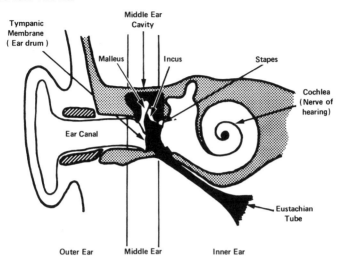

watery fluid. Part of this arrangement, the cochlea, is concerned with hearing and part, the utricle and semi-circular canals, with our sense of balance. The cochlea lies just beyond the middle ear cavity and is shaped like a snail shell of two and a half turns. The oval window is situated in the outer wall of its bony casing. The cochlea is divided into three chambers, scala vestibuli, scala tympani and cochlear duct. The two scalae are in effect parallel circular stairways within the spiral, the upper-scala vestibuli, the lower-scala tympani. Both contain a fluid, perilymph, which resembles cerebrospinal fluid. They join at the helicotrema at the top of the spiral. The upper scala connects to the oval window, the lower scala to the round window, a second membrane in the party wall between middle ear and cochlea. This membrane is slightly smaller and more compliant than the oval window.

The cochlear duct is a wedge-shaped compartment lying between the scalae. It contains the fluid endolymph which resembles intracellular fluid. There is no direct connection between the perilymph and endolymph. The cochlear duct contains the sensori nerve endings of the auditory nerve embedded in two membranes — the basilar and tectorial membranes. It is generally agreed that the nerve fibres constituting the auditory nerve (of which there are thought to be up to 30,000) are sensitive to sound of particular pitch. Those fibres that are sensitive to high pitch sounds are thought to lie towards the outer end of the spiral near the oval window, while those sensitive to low pitch lie in the innermost part near the apex. All of the fibres come together in a bunch as they leave the cochlea and constitute the nerve of hearing which conveys information to the cortex.

If one imagines a sound-wave travelling from source, for example, a musical instrument to receiver, that is, the ear, it becomes possible to appreciate the marvellous way that nature has equipped man so that he is able to perceive such sounds and derive pleasure from them. When a source emits sound it basically sets up vibration in the surrounding medium. Sound is in fact energy produced whenever an object is set into vibration. In our world this medium is the gaseous medium of air and it is via the air molecules that sound energy (that which produces vibration) passes from source to receiver. The vibrating source sets up tiny disturbances in the surrounding medium — these disturbances being rises and falls of air pressure relative to the normal ambient pressure. The pressure changes are tiny — for example, the pressure change produced by a 'just audible' tone in the mid-frequency region ($\sim$1500Hz) is 0·00002Pa, while we live under an air pressure of 100,000Pa. Very painful sounds have a pressure of about 20Pa.

As the sound-wave travels through the medium, the sound energy is being passed on by the air molecules via vibration. Eventually, the sound-wave will arrive at a listener. From the viewpoint of the sound-wave it simply impinges upon a funnel (the pinna) which acts to feed the sound-wave down a natural tube (the ear canal) to a terminating membrane (tympanic membrane) which is able to vibrate in response to the sound pressure variation and hence 'pass on' the sound energy via mechanical vibration.

The sound-wave is enhanced on arrival at the eardrum. This is a result of head baffle and ear canal resonance. These combine to produce a 10-15dB enhancement in the frequency region 1·5 to 7kHz (Von Bekesy, 1960; Littler, 1965). The head baffle effects are centred around 5000Hz, the ear canal resonance around 2600Hz.

If a person is to perceive a stimulus it will be necessary to translate the molecular sound energy to fluid vibratory energy in the cochlea, which will in turn produce the electrical potentials of the auditory nerve fibres. This can only be achieved effectively in man by means of the conductive pathway of the human ear. The role of the conductive pathway is therefore an important one — to facilitate the efficient transfer of acoustic vibratory energy into fluid vibratory energy, with the resultant generation of electrical potentials in the auditory nerve.

One may ask why it is necessary to have a conductive pathway? Why not simply place the cochlea with oval and round windows at the entrance to the ear canal and let the air molecules pass on their acoustic energy to the perilymph via the oval window? The problem would be that very little energy would pass to the fluid molecules. It would be much like trying to set a trampoline into vibration by hitting it with a balloon. Most of the energy would be reflected. The basic problem stems from the fact that the air molecules are very light inelastic particles, while perilymph molecules are much denser and highly elastic. It is necessary to boost the incoming sound-wave (sound pressure) so that an effective transfer of energy to the fluid medium is achieved. In effect, an acoustic transformer is required to match the low impedance air medium with the high impedance fluid medium. These differ by a factor of approximately 300 (Haughton, 1980). The conductive pathway is designed to achieve this objective.

It has already been shown that the sound pressure at the tympanic membrane is enhanced relative to that at the entrance to the pinna by the resonance effects of concha and ear canal. This sound pressure acts upon the tympanic membrane and causes vibration. Two-thirds of the membrane area is involved in sound pressure transfer to the manubrium of the malleus — a passage of sound energy transfer from tympanic membrane to stapes footplate being achieved via mechanical vibration of the ossicles. The effective area of the tympanic membrane involved is approximately $55\,mm^2$. The sound pressure acting on this area is then concentrated upon the much smaller area ($3\,mm^2$) of the stapes footplate. Now by definition:

$$\text{Pressure} = \frac{\text{Force}}{\text{Area}}$$

$$\text{if } P\text{ drum} = \frac{\text{Force}}{\text{Area drum}}$$

$$P\text{ footplate} = \frac{\text{Force}}{\text{Area footplate}}$$

$$\therefore \ P\text{ footplate} = \frac{P\text{ drum} \times \text{Area drum}}{\text{Area stapes}}$$

$$P\text{ footplate} = P\text{ drum} \times 18$$

The sound pressure at the stapes footplate is therefore enhanced by a factor of ~ 18, relative to that at the tympanic membrane.

Furthermore, the ossicles may be considered as a series of levers. Since the length of the manubrium and neck of the malleus is longer than the long process of the incus, a mechanical advantage of $1\cdot3$ results. This increases the pressure at the stapes by a further factor of

1·3 so that the overall boost to sound pressure at the stapes footplate is approximately a factor of 23 (i.e. 18 × 1·3). In decibels this is equivalent to a factor of approximately 27 dB.

Overall, therefore, the pressure at the stapes footplate is enhanced so that a reasonable degree of impedance matching occurs. It is of interest to note that work on the transfer function of the conductive pathway (Zwislocki, 1975) using equivalent circuits suggests that the frequency dependence of our auditory thresholds is determined principally by the transfer function of the conductive system. This is why for free field listening our ears are most sensitive in the mid-frequency region (Robinson and Dodson, 1956).

Vibrations that are transmitted to the oval window by the footplate of the stapes set up vibrations in the perilymph which surrounds the membranous labyrinth containing the end organs of hearing and balance. The vibrations spread upward in the scala vestibuli, are transmitted through Reissner's membrane to the endolymph and thence through the basilar membrane to the scala tympani where they pass downward to the round window. The vibrations of the round window therefore occur a fraction of a second later and in the opposite direction (opposite phase) to that of the oval window. The vibrations of the basilar membrane cause a pull or shearing force on the hair cells attached to the tectorial membrane. This action transforms the fluid vibratory energy into electrical impulses that stimulate the fibres of the acoustic nerve (eighth cranial nerve).

References

Bekesy, G. von (1960) *Experiments in Hearing*, trans. and edited by E.G. Wever, McGraw-Hill, New York

Haughton, P.M. (1980) *Physical Principles of Audiology*, Medical Physics Handbooks 3, Adam Hilger Ltd, Bristol

Littler, T.S. (1965) *The Physics of the Ear*, Pergamon Press, Oxford

Robinson, D.W. and Dodson, R.S. (1956) 'A redetermination of the equal loudness relations for pure tones', *British Journal of Applied Physics*, May, 66

Zwislocki, J. (1975) 'The nervous system' in D.B. Tower (ed.), *Human Communication and its Disorders*, Raven, New York

2 DIAGNOSIS OF HEARING—IMPAIRMENT IN CHILDREN

It is now widely accepted that it is advantageous to detect sensory handicap as early in life as possible. In no handicap could this be more important than in hearing-impairment where failure to detect may result in massive language deficit and damage to the child's developing personality. Indeed, too often detection results upon concern at the lack of language development. The child fails to hear and therefore fails to develop understanding and ultimately fails to learn to talk. It is of interest to note that in a very high proportion of cases parents are convinced that there is a hearing problem well before it is confirmed by the audiologist. We have noted this in our own clinics and Wallace (1973) reports parental detection to be 70 per cent. All audiological and/or medical practitioners faced by a mother who thinks that her child has a hearing-impairment should treat such comments seriously and take steps to resolve the situation, either by application of an appropriate test or referral to others competent in paediatric audiology – regardless of whether the child has been screened for hearing.

In the recent study of childhood deafness in the European Community (Martin *et al.*, 1981) details were presented on all children born in the Community in 1969 who had an average hearing loss of 50dBHL or worse in the better ear. Most of these children were enumerated in 1977 at eight years of age.

The results clearly demonstrate that there is no room for complacency in the area of diagnosis in any part of the European Community. Twenty-four per cent of the hearing-impaired children were *suspected* of being in difficulties with regard to hearing before one year of age and approximately two-thirds by the time they reached their third birthday. Yet slightly less than half of what are markedly hearing-impaired children had had their hearing loss *confirmed* by their third birthday. Even more disturbing was the finding that following diagnosis, which for many of the children can be considered nothing other than late, 37·8 per cent then had to wait up to a year before hearing aids were fitted. The conclusion of the study that these delays could 'have a deleterious effect on the ability of the deaf children to learn adequate speech' would be one with which anyone concerned with hearing-impaired children would concur.

Whether or not one subscribes to a critical period view of language development, that is, the view that if the child does not have the opportunity of developing spoken language at the appropriate time, then there will be longstanding damage to his capacities to learn language (a hearing-impairment which is undetected will have this effect), one is struck by the fact that even very bright hearing-impaired children who are detected late can fail to make the rate of progress necessary to enable them to start in the education system in the place where early diagnosis may have put them. They progress, but not fast enough to close the already enormous gap between them and their hearing peers. In practical terms late diagnosis can mean the difference between attending an ordinary school with professional support and attending a special school for hearing-impaired children. Bench (1978) has suggested that though the critical period theory is too strong, that is, if one person is deprived totally of language but learnt it at a later age then the theory fails, it may be possible to accept a concept of a 'specially sensitive' or 'vulnerable period'.

We conclude at this stage that only by early detection does the professional have a real opportunity of minimising the adverse effects of hearing-impairment. From our own clinical experience we are certain that the earlier habilitation is started the better the ultimate educational prognosis. Early diagnosis, therefore, is that first vital step on the road to a successful habilitative programme.

How Do We Detect Hearing-impairment in Children?

During the first five years of a normally hearing child's life it is usual for two tests of hearing to be applied — one in the first year of life and the other around the time the child enters full-time education. It is remarkable that during such a relatively short time period the child will have progressed from a test which may have been based solely on physiological reactions to sound (Blair-Simmons *et al.*, 1979) to a test requiring subjective responses which indicate perception of a test stimulus, that is, Pure Tone Audiometry. In fact by the age of five years the vast majority of children are able successfully to carry out the 'adult' test of hearing for pure tones.

It is vitally important at the outset of this section for the reader to be aware that there are two distinct categories of test employed in the assessment of hearing in children — SCREENING and DIAGNOSTIC.

The SCREENING test of hearing is a test of limits. It seeks only to set on one side for further investigation, a not inconsiderable (possibly 10 per cent) proportion of the total being screened, who for a wide range of reasons, hearing-impairment being only one, fail to respond in a totally 'normal' way. No attempt is made to actually measure a child's *thresholds* of hearing. The test stimuli are presented at a fixed level and should elicit a particular response from the child (this will be a function of the test being applied) if the child is to pass.

For example, in the Ewing (Ewing, 1957; Taylor, 1964; Sheridan, 1976) type sound field screening test of hearing used with all six- to nine-month-old babies in the United Kingdom (the DISTRACTION test described shortly) the stimuli are presented at 25/30dBA — the level at which normally hearing babies would 'just hear' in the typical test environment. The baby's response would be to turn and accurately locate the stimulus. If a baby responds at the screening level it is considered to have no significant hearing-impairment and has therefore sufficient hearing for normal language development. This must be the criteria which any screening procedure satisfies. A screening procedure must demonstrate a very low false negative detection rate. As mentioned earlier, for a variety of reasons a much higher false positive detection rate ($\sim$10 per cent) is to be expected.

If a child fails a screening test of hearing then that child has been identified as 'at risk' as regards hearing. No firm conclusion would be drawn on hearing acuity, quite simply because no measure of hearing threshold will have been made. The normal procedure in such cases as this would be a retest or rescreen of the child within two weeks. If the child failed to satisfy the test criteria on that occasion it would be referred for a DIAGNOSTIC test of hearing. Usually the rescreen would exclude a significant proportion of false positive babies (that is, babies who have normal hearing but who failed to satisfy the original screening criteria). The rescreen failures would require detailed investigations to clarify the position regarding their auditory acuity. This would involve DIAGNOSTIC procedures.

We stated at the outset of this chapter that our goal should be early identification of hearing-impairment. This can only be achieved by an EFFECTIVE screening programme.

Screening Hearing in Children

At the present time the most commonly used screening test of hearing of babies is the distraction test or sound field test. This test is behavioural — the child is expected to locate accurately a test stimulus presented out of vision at a minimal screening level (described in detail shortly). It is usually applied to six- to nine-month-old babies — an age when they are sitting unsupported and have good back and neck control, that is, optimal for the test. Other behavioural screening tests have been devised for use with older children (Ewing, 1957) and by the age of four years screening is achieved by pure tone audiometry.

A second group of screening tests which may be loosely described as 'objective' have evolved and are continuing to be developed. Many of these tests are intended as a means of identifying children as 'at risk', as regards hearing, very early on in life (neonatal period). These tests are not as widely practised or (for certain tests) as practical to apply for mass screening. However, the most recently developed 'computer-based crib' approaches, which are still undergoing validity trials, may find more general application as part of an ongoing audiological screening programme. None of the tests in this category can be considered truly objective because of the subjectivity in test design and in the interpretation of the test results. Furthermore, subjectivity on the part of the baby also plays a significant role.

Neonatal Screening (Objective Tests)

Testing the baby at birth might be regarded as the optimal situation, since the great majority of babies are born in maternity wards and are thus captives there for at least two or three days following birth.

The cluster of physiological responses provoked in a new-born baby (neonate) by a sudden sound involves changes in heart beat rate, respiration rate, head movement, body activity, muscle tone, head jerk and eye blink. These responses have been advocated for use as a means of screening hearing in new-borns.

Before the development of microprocessors the tests were administered by one or two clinicians. One clinician, the operator, administered the test stimulus (usually a relatively loud 90 dB SPL sound) while the other acted as observer and noted the baby's response (eye blink, limb movement, etc.) to the stimulus (Redell and Calvert, 1969).

Test Pitfalls

It is relatively simple to get inter-observer agreement on what is considered to be a response to sound. Unfortunately, the baby has all the possible patterns in its natural behaviour. The basic problem is distinguishing genuine from spontaneous responses. Furthermore, testing time required of personnel may be long and impractical in a busy hospital nursery. Clearly, trained personnel are required to apply such tests and as a result the efficiency of the test will depend on the skills of the observers.

Reflex Responses. A very commonly observed reflex response to sound is the auropalpebral reflex (APR) or eye blink response. This reflex was first noted by Wedenberg (1956) after tests on 20 children aged one to ten days. All normally hearing children in his sample exhibited the reflex in the frequency range 500 Hz to 4000 Hz to pure tones of 105 to 115 dB SPL.

The auropalpebral reflex (APR) shows similarity with the stapedius reflex threshold and anatomically there are similarities between the two. The afferent part (*n. acusticus*) and the efferent part (*n. facialis*) of the reflex arc are common to both, though the reflex centre of the stapedius is at a lower level of the brain stem (pons) than the APR (formatio reticularis). More recently a very large investigation by Froding (1960) on 2000 subjects all under the age of 30 minutes showed the APR to be a reliable response. Those who consistently failed to exhibit the APR were found to be neurologically impaired.

In view of the fact that eye blinks occur frequently anyway, it might be thought that clinically it would be difficult to distinguish random from stimulus-based responses. In fact, it has been suggested that spontaneous 'responses' giving a false positive can occur in up to 20 per cent of tests and there is a high rate of false negatives necessitating repeated testing (Bench and Boscak, 1970). Despite this many centres do make use of this reflex. Such centres use at least two clinicians to observe the subject's response either to a voiced plosive-vowel 'Ba' signal or to intense sound from a signal generator. The baby is usually in a relaxed state when the signal is delivered at a fixed screening level, of for example 90 dB SPL for plosive-vowel 'Ba'.

Recent developments of this principle have allowed automated recording of motor responses in babies.

Microprocessor-based Systems. It has proven possible to replace the operator and observer in neonatal testing by microprocessor-based auditory cradles or cribs. These devices seek to screen hearing on the basis of physiological reactions to sound in much the same way as the 'clinician' applied test. The most appropriate time to apply this type of test is about three to four days of age.

(i) The Crib-o-gram. The Crib-o-gram system employs a motion-detecting transducer attached to each crib or cot. The baby is stimulated by bursts of 92 dB SPL narrow band (2-4 kHz) noise and a microprocessor-based decision analysis system assesses motor activity from the highly sensitive motion detector in response to a series of 30 stimulus trials. Testing time is quoted as averaging 2½ hours but interruptions are permissible without affecting the screening process. The signal is delivered by a loudspeaker situated at the end of the child's cot (Blair-Simmons *et al.*, 1979).

(ii) Auditory Response Cradle. The Auditory Response Cradle (ARC) is a microprocessor controlled system which seeks to examine a baby's head turn, startle or head jerk, body activity and respiratory signals in response to sound stimulation. The system is automatic and takes three to ten minutes to complete a screen. The baby lies in the cradle which incorporates the non-contacting head turn, startle, body activity and respiratory sensors. Ear probes are used to deliver the test sound — a high pass broad band noise at 85 dB SPL acts as test stimulus (Bennet, 1979).

High pass noise is considered optimal for screening purposes because the vast majority of congenital deafness involves high frequencies.

Early results from ongoing validity trials of these systems are encouraging (McFarland *et al.*, 1980; Telsensory Systems Inc., 1982; Bennet and Wade, 1980).

It is important to remember that all of the neonatal tests described are screening tests. There is no quantification of hearing capacity nor determination of the site of the problem if one exists. Furthermore, there will inevitably, for a variety of reasons, be some degree of false negativeness in such testing, that is, hearing-impaired babies passing the test criteria — perhaps because a very moderate degree of hearing loss or the phenomenon of recruitment (abnormal growth in loudness) with a more severe hearing loss, enabled the babies to exhibit 'normal' responses to sound stimulation. As a matter of interest the minimal hearing loss detected by the Crib-o-gram is reported as 45 dB HL (McFarland *et al.*, 1980). There will also be some degree of false positiveness, whereby normally hearing babies will fail the test criteria. This will be a function of the baby's condition at birth and may rise to 20 per cent in 'sick' new-borns. While microprocessor-based tests in particular have potential for identifying hearing-impairment early in the life of some children, they will only prove effective if, and in many cases when, the subsequent follow-up DIAGNOSTIC programme is efficiently organised and appropriately staffed.

High-risk Registry. An alternative method of identifying babies in the neonatal period as being 'at risk' with regard to hearing is by means of an 'at risk' or high-risk register (Downs and Silver, 1972). Such an approach does not involve any screening of hearing function as such, more a by-medical-history-odds-type recognition of 'at risk' for deafness. The major pitfall of this approach is that it presupposes we know the predominant causes of neonatal deafness. The work of Taylor (1980) would seem to indicate that a yield of no more than 50 per cent can be expected using this register. Further, it is apparent that the incidence of hearing-impairment in certain types of 'at risk' category, particularly related to factors occurring around birth, will depend upon the quality of neonatal care (De Souza *et al.*, 1981). Table 2.1 lists the five features of the classical high-risk registry, together with others that have been suggested in the literature.

Table 2.1: Factors included in an 'at risk' register

1.	Positive family history of deafness
2.	Rubella, CMV, or other viral infection
3.	Premature delivery
4.	Hyperbilirubinaemia
5.	Maxilla facial anomalies
(a)	Bleeding
(b)	Foetal distress
(c)	Difficult delivery
(d)	Respiratory distress
(e)	Ototoxic drugs
(f)	Meningitis
(g)	Anomalies other than maxilla/facial
(h)	Sepsis
(i)	Low Apgars $\leqslant 6$ (5 minutes)

Source: after Blair-Simmons *et al.*, 1979.

Certain audiological services advocate a policy of follow-up and screening at six to nine months of age of only the high-risk registry babies. This policy is totally unsatisfactory because it will miss at least 50 per cent of the hearing-impaired babies in that authority at any one time.

General Comments Regarding Neonatal Testing

While the aim of a neonatal screening programme is early identification of children 'at risk' with regard to hearing, the programme must not, in the case of 'screen passes', be seen as the 'final pronouncement' on a baby's hearing capacity. It is not known, for example, how many babies have a progressive deterioration in hearing or acquire a sensori-neural hearing loss in the first year of life, or what is the precise incidence of secretory otitis media during early life. Neonatal screening must always be subjected to the scrutiny of what is arguably the most useful and effective screening procedure — sound field testing as pioneered by the Ewings (Ewing, 1957). Hence, all babies must be screened for hearing at six to nine months of age regardless of earlier test results. Because neonatal testing as described is a screening procedure, following rescreening it will be necessary to apply DIAGNOSTIC procedures to the rescreen failures, before any conclusions can be drawn about hearing capacity. It will therefore take time for the audiologist to acquire sufficient information on which to base the management programme. This is the very reason why the effectiveness of neonatal screening will only be as good as the subsequent follow-up programme.

When one considers that about one infant per thousand has a profound hearing loss (Ruben, 1972) and tests such as Crib-o-gram have a false positive rate of approximately 8 per cent in 'well' babies (McFarland *et al.*, 1980), it is obvious that great care must be taken not only in clarifying the hearing capacity of a baby, but also in the management of that baby's family. If neonatal screening becomes more universally practised, audiologists are going to have to face up to the particular dilemma of — 'how much information to give to parents?' It is vitally important not to alarm or seed doubts as to the 'perfectness' of a baby purely on the basis of a neonatal screen. If any information is to be given it must be based on the facts of a full diagnostic investigation and not simply on the possible inference of a screening test. This is of particular importance in cases where babies are not diagnostically assessed until sound field audiometry at six months of age. Parents would otherwise be left to get ever more anxious about a problem for which to them there seems to be no cure. Parental bonding and mother-child interaction could be seriously affected. The importance of good follow-up support and careful counselling for families is seen as a primary requisite in such a situation.

Electric Response Audiometry (ERA)

Electric response audiometry is a term that is used to encompass a collection of testing procedures that involve the recording of tiny electrical responses (potentials) that occur along the auditory pathway in response to acoustic stimulation (Gibson, 1978). There are in fact many different responses and each is classified according to the 'time after the stimulus' at which it occurs. This parameter is known as the latency. While many of these tests are particularly applicable to adults for identification of neurological disorders and objective measurement of hearing, some have been advocated for use in screening and diagnosis of hearing-impairment in children.

Such testing warrants the use of relatively sophisticated and expensive equipment operated by specially trained technicians. As a result it is not normally available for routine screening and is more usually found in specialist audiology centres where it may be employed in diagnostic procedures following screening failure or in assessing difficult to test children.

The PAM Response

It is of interest to note, however, that an instrument has recently been developed for screening of hearing based on the post-auricular myogenic (PAM) response (Flood *et al.*, 1982). This response is a reflex response to sound of the muscle behind the pinna (Kiang *et al.*, 1964). It is characterised as having a latency of about 15 msec and a large amplitude (see Figure 2.1).

As with all electric response audiometry measures, measurement is facilitated by the placement of three tiny electrodes, in this case one on the forehead, one on the scalp and one behind the ear on the mastoid bone. These electrodes sense the tiny electrical signals from the muscle in response to sound stimulation and a computer sorts and averages the results.

The test stimulus is a series of 60 dB SL clicks at the rate of ten per second with a maximum of 2000. The machine, which is portable, analyses the results and if the baby's response meets the programmed 'pass criteria' — latency 14-20 msec, D/S ratio less than 50 per cent, it passes the test and is considered to have sufficient hearing for development of normal language. Although the machine has facility for 80 dB SL clicks it would seem sensible for any child failing twice at the 60 dB SL level to be investigated by diagnostic procedures.

Testing may be carried out in any room with low background noise. The test is non-invasive, placement of the three electrodes

Figure 2.1: Measurement and resultant waveform of PAM response.

(a)

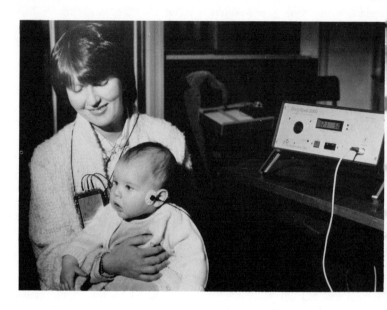

(b)

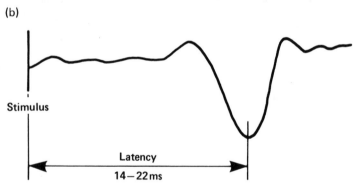

Stimulus

Latency

14–22 ms

on the head being the only contact with the child. The child is seated on the mother's knee and the sound is delivered from a loudspeaker built into the test unit. Testing time is approximately ten minutes.

The PAM response is myogenic and because of this it is necessary for the baby to have a high degree of muscle tone. This is why the optimal position for the baby is upright on mother's knee. It may often prove possible to test restless children because the muscle tone will be achieved fairly easily.

The main drawbacks of this approach relate to the variability in PAM response as a function of neck muscle tension. It can prove difficult to obtain even in subjects who have been instructed to tense their neck muscles. Absence of response is therefore not necessarily abnormal. It is not possible to obtain the response in sleeping children. The response provides no information on the baby's cortical response to sound.

The published results to date on screening by this approach are interesting (Flood *et al.*, 1982). The test is by no means absolute having both false positive and false negative aspects. The majority of false negatives in the Flood study were reported as not suffering sensori-neural deafness but secretory otitis media. This may have arisen after the PAM test. However, two 'false negative' children were subsequently found to have a high frequency sensori-neural hearing loss which was reported as 'not deafness for the speech frequencies'. Unfortunately, the follow-up sample of only 101 infants is much too small for firm conclusions to be drawn on the suitability of this approach for mass screening. It may find use in a screening service particularly in view of the fact that the test is recommended for use at the same age (six months) as the distraction test. Some degree of dual approach in screening may help to reduce the number of hearing-impaired babies who slip through the screening net.

Behavioural Tests of Hearing

The Distraction Test

In the United Kingdom behavioural screening tests of hearing are carried out routinely on *all* children (who attend child health clinics) by specially trained Health Visitors (nurses with additional qualifications in community nursing) or medical officers. In the main this job is the responsibility of the Health Visitor — in a Health Visitors' Association Survey (1977) 90 per cent of districts reported that Health

Visitors were responsible for hearing screening.

The first screening test is normally applied when the child reaches the age of six to nine months. Early work in the Department of Audiology at Manchester University showed that by this age normal babies have gained good back support and head control and are able to localise sounds provided these are delivered on a horizontal plane level with the child's ear. The response is so constant at this age that it is almost automatic and therefore provides a very convenient testing procedure. The test — the DISTRACTION test, is in fact used with children between the ages of six to eighteen months both as a *screening* test and *diagnostically* with screening failures. The closer the baby gets to the top end of the age range the more difficult the application and reliability of the test.

Figure 2.2: Layout of test for distraction procedure.

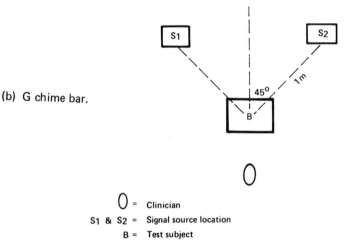

(b) G chime bar.

O = Clinician
S1 & S2 = Signal source location
B = Test subject

The mass screening of hearing in babies in the United Kingdom is carried out using behavioural techniques. The organisation of the test is such that when a baby reaches the age of 6 to 9 months the mother is sent an appointment asking her and baby to attend the local health centre where hearing tests are carried out. Since the test is a screen of hearing it is simply a pass-fail one. It is normally applied by two health visitors who have received training in the screening of hearing in young children.

The usual format of the test is to screen the baby for low, mid and high frequency stimuli. The screening level is set at 30 dBA. The child is required to respond by localising two separate signals from each frequency range at each ear if it is to pass the test.

The test layout is shown in Figures 2.2 and 2.3. The baby is seated on mother's knee in a slightly forward position with support at the waist. Babies who require a great deal of support, and this should not be the case at 6-9 months, are developmentally immature for the test and test results from such babies would be regarded with suspicion. In such children great effort would be being put into the physical requirements to turn, and signal levels required to elicit a turn would tend to be higher. Hence, screening failure would probably result. In summary, a developmentally ready child would be capable of sitting largely unsupported, with good head control, being capable of turning the head to each side without difficulty in order to locate signals of different frequency. The tester who is positioned in front of the baby gains his attention using, for example, a small toy. Meanwhile the second tester moves into position at the rear as in Figure 2.3, one metre from the child, at an angle of 45° and level in height with the child's ears. At the front the tester will relax the child's attention, perhaps by covering or removing the toy and at that point the sound stimulus is presented from behind. In order to be credited with a response the baby must hear the signal, turn and locate its position. The signal presentation level for screening is, as already mentioned, 30 dB A.

The tester who is positioned at the front is the judge of what is, or is not a response to an auditory signal. Various researchers (Moncur, 1964, 1968) have shown that there is very little difference between trained and naive judges as to what is a response. Chalmers *et al.* (1974) have suggested that a degree of observational skill in evaluating infants' behavioural responses to sounds is acquired rapidly at the very beginning of such work and that subsequent training or experience confers rather little additional expertise. It does not seem unreasonable to suggest that a careful observer will spot when a baby is responding to a sound signal. The real skill in the distraction test is for the front tester to manipulate the child to an appropriate attention state for him to be responsive to the signal. This involves the use of small, relatively uninteresting toys to first gain attention and then for that attention to the front to be plateaued when the rear tester is in position. It is important to remember that the activity need only be some- thing simple such as spinning an object on the table, or throwing a coin or ball into the air. A good working relationship between testers is vital since the rear tester must be ready to deliver the signal immedi-

Figure 2.3: The distraction test: (a) high frequency rattle.

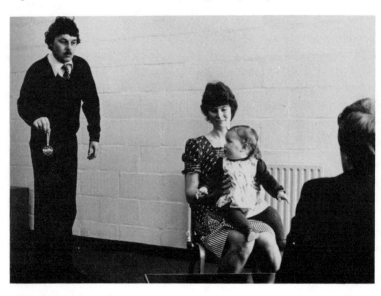

(b): g chime bar

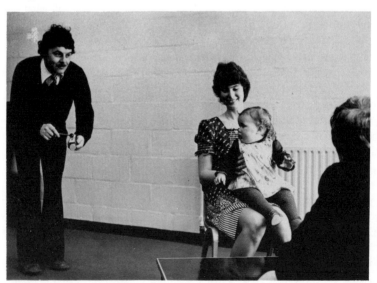

(c) warble tone.

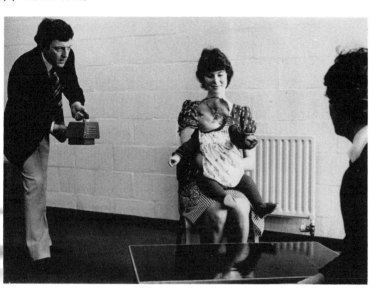

(d) voice.

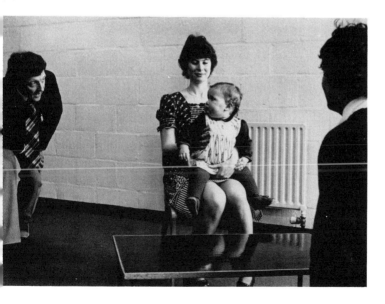

ately attention to the front is plateaued. The signal must be delivered from the right place, that is, three feet from the ear, on a horizontal plane which passes through the child's ears and outside the child's field of vision. The signal must be delivered at the right time — fractionally after the activity has been phased out at the front. The signal must also be delivered at the right level (30 dBA). It is important that the test design is such that normally hearing babies have every opportunity of satisfying the pass criteria. If signals are presented outside the horizontal plane this can lead to difficulty for the baby in localising the sound. For example, a sound presented above the head would almost certainly not be located until the baby was older, possibly 12-16 months.

Correct test application is vital for an effective screening programme.

The test must be carried out in reasonably quiet conditions (30/40 dBA) with little interference from visual distractors or from noise generated either within (for example, dental surgery above test room) or outside the building (for example, traffic noise).

Test Stimuli-frequency Specificity

One of the biggest drawbacks of the 'objective' screening tests so far considered relates to the test stimuli. It will have no doubt been noted that most of the tests used relatively intense, predominantly high frequency emphasis rightly resulting because of the fact that the vast majority of congenital hearing problems include at least high frequencies. However, it would seem desirable to ensure that a baby has sufficient hearing across the whole speech frequency region by using 'quiet' sounds so that even moderate hearing losses (<45 dBHL) are identified. This desire has influenced audiologists in their choice of stimuli for the distraction test. The most useful frequencies from a speech perception point of view range from 100 to 8000 Hz and the distraction test has therefore been designed to assess hearing in specific regions across this frequency range. Test items have therefore been developed in the low, mid and high frequency parts of this range. Robson (1970) has shown that *pure tone* signals require a higher signal presentation level than wider band more meaningful signals such as the human voice and rattles, etc., the latter being more emotive. For example, if the vowel 'oo' (as in shoe) is gently made and rhythmically presented, practically all of its sound energy is in the region below 500 Hz. A 'G' chime bar gently tapped with the knuckle is a good mid frequency item with most of its energy in the region of 1600 Hz. High frequency is tested by use of the consonant 's' where air is gently blown over the tongue and between the teeth with no voicing. This signal is presented naturally in a rhythmical fashion. Most of the energy of 's' when natural is in the high frequency speech region above 3000 Hz. A specially developed high frequency rattle which is available from the Department of Audiology, University of Manchester, is used on a very wide scale for screening. The sound energy is concentrated in the 8000 to 10,000 Hz region.

Figure 2.4: Bruel and Kjaer 2033 real time analyser.

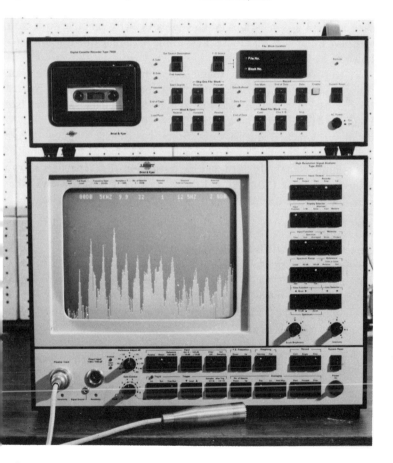

It is necessary for the stimuli of the distraction test to be frequency specific. There is no point in using sounds with a wide band width, that is, sounds containing a broad range of frequencies. Such sounds may be heard at the screening level by children with significant hearing-impairment. This may be best illustrated by recalling that the vast majority of congenitally deaf children have hearing-impairment in at least the high frequency region. While hearing in the mid and low frequencies will show differing patterns of severity, it is not unusual to see children with relatively normal hearing for low frequencies. If a wide band noise such as rustling tissue paper were used to assess hearing in such a case it would be possible for the child to hear the low frequency component of this sound at the screening level and pass the test. The only exception to the use of such a stimulus is the 'cup and spoon'. This stimulus is particularly emotive to a baby and may be used as an arousal item at the beginning of a test. It is not, however, counted as a test item.

It is possible to record sound and obtain a visual representation (image) of the frequencies constituting that sound. This is achieved by the use of a Sound Spectrograph or a Real Time Analyser (see Figure 2.4). It is therefore possible by looking at these images to determine which frequencies constitute a particular stimulus. Figure 2.5 has been designed to show the frequency specificity of some of the stimuli commonly used in the distraction test. They are shown at both screening (30 dBA) and raised levels. Figure 2.6 shows other stimuli which are used, but which are totally non-frequency specific.

Some Common Pitfalls and Problems of Distraction Testing

The major pitfalls relate to the introduction of 'signals' which should not be present, and which can lead the testers to believe the child is responding to the auditory signal when in fact he is responding to something else. These are:

1. Visual cueing — where the rear tester or his shadow moves into the peripheral vision of the child.
2. Tactile cueing — this can be the breath of the tester when delivering a signal or it can be a mother squeezing the child to encourage a response.
3. Auditory cueing — can be the introduction of a non-test sound by wearing creaky shoes or being heavy footed on hard floors, or from clothes' noise.
4. Olfactory cueing — using strong perfume or aftershave can invalidate the test, when the child responds to smell rather than sound.

Figure 2.5: Frequency composition of 'free field' sound stimuli (30 and 60dBA) which are frequency specific at the screening (30dBA) level.

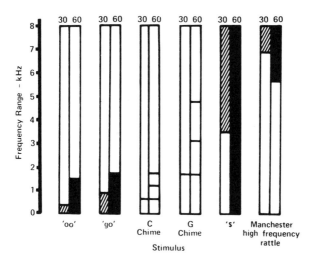

Figure 2.6: Frequency composition of 'free field' sound stimuli which are not frequency specific.

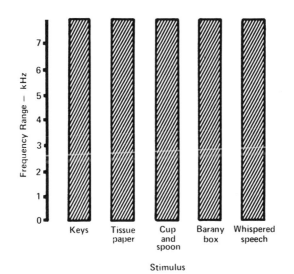

Figure 2.7: Distraction test — bad test set-up. (a) Tester too close, too far forward (danger of being in vision), stimulus too high. (b) Child sat incorrectly 'between' father's legs, held incorrectly and seated too close to father's chest.

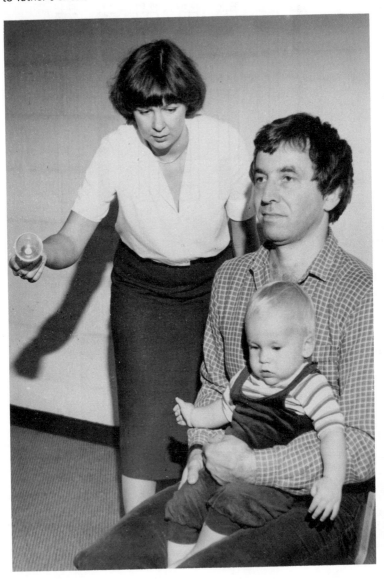

Testers also have difficulty in maintaining the correct attention levels, some do not vary the signals in order to maintain interest. It is also very important to set up the test situation carefully with the child sitting squarely on the parent's knees, being erect and not just resting back on the parent's chest (see Figure 2.7). Perhaps the greatest single difficulty is for the two workers to synchronise the attention state of the child and the signal input. If the signal is delivered too late the child may well become restless and start searching for other areas of interest, by turning towards the parent or trying to reach the toy. Experience of working together helps the testers in this respect. Where the child shows no interest in a particular test stimulus it is often useful for the person at the front to incorporate the same or similar sound in the activity he is using to control the child's attention. Beyond the age of one year some babies may quickly lose interest in the test sounds, turning once and then ignoring the stimuli if presented again. It is often helpful in these situations to vary the order of presentation of signals to each ear.

Finally testers should be aware of possible problems when other relatives are in the room. These should be seated in front of the child so that the child is not searching for them, but if there is any question of them providing distraction or other problems in the test they should be asked to leave and wait elsewhere.

If a child does not respond in the expected fashion on each side separately, if he persistently turns to one side only, or if he shows by moving his eyes and head from side to side that he is uncertain of the sound's location then he must fail the screen. The latter described behaviour may be observed in unilateral hearing loss. However, the fact that the test is free field means that information on unilateral acuity is difficult to obtain. Children with unilateral problems often do behave in a totally normal manner. The main point of note here however, would be, that by passing screening due to having one 'good' ear, the unilateral baby does have sufficient hearing for normal language development.

It will have been noted from a consideration of the stimuli normally used in distraction testing that these are non-electronically produced. There are good reasons for avoiding the use of electronic devices for mass screening. In particular, problems of reliability, calibration and consistency of product are of primary importance. The screening tests are applied by staff with little or no technical skill in maintenance of electronic equipment and backup support is often very limited indeed. Electronically generated stimuli are more useful in diagnostic

Figure 2.8: Variation in sound pressure level of a pure tone with increasing distance to sound level meter.

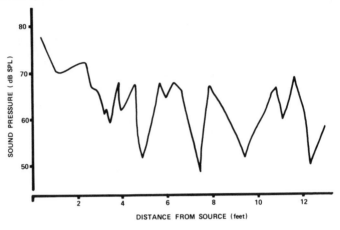

Source: after John, 1957.

setttings where technical backup and effective calibration services should be in evidence. There are additional factors that also militate against the use of such stimuli in free field screening. While pure tones are by definition 'frequency specific', they are not normally employed in free field hearing tests. This is because interaction of direct and reflected sound-waves may produce considerable variability of sound pressure at different locations in the vicinity of the child. This variability will be a function of the test environment (John, 1957; Dillon and Walker, 1982). In the light of the acoustics of typical test rooms used for mass screening, and from a consideration of Figure 2.8, it should be obvious why such sounds should not be employed in screening. To overcome the deleterious effects of standing wave patterns produced by pure tones in a test enclosure, warble tones and narrow bands of noise have been recommended for use (Reilly, 1958; Staab and Rintelmann, 1972; Dockum and Robinson, 1975; Robinson and Vaughn, 1976; Morgan *et al.*, 1979; Sanders and Josey, 1970; McDermott and Hodgson, 1982). Such sounds are frequency specific and because they are produced electronically, are not subject to the 'skill' of the tester factor involved in accurately producing many of the typical sounds of a distraction test. However, while such sounds appear to be suitable for screening application it is important to remember the earlier made points related to electronic equipment. In addition, both of these stimuli will be affected by the test enclosure and test set-up in relation to the interference factor. Overall, it is our considered opinion that at present such stimuli have more potential in diagnostic procedures related to hearing aid use than in mass screening of young children.

When a baby responds to a test stimulus of the distraction screen the response is almost automatic and will often be accompanied by a delighted smile upon localising of the stimulus. The tester in the rear will reward the child with a friendly smile and overall the baby receives both auditory and visual reward. Testing which employs the use of loudspeakers for signal presentation may lose the warmth and friendliness of the conventional screen — the baby would simply localise to a meaningless source upon hearing the sound.

It has proved to be advantageous both for achieving visual reward in screening, when such an approach is applied, and in conditioning training for diagnostic procedures related to hearing aid fitting, to make use of chasing lights around the speaker cabinet or smoked glass light boxes which contain small toys or cartoon-strip character slides. The boxes are situated on top of the speaker cabinets and are illuminated in response to a correct localisation on the part of the baby (Suzuki and Ogiba, 1960; Moore *et al.*, 1975, 1977).

The Co-operative Test of Hearing

This test is employed in the approximate age range of 18-30 months. Children at this age would be much more difficult to screen by distraction, because they will be developing powers of inhibition, that is, they will be capable of selectively ignoring the signals being presented to distract them. The child's motor development should be such that he has left behind problems of head control and sitting posture, in fact he should have good stability in the standing position and be able to pick up objects from the floor without falling.

In terms of the normal child's development of language the peak of jargon is at about 15-18 months. Even as late as 18 months 'talking' is largely a form of play or the accompaniment of play and this can be used to good effect in the co-operative test which only requires the child to understand language and carry out prescribed actions with simple toys. Unfortunately, this can also be a period of marked negativism which may manifest itself in the clinic by distinct *lack of co-operation*. However, experience has shown that handling can be crucial to the successful application of the test. Being positive and outgoing to a negative child is much more successful than being deferential. 'Would you like to . . .?' is much more likely to meet with a resounding 'No!' than 'Hey give that to your mummy' which is positive and includes the mother at a time when the child may feel strange in the clinic.

The test is again a test of limits (40 dBA) and involves the tester using toys (for example, men in a boat or wooden balls and a large egg box) to gain rapport with the child and then giving him a few simple instructions to follow such as 'give him to mummy', 'put him in the boat', 'put him on the table', as shown in Figure 2.9. The tester is positioned in turn on each side one metre from the child's ear. The child must respond to two commands at minimal level in order to pass that part of the test (see Figure 2.9).

Figure 2.9: The co-operative test. The child has been asked to 'give it to mummy'.

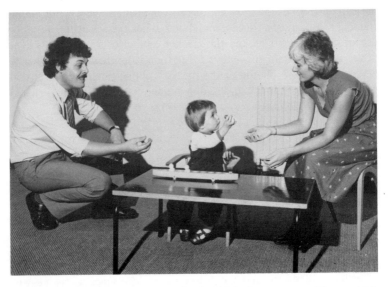

The child is then tested with the high frequency rattle or high frequency sibilant 's' as in the distraction test, but possibly with the child still seated at the table as in the co-operative part of the test rather than formally on mother's knee. The application of this part of the test would otherwise be the same. This approach sometimes reduces the problem of inhibition reported earlier. The child's ability to locate sound at a distance would be assessed using raised sound levels from a chime bar or other noise-making toy. This is done so as to try and identify unilateral losses. Because the test is free field and the ears are not effectively isolated it will often be possible for a child with such a loss to respond in the correct manner in the screening test. Such children may show more difficulty in accurately locating sounds from a distance — which should alert the tester to the possibility of unilateral loss. There is little doubt that this is the most difficult of the early behavioural tests to undertake from the clinician's point of view because child handling can be difficult. However, it is very important to attempt this test in the post-18 month age group because of the danger of the child inhibiting to distraction stimuli.

Failure in the high frequency part of the test alone would still be regarded as failure. With some hearing problems where hearing is relatively normal in the low frequencies it may be possible for the child to carry out all the simple tasks of the first part of the test, but still not be capable of hearing the high frequency consonants such as 's', 'p', 'f', 't', 'k', etc. All failures in the screening test should result in referral for full audiological investigation.

The Performance Test of Hearing

By the time the child is about 30 months he is often capable of waiting for a particular signal and then performing an action which indicates that he hears the signal. In this test a play situation is developed so that when the child hears the voiced command 'go' he puts a small wooden man in a boat, or a ball on a stick, or a peg in a board. Referral to Figures 2.5 and 2.6 on the frequency composition of the test stimuli will show that 'go' is a good low frequency stimulus. The 'go' signal is presented at minimal level, 30 dBA, at one metre from the ear with the tester out of vision (see Figure 2.10). Being out of vision in this test is most important. It is not satisfactory merely to cover one's face, since some facial movement is bound to occur and this will act as a signal to the child. The child, to pass the screening test, must respond to two minimal 'go' signals at each ear. The child is then trained to respond to the signal 's' as a test of the higher speech frequencies. The tester might ask the child to 'listen for sammy snake' or 'listen for the little whistle' and he is, on hearing these signals, encouraged to put a man in the boat or some such action, thus maintaining the play nature of the task. When the tester is convinced the child can respond in such a way to the signal he retires out of vision to three feet from the ear and screens each ear in turn for 'go' and then 's'. It is worthwhile remembering that for shy children it is a good idea to get mum to try the task first and for the child to then follow by example. It is also worth noting that the test can sometimes fail

Figure 2.10: The performance test. The child is responding to the stimulus 'go'.

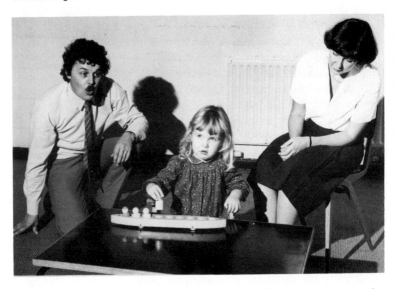

because the tester uses too complicated an instruction pattern for the child to cope with. It is often quite simply a matter of giving the child a little wooden man, then holding his hand, saying 'go', and guiding his hand to put the man in the boat. Thus, the child is conditioned to the task before he is expected to do it on his own. Alternatively, if the child is secure and confident, the tester might say 'Listen for "go" and when you hear it put the man in the boat.' The same applies to 's' but with children on the borderline of being mature enough for this test, it is at the point of change from 'go' to 's' that there may be a breakdown and then it may be necessary to distract for the high frequency.

Once the child is capable of confidently undertaking the performance test he is well on the way to carrying out the adult test of hearing pure tone audiometry. In fact at 'performance level', clinicians will introduce pure tone stimuli via the free field audiometer to assess whether the child will readily respond to pure tones as signals.

Diagnostic Procedures

If a child fails a screening test of hearing it is our opinion that he should be retested within two weeks and if still failing should be referred on for a full diagnostic investigation.

The aims of the DIAGNOSTIC test of hearing are twofold.

1. Quantify the hearing levels at distinct points across the speech frequency spectrum.
2. In conjunction with other components of the diagnostic test battery (for example, impedance, speech tests) classify the hearing problem.

The clinician having applied the diagnostic procedures should ideally be in a position to provide information on: (a) the degree of hearing loss, if any, across the speech frequency spectrum; and (b) where along the auditory pathway the problem is situated. This is a most important piece of information because it distinguishes between problems lying in the conductive pathway and those that are sensori-neural in origin (Figure 1.1). This distinction is vital because it will influence the procedures of the management programme. Problems lying in the conductive pathway can very often be cured by medication or ENT surgery. Sensori-neural problems must be seen as permanent and therefore if the loss is significant enough to affect language development hearing aids must be fitted at the earliest opportunity.

At the present time the vast majority of hearing-impaired children are screened for hearing at 6 to 9 months of age by distraction type sound field techniques based on the early pioneering work of the Ewings. Screening failures are then further assessed using distraction techniques at a diagnostic level.

A very small percentage of children are being screened in the neonatal period. Screening failures at this age present as a new challenge to audiologists who attempt to clarify the audiometric picture. It has, for example, already been pointed out that children are not developmentally ready for the distraction test until about six months of age. There will therefore be a danger of a 'gap' between failure of a neonate and firm clarification of the auditory picture if the follow-up programme is designed around the diagnostic distraction test. This is why we consider the value and effectiveness of early screening to be totally dependent on the follow-up programme. This is also the reason why we are concerned about the adoption of mass screening of neonates without consideration, thought and planning being put into the follow-up programme, particularly in view of the number of false positive babies whose parents may be otherwise put under unnecessary stress. At the present time those centres who employ neonatal screening include electric response audiometry in the early follow-up diagnostic sessions. The most appropriate procedure must be non-invasive and as a result Brain Stem Electric Response Audiometry (BSER) is generally practised (Barratt, 1980). The test requires expertise in application and only provides information on hearing in the higher speech frequencies. It can nevertheless provide a basis for early intervention particularly in very severe losses – the authors themselves having fitted hearing aids at 3 months of age partly on the basis of BSER information. It is true to say, however, that information from a distraction diagnostic procedure at 6 months is of vital importance for such children.

Electric Response Audiometry

There are four widely used tests (Gibson, 1978) that involve the recording of tiny electrical potentials that occur in the auditory system in response to sound stimulation:

(i)   Electrocochleography (E Co G, E Coch G)
(ii) Brainstem Electric Response Audiometry (BSER)
(iii) Post-auricular myogenic response (PAM)
(iv) Slow Vertex Cortical Potential

E Co G is an invasive procedure – a needle electrode normally being placed through the eardrum on to the promontory of the cochlea. This means that the child will require a general anaesthetic for the measure to be made. The process is therefore not practically suitable as a routine diagnostic procedure for screening failure.

The PAM response has already been discussed under screening of hearing and is not considered as sufficiently sensitive for diagnostic purposes.

Cortical electrical responses are unreliable and difficult to elicit in infancy.

BSER

The BSER response test involves recording from the scalp of tiny electrical potentials that are generated in the cochlear nerve and the auditory pathway up to the inferior colliculus in response to sound stimulation. In order to 'recover' the potentials from the ongoing random noise of the brain, it is necessary to deliver a large number of sound impulses in a relatively short time period. Clicks are therefore used to elicit the response. The potentials are recovered by three electrodes, placed on forehead (earth), vertex and behind each ear on the mastoid process. The information from the electrodes is processed by an averaging computer and the response appears on a visual display as a characteristic multiwave complex (Figure 2.11). The test is applied with the child sitting on mother's knee or more appropriately with young babies, during natural sleep — the child must be quiet and relaxed. The signal is presented via a circumaural headphone held against the ear.

Attention has been drawn to a relatively small group of children in the 'difficult to test' category who produced discrepancies between BSER and impedance thresholds (Mokotoff *et al.*, 1977), or BSER and E Co G measures (Ryerson and Beagley, 1981). Both studies recommended a thorough assessment of these children using other objective measures before firm conclusions were made about hearing levels. This is one reason why BSER information must be considered together with other information of the diagnostic investigation before any firm conclusions are drawn. The main limitation as regards management on the basis of BSER information relates to the fact that the test only provides threshold information for higher speech frequencies. Information on which to base a hearing aid prescription will therefore be very limited.

Research has shown that the BSER in young babies differs from normal adult response (Mecox and Galambos, 1974). The amplitude of the response is smaller, the wave complex is less well defined with only two or perhaps three waves, instead of the full five wave complex being present, and the waveforms occur slightly later in time. The response is present at 26 weeks gestation and then undergoes maturation process so that by about 18 months of age the normal adult latencies are present. Application of the test and, in particular, interpretation of test results requires the experience and expertise of specially trained staff.

Diagnostic Testing using Behavioural Responses

The behavioural tests of hearing employed in screening are also used

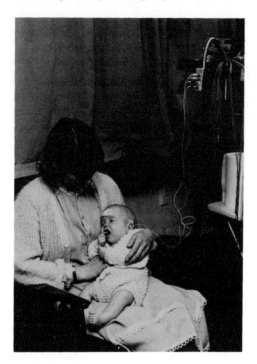

Figure 2.11: BSER testing. (a) Child being prepared for test — electrodes in place. (b) Measuring equipment. (c) Examples of resultant waveforms.

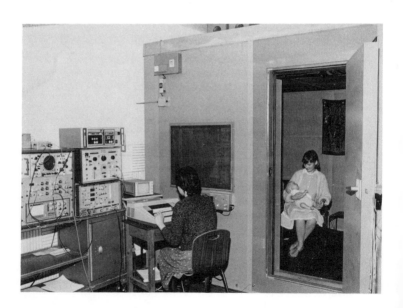

(c)

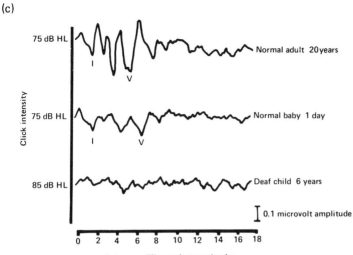

Source: After Barratt (1980).

at a diagnostic level. Whereas screening tests are applied by Health Visitors, diagnostic tests are normally carried out by audiologists who have received training in paedo-audiological assessment. The tests are applied in specially equipped audiology centres which are part of the hospital service or based in university establishments.

In the diagnostic test the signal levels must be raised until the baby responds reliably. The level of the signal should then be measured using a sound level meter mounted on a tripod, the stimulus being at the same distance from the meter as it is from the ear. The vast majority of sound level meters measure sound pressure level in dBA. It is necessary to state the decibel scale employed when quoting results — otherwise confusion may occur.

Frequency Specificity and Signal Presentation Level

It is important to realise that signals which are frequency specific when delivered at a screening level may not be specific when levels are raised. Examples of this are shown in Figure 2.5. It will be readily seen that 'high frequency' stimuli become broad band with a significant low frequency component when raised. This can have the effect that the child responds to the lower frequency component rather than the 'high frequency' stimulus and as a result an underestimation of high frequency hearing-impairment occurs. For example, when the performance test is carried out diagnostically, 'go' retains its frequency specificity to high sound pressure levels but 's' can only be raised to 50dBA before its frequency content becomes non high-frequency specific and spreads into the low frequencies.

It is advisable, when applying diagnostic procedures at moderately raised levels to move in closer to the child's ear – move to 15 cm rather than staying at 1 metre. This has the effect of increasing the sound pressure level at the ear and gives a better chance of obtaining frequency-specific information, particularly with partially hearing children. Great care must be taken, however, to ensure that the child does not respond by sensing the presence of the tester through visual, tactile or olfactory channels.

Warble Tone and Narrow Band Noise. In the case of severe and profound hearing loss it is not possible to elicit responses to the higher frequency stimuli before the upper sound pressure limit is reached. In such cases it may prove possible to obtain frequency-specific information by use of warble tones or narrow bands of noise. Such information should be interpreted with caution, however, unless the test stimuli have been thoroughly assessed by a Real Time Analyser. This permits a check of the frequency composition of the test stimuli. There is a danger, particularly at high output, of harmonic distortion and of low frequency contamination of a supposed high frequency signal. This 'real time' information will clarify the situation.

The ideal test set up is one where the loudspeaker is positioned directly in front of the child at 1 metre (see Figure 2.12). This helps to control the variability in the sound field at the child's test position. This format is suitable for application to children who are at the 'performance level' of hearing tests. However, it is not satisfactory where younger children are concerned (for example, distraction, co-operative test age-group categories). In such cases a localisation response is required and two speakers (again set up in a well defined reproducible format) are therefore required. These should be placed at a distance of 1 metre on a plane level with the ear, either at 45° to either side front on, or 45° to either side at the rear as in the format of the conventional diagnostic test (see Figure 2.13). Sound pressure at the child's test position must be measured by means of a sound level meter. A 'normal' threshold curve across frequency should be obtained for the test rig. This will help in equating the child's diagnostic response level to that to be expected when subsequent tests under headphones are applied. Use of a 'normal population' of young children in the distraction, co-operative and performance category is

Figure 2.12: Sound field testing using warble tones — aided and un-aided (performance approach).

(a)

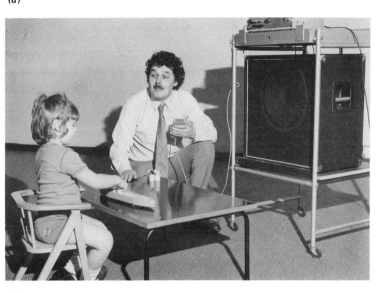

(b)

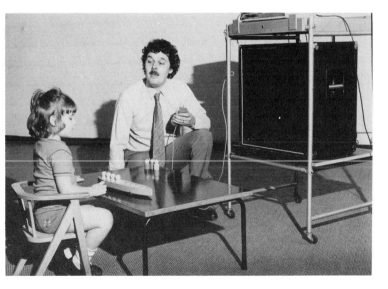

Figure 2.13: Sound field testing using warble tones (distraction approach).

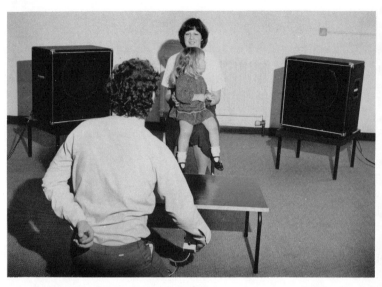

therefore desirable in obtaining this information. The test set-up may also prove valuable in estimation of 'real ear' performance of hearing aids and in investigation of children's dynamic range, as will be discussed later.

The Warble Tone. A warble tone is a sound of continually changing frequency — sweeping to and fro between upper and lower frequency limits. The warble tone has three parameters of importance, the bandwidth, modulation frequency and modulation waveform. The bandwidth is the difference between upper and lower frequency limits. The modulation frequency is an expression of the rate at which the tone sweeps to and fro. There are as yet no agreed standards on the required parameters of the warble tone for hearing assessment. However, bandwidths of 5 to 10 per cent of the centre frequency and modulation rates of 5-10Hz are commonly used with young children. Such parameters should be defined when reports of hearing levels are being made. If, for example, a test was carried out with a '1000Hz warble tone having a 5 per cent bandwidth and 10Hz sinusoidal modulation' this would mean that the tone was centred on 1000Hz, was modulated in a sine wave format, swept over a 50Hz frequency range (5 per cent of 1000Hz) and achieved 10 complete sweeps per second.

t is of interest to note the work of Walker and Dillon (1983) who ecommend a 10 per cent bandwidth and a modulation frequency f 20 Hz for use with the hearing impaired.

Management Foundations

t is true to say that at an early age great emphasis is placed upon ehavioural tests of hearing. Such tests provide the foundations upon vhich all management strategies are based. The results must there- ore be accurate and this will only occur if the tests are applied by killed professionals having a knowledge of the pitfalls and limitations f the procedures.

Asymmetric Loss

The behavioural tests are free field in nature and it is because of this hat it can prove difficult to quantify or even identify asymmetrical osses until closed-circuit pure tone audiometry under headphones s successfully applied.

It has been shown (Forse, 1980) that the optimal distance in the ehavioural tests which gives clinicians the best opportunity of identify- ng asymmetry in hearing is 1m for screening. For diagnostic purposes t is proposed that once the signal level is raised to 50 dBA at 1m the ester should move to 15 cm. While it is difficult to isolate the test from the non-test ear in free field tests, this can be attempted by occluding the non-test ear either with one's thumb or a commercially produced mould such as is used for swimming or in noise protection. Such an approach will only be practical with children at the perform- ance age level.

Severe Hearing Impairment

As hearing-impaired children mature their hearing is assessed by co- operative and subsequently performance procedures, before pure tone audiometry is eventually applied. When testing severely hearing-impaired children on the performance test it is a good idea to condition the child in vision and with his aids on (if he has them) and only when confident he is responding, first remove the aid and continue, then retire from vision and continue the test. In this way responses to 'go' can be obtained up to 110 dBA.

Pure Tone Audiometry

When children reach the age of three years it is generally possible with skilful handling to train them to carry out a pure tone audiometric test of hearing. This test can be treated as a natural development of the performance test — in fact once a child has developed sufficiently to the stage of waiting for the command 'go' and then performing a task in response, it is a relatively short step to performing the same action in response to a pure tone via a headphone. The child is therefore required, in play audiometry, to listen for pure tone signals usually at frequency stations in the range 125 Hz to 8000 Hz and respond by an action such as putting a little man in a wooden boat. It is very important with young children to retain the 'play like' nature of the test — the test being in fact a game as far as the child is concerned. The pure tone is by definition a signal of one frequency. The test can therefore provide clinicians with detailed information on the child's ability to hear in each ear separately across the speech frequency range (Figure 2.14).

Pure tone audiometry at a diagnostic level seeks to define the level where the patient can just hear the signal (threshold) in comparison with accepted norms. The signals are presented via headphones from a signal generator known as an audiometer. This device is built to stringent specifications and must be regularly calibrated (BSI, 1969). Basically, when the signal level of the audiometer is set to 0 dBHL, the output from the headphone will be at the normal threshold of hearing. A large number of normally hearing people have been tested via this 'standard' headphone (TDH39 in an MX41AR cushion) and 'normal' thresholds of hearing determined. The sensitivity of the normal ear in terms of frequency, when listening via the standard headphone is shown in Figure 2.15. It may be seen that our hearing is not equally sensitive over the speech frequency range. The audiometer takes this fact into account, automatically delivering each test frequency at the 'normal' sound pressure level when the signal level dial is set to 0 dBHL. A diagnostic test of hearing is therefore an expression of a subjects hearing levels in comparison with the accepted norm. If a child is reported as having a 40 dB hearing loss, this means his hearing is 40 dB worse than the norm at that frequency.

Screening

In 'screening' by pure tone audiometry the signal is set at a fixed screening level (~25 dBHL) and the child is tested under headphones for each ear. If the child fails to respond he must be rescreened within a fortnight and if still failing then referred on for diagnostic procedures.

Figure 2.14: Pure tone audiometry using play technique.

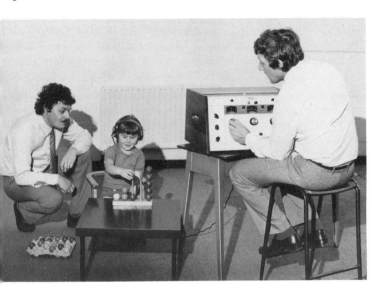

Figure 2.15: Sensitivity of the normal ear when listening through the TDH39 earphone in an MX41AR cushion (dB SPL) (BSI, 1969).

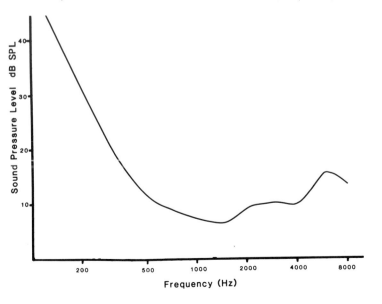

Diagnosis. In a diagnostic procedure involving the use of an audiometer a child will hear pure tone signals in the same way as in screening, that is, via headphones. Each ear should be tested separately. The tester should begin by giving the child a signal he believes the child will hear and the child should respond by performing a play activity (ball in an eggbox). The signal level should then be reduced in 10 dB steps until the child no longer responds. When the child no longer responds the signal is raised in 5 dB steps until he responds again. The signal level is again reduced in 10 dB steps to no response and up in 5 dB steps to a response. Threshold is defined as the lowest level at which responses occur in at least half of a series of ascending trials with a minimum of two responses required at that level (BSA, 1981). The resulting level is then plotted on a record form – an audiogram (Figure 2.16). This form comprises a horizontal axis on which the test frequencies are listed and a vertical axis corresponding to the reading of the sound level dial of the audiometer. The thresholds of hearing are recorded on the audiogram using a symbol O for right ear and X for left ear.

When a pure tone is produced by a headphone the signal travels down the ear canal and sets the eardrum into vibration. The vibrations are then conducted across the middle ear by the ossicles to the cochlea where conversion into electrical impulse occurs. This impulse then travels along the auditory nerve to the cortex. Testing under headphones therefore assesses the integrity of the whole hearing mechanism. Such tests are termed air conduction and measure a child's total hearing. If the test is carried out flexibly and includes play build-up, then children as young as 2½ years can be tested. If it is carried out without regard for child developmental features then it may still be impossible for children who are four or five. Play techniques with mum close at hand as in the earlier test are vital if reliable results are to be obtained. It would be hoped to test frequencies 125, 250, 500, 1000, 2000, 4000 and 8000 Hz but in young children whose attention span may be short, it would be better to gain information on a more restricted range of frequencies – but for each ear – than the whole range on just one ear. Where a compromise needs to be made the clinician should attempt to gain information in the low, mid and high frequency regions, for example, 250, 1000, 4000 Hz.

All the tests so far described have used air conducted sound signals. This means that results obtained are the sum total of the hearing loss, including loss through the conducting pathway of the ear canal, the tympanic membrane and middle ear as well as any sensori-neural loss

Figure 2.16: A normal pure tone audiogram.

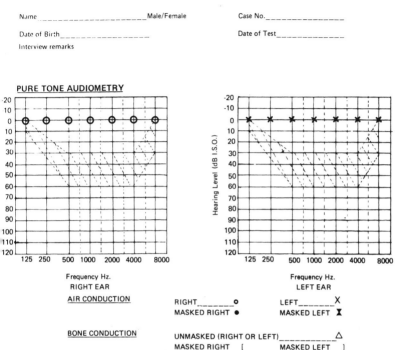

UNIVERSITY OF MANCHESTER
DEPARTMENT OF AUDIOLOGY AND EDUCATION OF THE DEAF

Name_____Male/Female   Case No._____

Date of Birth_____   Date of Test_____

Interview remarks

PURE TONE AUDIOMETRY

RIGHT EAR / Frequency Hz.
LEFT EAR / Frequency Hz.

AIR CONDUCTION

RIGHT_____ o   LEFT_____ X
MASKED RIGHT ●   MASKED LEFT ✗

BONE CONDUCTION

UNMASKED (RIGHT OR LEFT)_____ △
MASKED RIGHT   [MASKED LEFT   ]

associated with the cochlea or auditory nerve from cochlea to the
auditory cortex in the brain. It is common to group losses into three
categories:

(a) conductive or relating to the conducting mechanism;
(b) sensori-neural relating to the cochlea and beyond;
(c) mixed – a mixture of (a) and (b).

Discovering the Site of the Hearing Problem

Pure Tone Audiometry

One of the major purposes of audiometry is to help define the *nature*
of a subject's hearing problem in each ear, this after the *degree* of the

problem has already been defined. There are good reasons for this, as mentioned earlier — conductive problems generally being amenable to treatment with a resultant improvement in hearing extent, while sensori-neural problems must be seen as permanent.

Bone Conduction Testing. Once the air conduction audiogram has been obtained the clinician should proceed to bone conduction audiometry. This test is similar to that used with headphones excepting the fact that the signal transducer is a small bone oscillator (Figure 2.17) which is placed on the mastoid bone behind one ear. The child will perceive the same tonal effect as in air conduction testing. The signals produced by the bone oscillator effectively bypass the outer ear and middle ear and as a result are interpreted as a measure of sensori-neural integrity. Although it is true to say that conditions arising in the outer and middle ear have been found to affect bone conduction sensitivity (Gatehouse and Browning, 1982) the effects are such that, clinically, bone conduction results may be correctly interpreted in the above manner. Hence, while air conduction is a measure of the total hearing loss, bone conduction is a measure of sensori-neural loss. A normally hearing person will therefore hear the air and bone conducted signals at the same 'normal level' on the audiometer signal level dial.

Figure 2.17: Example of a bone oscillator as used in pure tone bone conduction testing (Radio Ear B71).

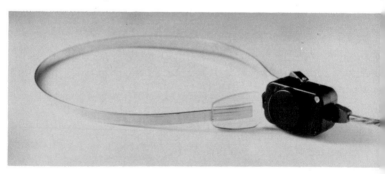

If a child displays a loss for air conduction and normal hearing for bone conduction the conclusion drawn would be that the inner ear pathway was normal and that the problem lay somewhere along the conductive pathway of the ear. This would be termed a CONDUCTIVE hearing loss.

If a child displays an equal loss for air and bone conduction the

onclusion to be drawn would be that there must be damage in the
inner ear pathway and the conductive pathway must be normal. This
would be termed a SENSORI-NEURAL loss.

If a child displays a loss for both air and bone conduction with a
more significant loss for air conduction, a MIXED loss would be concluded.

Table 2.1 illustrates examples of how different hearing losses are
interpreted from the results of air and bone conduction audiometry.

Table 2.1: Example of how different hearing losses result.

	OUTER-MIDDLE EAR LOSS	INNER EAR LOSS	TOTAL LOSS
AIR CONDUCTION	a	b	a + b
BONE CONDUCTION	—	b	b
NORMAL HEARING	a = 0	b = 0	
CONDUCTIVE LOSS:	a = 30 (e.g.)	b = 0	
AIR CONDUCTION = 30 dB			
BONE CONDUCTION = 0 dB			
SENSORI—NEURAL LOSS:	a = 0	b = 40 (e.g.)	
AIR CONDUCTION = 40 dB			
BONE CONDUCTION = 40 dB			
MIXED LOSS:	a = 20	b = 40	
AIR CONDUCTION = 60 dB			
BONE CONDUCTION = 40 dB			

Audiometric Problems

Whilst audiometry can be useful in helping a clinician to determine
the nature of a hearing problem, it will often prove to be of very
limited value in this respect, particularly where young children are
concerned. The audiometric problems relate to three factors listed
below:

a) Age of Child. Children must be developmentally ready to carry out
the tests and therefore audiometric information will not be available
on the pre three year olds.

b) Vibrotactile Thresholds. It is important to note that a very deaf
subject will respond by feeling rather than hearing to signals at lower
levels than his true hearing thresholds. These levels of response to

vibration have been quantified (Bayne, 1968) (see Table 2.2).

Table 2.2: Vibro-tactile thresholds in dB re Clinical Zero (dBHL).

	Frequency (Hz)				
	250	500	1000	2000	4000
Bone Conduction dB	30	60	80	—	—
Air Conduction dB	95	115	125	130	—

Source: after Bayne, 1968.

An example of a severe hearing loss with the vibro-tactile bone conduction thresholds is shown in Figure 2.18.

Figure 2.18: Example of an audiogram for a subject with a bilateral severe sensori-neural hearing loss, responding to bone conduction at vibro-tactile levels in the low-mid frequencies.

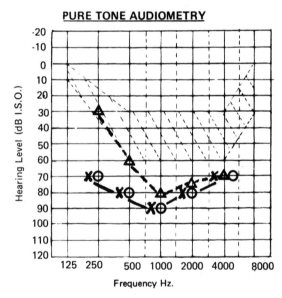

AIR CONDUCTION   RIGHT_____ o   LEFT_____ X

    MASKED RIGHT ●   MASKED LEFT

BONE CONDUCTION   UNMASKED (RIGHT OR LEFT)_____ Δ

    MASKED RIGHT   [MASKED LEFT

The unwary might be led to believe that there is an air-bone gap and therefore some conductive element in the hearing loss, when in fact the loss is totally sensori-neural in nature and the gap is caused because of the low bone vibro-tactile thresholds at 250 Hz and 500 Hz.

(c) Signal Cross-over. It is difficult to test each ear separately. There is a danger in both air and bone conduction testing that the non-test ear will hear the stimulus (the cross-over effect) before the test ear, that is, at a quieter level. As a result audiometric information may be uncertain and the unwary clinician can misdiagnose or underestimate the total hearing loss. The example shown in Figure 2.19 illustrates this point.

Figure 2.19: Example of an unmasked audiogram for a subject with a 'dead' right ear.

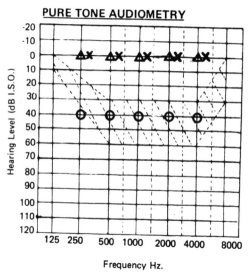

PURE TONE AUDIOMETRY

AIR CONDUCTION		
	RIGHT_____o	LEFT_____X
	MASKED RIGHT ●	MASKED LEFT **X**

BONE CONDUCTION	
	UNMASKED (RIGHT OR LEFT)_____△
	MASKED RIGHT [MASKED LEFT]

The results of air and bone conduction testing (vibrator behind right ear) indicate a 40 dB conductive loss. However, the ear is really a dead ear and the results are due to the test stimuli being heard in the normal non-test ear. Although steps can be taken to overcome this problem it can prove to be extremely difficult with young children.

In air conduction testing, the problem of cross-over can arise once the stimulus level is 40dB above the bone conduction threshold of the non-test ear (Zwislocki, 1953).

In bone conduction testing both ears are stimulated equally regardless of where on the head the bone oscillator is placed (Studebaker, 1964). This means that the clinician cannot simply place the vibrator behind the right ear and test this ear, and then repeat for the left ear as is possible, at least up to 40dBHL, with air conduction testing. The bone conduction test as described simply indicates the sensitivity of the better cochlea.

Masking

A technique known as masking has been devised so that clinicians can in many cases effectively isolate the test ear and determine true hearing thresholds (Sanders and Rintelmann, 1964). This removes the worry about the influence of the non-test ear on the test results. This technique involves the introduction of a continuous noise into the non-test ear while the testing technique for pure tones is applied to the test ear. Unfortunately, young children find this procedure very difficult and many are unable to perform reliably until the age of about seven years.

Comments Relating to the Need for Masking

Air Conduction Testing

In air conduction testing a TDH 39 earphone (the transducer) in an MX41 AR cushion delivers the signal to the test ear. By its very nature the transducer is in contact with the skull and it therefore gives sound energy to the skull. The amount of energy is a function of the contact area between transducer and skull. This energy causes skull bone vibration and as a result the signal can cross the head and stimulate the non-test ear by BONE CONDUCTION. It is therefore possible for sound delivered to one ear by air conduction to cross over the head to the other ear where it is perceived by bone conduction.

There is a difference in the intensity level of the signals reaching the two cochleas − the difference being due to the amount of energy lost by the signal in crossing over the skull. This factor is known as

TRANSCRANIAL or INTERAURAL ATTENUATION and varies between individual subjects. Research has shown that the factor ranges from 40 to 80 dB when using the standard headphone (Zwislocki, 1953). It is not possible clinically to be sure of the absolute value for a particular subject and so all subjects are assumed to have the same value of 40 dB (that is, the minimal value found).

An Example

The example in Figure 2.20 may help in understanding the situation. The subject has a dead right ear and a normal left ear. Transcranial attenuation is 40 dB. Using basic audiometric testing the audiogram suggests a normal left ear and a 40 dB HL conductive loss in the right ear. Why is this so? When testing the right ear by air conduction no response was observed until the signal reached 40 dB. When the signal reached this level a bone conducted signal of 0 dB was present at the non-test ear, that is, the 40 dB air conducted signal in the test ear lost 40 dB (transcranial attenuation) crossing over the head and therefore presented at the test ear at 0 dB by bone conduction. (40 dB in test ear − transcranial attenuation 40 dB = 0 dB = signal level by bone conduction at non-test ear.)

Figure 2.20: Production of a shadow audiogram, when testing by air conduction.

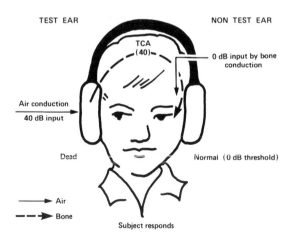

The subject therefore heard the signal and responded. A shadow audiogram (non-test ear response) was obtained for air conduction testing which was not a true indication of hearing in the test ear (Figure 2.19). The skull is stimulated directly when testing by bone conduction and both cochleas are given the same amount of energy regardless of the position of the bone oscillator. Hence, placement of the oscillator behind the right ear does not necessarily tell us anything about the integrity of the right cochlea. As the left ear was normal, responses at normal threshold levels were to be expected.

Masking Stimulus

The above comments highlight the fact that in certain test situations it is not possible to isolate the two ears acoustically. It is therefore necessary, if we are accurately to determine the hearing loss in each ear, to reduce the sensitivity of the non-test ear, so enabling the test ear to respond to the stimulus. The method of masking, whereby narrow bands (NB) of noise centred around the test frequency are continually presented to the non-test ear, achieves the necessary de-sensitisation of the non-test ear (Denes and Naunton, 1952; Liden *et al.*, 1959a; Studebaker, 1962; Barratt and Rowson, 1982). The narrow bands of noise are of such a width (that is, contain a certain range of frequencies) that they produce the greatest shift in threshold for the least amount of energy (Fletcher, 1940). All audiometers are designed with such masking noises available for all the test frequencies used in audiometry. An NB masking noise is said to be *effective* (that is, effectively shifts threshold sensitivity in the non-test ear) when a 1 dB increase in masking produces a 1 dB increase in threshold for the pure tone. The level at which masking becomes effective varies with individual subjects — masking is not therefore necessarily effective immediately above threshold.

Rules of Thumb of Deciding When to Mask

Air Conduction

If the signal presented to the test ear exceeds the bone conduction sensitivity of the non-test ear by more than 40 dB then masking should be applied to the non-test ear.

The decision as to 'when to mask' for air conduction is based on three factors:

Figure 2.21: (a) Example where the criteria for masking for air conduction are satisfied but where the child did actually hear in the test ear. Masking would be applied here. (b) Unmasked audiogram in this case.

(a)

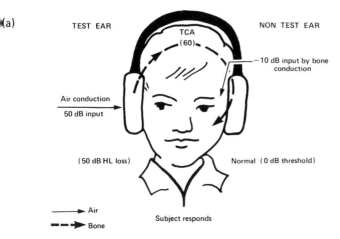

(b)

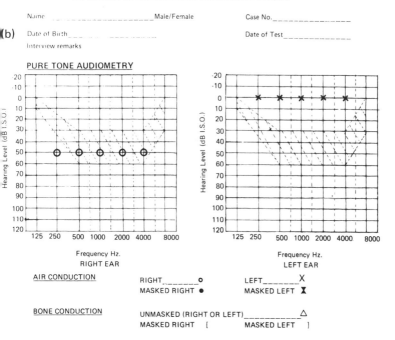

1. Test signal intensity.
2. Bone conduction sensitivity of the non-test ear.
3. Transcranial attenuation factor.

It is assumed that everyone has a transcranial attenuation of 40 dB and so masking may be applied unnecessarily on some occasions. This may be illustrated by reference to the example in Figure 2.21. The air conduction audiogram without masking is in fact accurate despite the fact that the criteria for masking are satisfied.

The reason for this is simply a result of a relatively high value for the subject's transcranial attenuation. Masking would be applied, however, because all subjects are assumed to have the minimal transcranial attenuation of 40 dB.

Bone Conduction

Masking for bone conduction should occur whenever there is a gap of 15 dB or more between the unmasked bone conduction threshold and the air conduction threshold for the test ear. This gap is generally defined as the air-bone gap. In the above example masking of the left ear would be necessary so as to determine the true bone conduction thresholds for the right ear.

Technique of Masking

It is very important for a clinician to use sufficient masking to allow determination of the true hearing thresholds of the test ear. Too little masking (undermasking) will lead to an underestimation of the loss and incorrect diagnosis of the nature of the loss (Figure 2.22), while too much masking (overmasking) will result in the masking noise crossing over the head to the test ear resulting in overestimation of loss and incorrect diagnosis of the nature (Figure 2.23). These examples highlight the fact that it is not good practice simply to mask at one level and redetermine threshold in the test ear. The most appropriate procedure of masking is that based on the proposals of Hood (1957). It is based on the fact that if increases of 10 dB in the masking level do not affect the threshold measurement obtained, then the ear responding is the ear under test.

Procedure

The same method is used for air and bone conduction measurements

Figure 2.22: Example of undermasking where the bone conduction thresholds, vibrator on right mastoid masking in left ear, were determined using only 15dB of masking. A sensori-neural loss was actually present in the right ear.

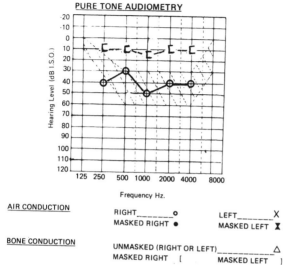

AIR CONDUCTION

RIGHT_____o   LEFT_____X
MASKED RIGHT ●   MASKED LEFT ✗

BONE CONDUCTION

UNMASKED (RIGHT OR LEFT)_____△
MASKED RIGHT [MASKED LEFT]

Figure 2.23: Example of overmasking where masked bone conduction thresholds were determined with 70dB of masking in the non-test right ear. The true loss was a 40dB conductive loss in the left ear.

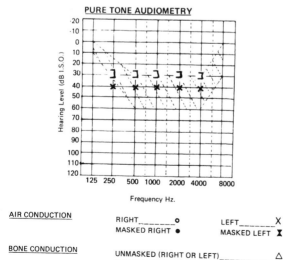

AIR CONDUCTION

RIGHT_____o   LEFT_____X
MASKED RIGHT ●   MASKED LEFT ✗

BONE CONDUCTION

UNMASKED (RIGHT OR LEFT)_____△
MASKED RIGHT [MASKED LEFT]

except that with bone conduction an insert receiver is often used. This frequently falls out with children but can be secured under the headband of the bone vibrator.

(1) Measure the unmasked threshold of the ear under test.
(2) Find the level at which the masking is just audible in the contralateral ear. Set the masking level 20 dB above this.
(3) Remeasure the threshold of test ear.
(4) Increase the masking level by 10 dB.
(5) Remeasure the threshold of test ear.
(6) Steps 4 and 5 above are repeated until for two successive additions of masking the pure tone threshold changes by 5 dB or less. This is then regarded as the threshold of the test ear. Measuring threshold in the conventional manner for each change in masking level is a lengthy process and impractical with children. It is sufficient to increase the signal in steps of 5 dB until the child responds, starting at the threshold value of the previous masking level (Brasier, 1974).

Child-oriented Technique

The manner in which the test is applied with young children is critical to a successful outcome. Children can become totally confused by 'noise in one ear and whistles in the other' and may respond inappropriately simply because they do not know what to do. The test should not begin with the introduction of masking and then an explanation to the child of what he has to do. It should begin by a procedure such as, 'lets see if we can hear the train coming, can you tell me when you hear it?' Then the masking is introduced and an attempt is made to determine the level of awareness. The child is then encouraged to forget about the train — 'lets listen for the whistle' — tone is introduced at supra-threshold level in the test ear and the child carries out play activity, that is, is encouraged to put ball in box in response to tone. Once the clinician is satisfied that the child is performing reliably he proceeds with the test, encouraging and observing the child at all times and taking particular care not to increase the masking and then immediately introduce the tone. Children often respond to this masking increase rather than the tone and a false picture of hearing for the test stimulus could occur.

The threshold determined by the masking procedure occurs when a 'plateau' is reached and further additions of masking do not alter the level responded to, that is, the ear responding is truly the ear under test. In cases where no plateau is found it is possible that there is no response to the sound limits of the audiometer, that is, a very profound loss. Another possibility is that the level of masking needed is such that it is already crossing over and affecting the ear under test. An example of where this might occur is where there is a bilateral unmasked air bone gap of 50dBHL or 60dBHL.

It may prove possible to obtain a clearer insight into the audiometric situation in such cases by means of the Rainville (1959) test. This test permits a more thorough investigation into the actual bone conduction levels, thus helping to differentiate between conductive and sensorineural loss. The format of the test is shown in Figure 2.24. Masking is introduced via the bone oscillator placed on the forehead. Each ear is tested for air conduction via headphones.

Taking an example as shown in Figure 2.25, the basic problem using conventional audiometry in this case would be the danger that once the masking signal became audible (~50dB) it could be of sufficient intensity to cross over and mask the test ear. This would make determination of a 'plateau response' impossible. The Rainville test is therefore applied to try and identify the true bone conduction levels in each ear. The procedure is as follows:

1. Introduce masking via bone oscillator and determine threshold for masking.
2. Measure air conduction threshold for test ear.
3. Increase masking in 10dB steps up to the original air conduction threshold (50dB in this example).
4. For each masking level redetermine threshold for air conduction. The manner in which the air conduction levels behave are indicative of bone conduction sensitivity in the test ear.

(a) Test Ear – 50dB Conductive Loss. In this case the test ear will hear the masking via bone conduction and therefore as the masking level is increased the threshold for air conduction will shift 1dB for each 1dB increase in masking once masking becomes effective. The results, assuming masking becomes immediately effective, may appear as:

Air Conduction Threshold dBHL	Masking Level dBHL
50	0
60	10

continued on page 61

Figure 2.24: Test set-up for the Rainville test, masking via bone oscillator on forehead.

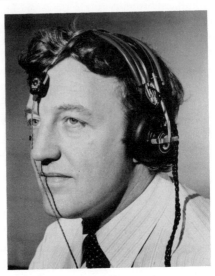

Figure 2.25: The 'difficult' unmasked audiogram where it may prove impossible to resolve the audiometric picture using conventional procedures.

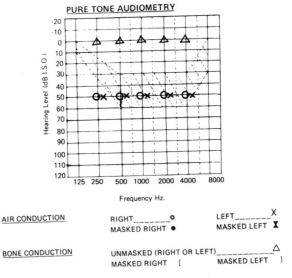

Air Conduction Threshold dBHL	Masking Level dBHL
70	20
80	30
90	40
100	50

(b) Test Ear – Sensori-neural Loss of 50dB. In this case the test ear will not hear the masking (the non-test ear being the one with normal bone conduction thresholds). Therefore, because no masking is heard in the test ear its air conduction threshold will remain steady as the masking is raised up to the air conduction level.

Expected results will be:

Air Conduction Threshold dBHL	Masking Level dBHL
50	0
50	10
50	20
50	30
50	40
50	50

(c) Test Ear – Mixed 50dB Hearing Loss. In this case assuming the conductive loss is 25dB, the bone conduction levels for the test ear will be 25dB. The masking will not be heard in the test ear until 25dB and from then on the test ear will be masked. Expected results will be:

Air Conduction Threshold dBHL	Masking Level dBHL
50	0
50	10
50	20
55	30
65	40
75	50

(d) Test Ear – Very Severe Sensori-neural Loss (>100dBHL). It is important to note that the same pattern of response may be seen when the patient has a very severe sensori-neural loss as is seen in the case of a pure conductive loss. In both cases the pattern of response

is one of a shift in air conduction threshold with increase in masking.

This results from the fact that in the audiometric test, the ear with the very severe sensori-neural loss was not responding, the responses being due to signal cross-over to the non-test ear. When masking is introduced via the bone vibrator it is perceived in the non-test ear. One must remember that the air conduction signal in the test ear is being perceived in the non-test ear by bone conduction. Therefore, as the masking level increases, it is necessary to increase the signal level to reach the threshold of the non-test ear. The signal level in the test ear is not sufficient to reach threshold in the test ear before being perceived in the non-test ear.

Expected results in this case are:

Air Conduction Response dBHL	Masking Level dBHL
50	0
60	10
70	20
80	30
90	40
100	50

(e) Test Ear – Less Severe Sensori-neural Loss of 75 dBHL. This example illustrates the pattern of response which may be seen in less severe sensori-neural losses. As in example (d) the patient's audiogram responses for air conduction are due to cross-over to the non-test ear. The masking via the bone oscillator will be perceived in the non-test ear and hence its threshold will shift. It will therefore be necessary to increase the level of the test ear signal. However, once this reaches 75 dB it will be heard in the test ear, and subsequent increases of masking will produce no effect on threshold of the test ear because masking will not be heard in this ear (bone conduction threshold 75 dBHL).

Expected results in this case are:

Air Conduction Threshold dBHL	Masking Level dBHL
50	0
60	10
70	20
75	30
75	40
75	50

While this test may prove useful, the impedance bridge test will be of paramount importance as part of the diagnostic procedure.

Unilateral Loss

The results that occur in a unilateral conductive and a unilateral sensori-neural loss of 35 dBHL when masking is applied to bone conduction audiometry are shown in Figures 2.26, 2.27 and Tables 2.3 and 2.4.

Table 2.3: Masked bone conduction right.

Signal Level (dBHL)	Masking Level (dBSL)
0	0
0	20
0	30
0	40
0	50

Table 2.4: Masked bone conduction right.

Signal Level (dBHL)	Masking Level (dBSL)
0	0
20	20
30	30
35	40
35	50
35	60

Unilateral Conductive Loss

The true audiogram and the apparent situation without masking are shown. The air conduction levels are accurate because the signal level in the test ear (right) is not sufficient to be heard in the non-test ear.

Why? Signal level in the non-test ear will be equal to signal level in the test ear minus transcranial attenuation.

Therefore, signal level in the non-test ear is equal to −5dB that is, 35-40dB). This is the signal level by bone conduction at the non-test ear. The bone conduction threshold at the non-test ear is 0dB. The signal of −5dB is too weak to be heard. Therefore 35dB is the true air conduction threshold for the test ear.

Figure 2.26: An example of a unilateral conductive hearing loss (see Table 2.3).

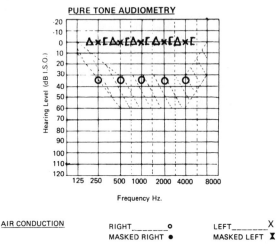

PURE TONE AUDIOMETRY

Frequency Hz.

AIR CONDUCTION   RIGHT_____o   LEFT_____X
                        MASKED RIGHT ●   MASKED LEFT 𝕏

BONE CONDUCTION   UNMASKED (RIGHT OR LEFT)_____△
                        MASKED RIGHT [MASKED LEFT]

Figure 2.27: An example of a unilateral sensori-neural hearing loss (see Table 2.4).

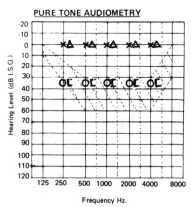

PURE TONE AUDIOMETRY

Frequency Hz.

AIR CONDUCTION   RIGHT_____o   LEFT_____X
                        MASKED RIGHT ●   MASKED LEFT 𝕏

BONE CONDUCTION   UNMASKED (RIGHT OR LEFT)_____△
                        MASKED RIGHT   [MASKED LEFT   ]

The bone conduction levels unmasked are normal. At this stage it is not clear what the thresholds in the test ear are because these responses could be due to the response from the non-test ear. Masking must be applied to the non-test ear. The application of masking shows that raising the masking from 20 dB to 50 dB does not produce a shift in threshold for bone conduction in the test ear. A plateau has been achieved. The level of 0 dB is the true threshold for the right ear and the loss is conductive, that is, air-bone gap of 35 dB.

Unilateral Sensori-neural Loss

The same comments apply here as with the conductive example with reference to air and bone conduction unmasked levels. Application of masking to bone conduction reveals a different pattern of response from the test subject in comparison with the previous example. The level at which a response is elicited increases with increasing masking. At a masking level of 40 dB a plateau response begins and the bone conduction threshold is confirmed as 35 dB. Hence the loss is sensori-neural — no air bone gap being present.

Electroacoustic Impedance Bridge

The electroacoustic impedance bridge is now established as an integral part of any diagnostic battery. The measurement may be applied to children from the neonatal period and has the great advantage of being objective. No subjective response or real co-operation is required of the child other than that he remains reasonably still and quiet. The impedance bridge test facilitates investigation into the way in which the middle ear at the plane of the tympanic membrane reacts to an incoming sound-wave. It is extremely useful in helping to distinguish between conductive and sensori-neural problems. Normally no firm conclusions will be drawn until all test procedures have been completed. The impedance bridge test is therefore one piece of the diagnostic jigsaw.

Concept of Impedance

The conductive part of our hearing mechanism is extremely important in ensuring that our hearing sensitivity is satisfactory for everyday functioning. Its role is efficiently to convey sound energy to the inner ear. When a sound-wave enters the ear canal it travels down to the tympanic membrane. There some of the energy is 'passed on' to the eardrum which is set into vibration and some energy is reflected. The vibration is transmitted across the middle ear by the movements of the ossicular chain. A normally functioning middle ear is extremely efficient, little sound is reflected by the tympanic membrane, the major part being conveyed by vibration to the inner ear.

The difficulty or hindrance to flow of acoustic energy along the conductive pathway is known as IMPEDANCE. Clinically, interest in impedance is focused on that presented to a sound wave at the plane of the tympanic membrane. This information is indicative of the 'well being' of the middle ear system.

Impedance basically comprises two components: *resistance* and *reactance*. Resistance is the component that takes away energy from the incoming sound-wave and therefore reduces its intensity. It occurs, for example, in the form of friction during the movements of the ossicles and wherever energy is converted from one form to another. The resistive component is small and fairly constant and not of particular interest clinically.

Reactance removes energy from the incoming sound wave stores it, and then returns it to the system at a later time. The resultant effect is that less energy reaches the inner ear. Reactance is made up of two elements – *stiffness* and *inertia* (mass). These elements combine by subtraction in determining the overall value of reactance. Their contributions differ as a function of frequency, stiffness being dominant for low frequencies, inertia for higher frequencies (greater than approximately 1500 Hz). Reactance is the dominant component of impedance and as a result the overall impedance of the conductive pathway can be said to be stiffness dominated for low frequency sound waves.

Clinically speaking, interest centres on determining how efficiently the middle ear conveys sound. Pathologically the diseases which cause a reduction in this efficiency, that is, cause conductive deafness, produce stiffness changes. Clinicians obviously wish to identify these pathologies and use is therefore made of a low frequency stimulus (probe tone) in the impedance test. The test assesses how efficiently a low frequency stimulus is conveyed by the middle ear.

Compliance

The mobility (inverse of stiffness) of the middle ear is of particular clinical importance. The term COMPLIANCE is used as an expression of this mobility or resiliance. COMPLIANCE is the inverse of stiffness – a highly compliant middle ear having a low stiffness.

The impedance of a hard walled cavity, which is effectively what the ear is during the impedance test, is inversely proportional to its volume. This means that for a low frequency stimulus the stiffness of the cavity is inversely proportional to cavity volume. The compliance, therefore, is proportional to cavity volume. The compliance is an expression of mobility in terms of an equivalent volume of air. The units are cc. A highly compliant system would have a large equivalent volume, while a very stiff system would have a small equivalent volume.

Equipment

The electroacoustic impedance bridge in its many forms basically comprises the system shown in Figure 2.28. A small probe unit, comprising three channels of input via plastic tubes, is placed at the end of the ear canal. A rubber cuff is placed over the end of the probe so as to facilitate an airtight seal between probe and canal wall. One channel provides the probe tone, a low frequency (220 to 275 Hz) continuous tone produced by a miniature earphone transducer, fed from an electrical oscillator via a variable attenuator (the COMPLIANCE control), so that the sound pressure level in the ear cavity between probe and tympanic membrane can be adjusted. The level of sound in the cavity is monitored by the second channel comprising a miniature microphone, the signal from which is filtered, rectified, amplified and directed to one side of a centre-balancing voltmeter. The other side of the voltmeter is supplied by a reference DC voltage such that when the voltmeter is balanced sound pressure level in the cavity is equal to 65 dB SPL.

Figure 2.28: The constituent parts of a typical electroacoustic impedance bridge.

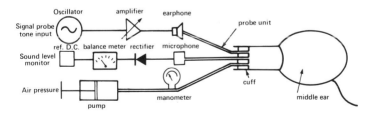

The third channel provides a means of applying small amounts of air pressure to the tympanic membrane by means of a pump connected to a manometer for the reading off of ear canal pressure. This channel enables the clinician to artifically stiffen the ear drum, and hence middle ear system and observe the changes that occur in the efficiency of sound transmission.

Although bridges do differ in layout and actual mode of operation they are all basically assessing how well the middle ear conducts sound energy to the inner ear.

Theory of Test

When the probe unit is placed in the ear canal and an airtight seal is obtained, it is, as far as the sound-wave is concerned, just as if the probe has been connected to a hard walled cavity. The level of sound in the ear canal will therefore be a function of two factors:

1. How much sound is being fed into the ear canal.
2. How much sound is 'absorbed' by the tympanic membrane and middle ear. If the absorption of energy is high, then for a given amount of input energy, only a low sound pressure level will be attained. If on the other hand the absorption is low – due to a stiff reflective system, then for the same energy input, a higher sound level will be attained.

Put another way, if the system is highly absorbent then it will be necessary to feed in more sound energy to attain a fixed sound level in the cavity, relative to that for a stiffer (less absorbent) system.

Tympanometry

The clinical measure involving the impedance bridge is known as tympanometry. This assesses the mobility of the middle ear system and expresses it as compliance in cc. This is achieved by stressing the middle ear at the tympanic membrane with air pressures ranging from $+200$ to -400 mmH$_2$O while simultaneously measuring the change in sound pressure of the low frequency probe tone.

Normal Ear Response

The air pressure in the middle ear cavity is equalised with that in the ear canal by means of the Eustachian tube. This tube momentarily opens when we swallow or blow our noses and lets a puff of air in to the middle ear cavity. Under normal circumstances, therefore, the middle ear pressure will be virtually the same as the ambient air pressure.

Figure 2.29: The application of typanometry using a clinical based manual (a) and a portable automatic (b) system.

(a)

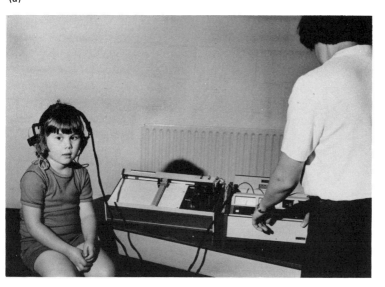

(b)

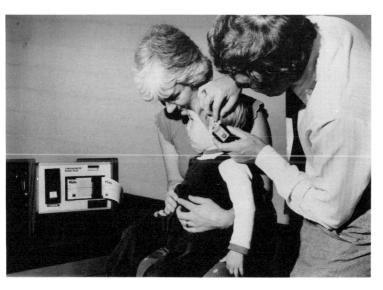

The eardrum will not as a result be under any unnecessary stress and will be in a relaxed and efficient state.

The test of tympanometry begins with the child being seated side-saddle on mother's knee (see Figure 2.29). The child's ear should be examined by means of an auroscope. If there is evidence of foreign body, very heavy deposits of wax or discharge then medical referral should precede the application of the test. If all is well the test may begin. A suitably sized rubber-cuff should be selected and a check then made that an airtight seal can be achieved. With young children it often proves advantageous to hold the headset and place the probe in the ear. The seal should be checked by applying a positive rising pressure observing whether this holds at 200 mmH$_2$0. With the pressure at 200 mmH$_2$0 the eardrum is very stiff and highly reflective and the cavity between probe and eardrum is effectively hard walled. It is therefore possible to obtain a reading from the compliance control of this cavity volume. This is achieved by centre balancing the bridge either manually, or automatically in the case of many modern bridges, a direct read-out of this volume being provided. This volume is of no real significance except in drawing the attention of the clinician to a perforation of the tympanic membrane or in assessing the function of grommets. This will be considered later. (Normal range for this volume is 0·2 to 1cc.) The canal volume reading can also indicate in 'tympanometer type' bridges that the seal is against the canal wall and not at the ear drum.

The tympanometry test proceeds along the lines that once the air pressure has been set to +200 mmH$_2$0 the sound level in the cavity is adjusted to a REFERENCE value, that is, a reference COMPLIANCE value is set. The amount of sound being fed into the ear is fixed at this level for the remainder of the test. The air pressure on the tympanic membrane is then smoothly swept either manually or automatically through to −400 mmH$_2$0. Usually the output of the impedance bridge is connected to an XY recorder so that a record of the result, a tympanogram, is produced. This record displays 'air pressure' along the horizontal X axis and 'compliance' (in relation to the reference value) along the Y axis. The test is therefore a measure of change in stiffness as a function of applied air pressure. The result for a normally functioning middle ear is shown in Figure 2.30.

Summary and Explanation

With the pressure at 200 mmH$_2$0 the sound level is set to a reference

Figure 2.30: Examples of tympanograms in (a) normal middle ear; (b) normal neonate; (c) Eustachian tube dysfunction; (d) middle ear fluid; (e) scarred flaccid drum or ossicular disruption; (f) perforated eardrum.

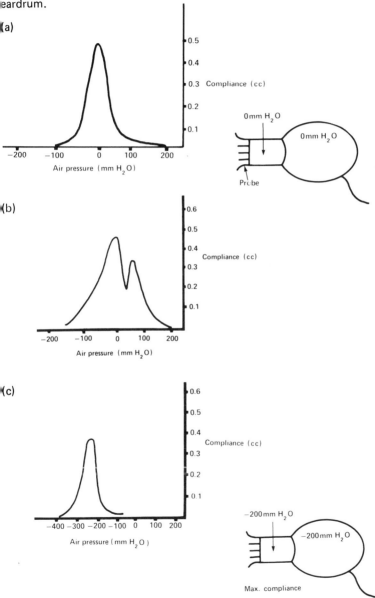

Figure 2.30 (cont'd)

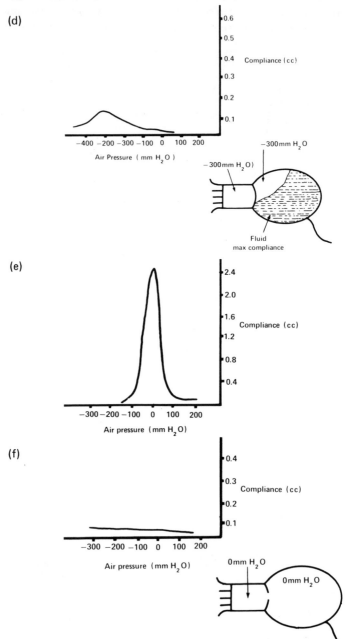

value. As the air pressure is reduced and approaches the value in the middle ear cavity (atmospheric, 0 mmH$_2$0 for this example), the tympanic membrane begins to relax. The sound level in the cavity therefore begins to fall (more sound is being absorbed) and the COMPLIANCE of the ear begins to rise. When the air pressure on both sides of the tympanic membrane is equalised, the middle ear will be in its most efficient state for absorbing sound energy and the sound level in the cavity will therefore be at a minimum. The compliance reading therefore peaks at this point. As air pressure is reduced below atmospheric (that is, −ve) a differential is again set up across the tympanic membrane the middle ear system begins to stiffen again and the sound level in the cavity begins to rise. A symmetrical curve is therefore produced.

Clinical Interest

Clinically, the interest focuses on two characteristics of the tympanogram:

1. The shape of the tympanogram.
2. The air pressure at which maximum compliance occurs — this is equal to the middle ear pressure.

Middle ear pressures in the range of −80 to +30 mmH$_2$0 are considered normal. The actual values of compliance are of little clinical value because of the wide range in normals (0·3 to 1·75cc) (Brooks, 1969). However, attention is paid to the height of the tympanogram in certain cases because when put together with other diagnostic information this can help effect a differential diagnosis. This will be considered in more detail shortly.

Understanding the Procedure

The measuring procedure described which permits a conclusion to be made regarding the mobility of the middle ear system through the parameter compliance may be best understood by reference to the following example (Figure 2.31).

With the drum stressed at +200 mmH$_2$0 the probe unit effectively 'sees' a hard walled cavity between the end of the probe and the tympanic membrane. This volume, when the bridge is balanced, is effectively the canal volume V_1 (equal to compliance C_1). As the pressure

Figure 2.31: Theory of impedance bridge testing.

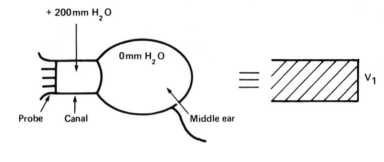

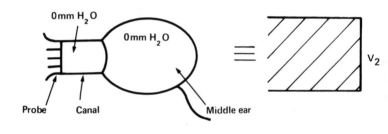

$$V_3 = V_2 - V_1$$
$$V_3 = C_3 = \text{Compliance of the middle ear}$$

differential across the tympanic membrane is reduced more energy is absorbed and as a result the sound level in the cavity falls. This is exactly what would happen if the volume of the cavity was increased and so the falling sound pressure is consistent with an apparent increase in cavity size. The point of maximum compliance occurs when the middle ear absorbs the maximum amount of sound energy — the sound level in the ear canal cavity being at a minimum. The effect is just the same as would occur if the cavity volume had been increased to a maximum value of V_2. Hence, at middle ear pressure, the middle ear has maximum compliance C_3 and this is equal to the apparent increase in volume of the cavity between probe and eardrum in going from a pressure of +200 mmH_2O to middle ear pressure (that is, $C_3 = V_2 - V_1$).

Neonatal Response

While the curve of the normal tympanogram is very stable and reliable

rom early in life, it is of interest to note that the normal curve in the
eonatal period may be somewhat different. The curve is characterised
y a deep notch between two peaks. This shape results primarily from
he flaccid nature of the new-born's tympanic membrane and is con-
idered normal (Shallop *et al.*, 1982). The value of compliance and
liddle ear pressure is in keeping with normal, the middle ear pressure
eing estimated from the pressure point of the notch rather than either
f the two peaks (Figure 2.30).

Pathological Conditions Causing Conductive Deafness in Children

1) Eustachian Tube Dysfunction

A very common problem that can result in a conductive hearing loss in
hildhood is that of Eustachian tube dysfunction. This condition
produces a characteristic tympanogram as may be seen by reference
o Figure 2.30. The striking difference between this and the normal
urve relates to middle ear pressure. In the case of Eustachian tube
lysfunction, middle ear pressure is found to be very negative. This is
. direct result of the fact that the middle ear is not receiving a regular
resh supply of air. As a consequence the oxygen content of air in the
middle ear falls, the air becoming 'thinner' and the tympanic membrane
ecomes stressed due to the abnormal pressure differential across it.

When the tympanometric procedure is applied, the situation is one
f a very stiff and immobile tympanic membrane until applied presure begins to approach middle ear pressure (Brooks, 1967, 1968;
Thomsen, 1955; Porter 1974). The tympanogram is then seen to be
imilar in shape to the normal. This is because once pressure is equal-
sed across the tympanic membrane the middle ear system attains
normal function and therefore absorbs a similar amount of energy
s in the normal ear.

2) Middle Ear Fluid

The condition of secretory or exudative otitis media is relatively
common in children (Porter, 1974). This condition gives rise to the
presence of fluid or exudate in the middle ear cavity. This has the
effect of stiffening the ossicular chain and tympanic membrane and
may result in a considerable hearing problem. Again as with Eustachian
:ube dysfunction it is usually characterised by a certain shape of tympanogram (Figure 2.30). The reason for this curve may be seen from
:he following.

The ear is in a state of maximal stiffness when a pressure of $+200$ mm H_2O is applied to the tympanic membrane. The situation in the middle ear cavity (that is, the other side of the tympanic membrane) will be one of a fluid-filled cavity or a partially filled cavity with a residual negative middle ear pressure.

As the applied pressure is reduced, the mobility of the middle ear system will be relatively unchanged, being stiff because of the presence of the fluid. Even when pressure equalisation occurs, the situation is still one of a very stiff (reflective) system and a low compliance reading is therefore achieved. This is why the curve is considerably different to the normal. There are in fact three marked differences between this curve and the normal:

1. The point of maximal compliance (if any) is shifted considerably towards the negative pressure side.
2. The curve is flattened with no sharp peak.
3. The difference between maximum and minimum compliance (C^3) is much smaller.

The flattening of the curve is very indicative of middle ear fluid and is generally not seen in other conditions affecting the conductive pathway.

(3) Ossicular Discontinuity, Scarred or Flaccid Tympanic Membrane

The tympanogram which may be seen in the above condition is shown in Figure 2.30. The middle ear pressure is again normal but now the compliance is much larger than normal, because the tympanic membrane and ossicles are able to move much more freely than in the normal ear. Compliance values may be four or five times the normal. It is important to note, as mentioned earlier, that absolute values of compliance are not of clinical value when taken in isolation. Tympanograms are therefore only one part of the diagnostic test battery and no firm conclusion would be drawn on pathology on the basis of tympanogram alone, particularly in this category.

(4) Otosclerosis

The condition of otosclerosis which causes stapes fixation is characterised by markedly reduced compliance and normal middle ear pressure. The fixation of the stapes by fibrosis results in a much stiffer middle ear system. The above description, however, must be treated with caution. Considerable overlap may occur between normal and oto

clerotic ears (Nueva Espana, 1979) and the tympanometric result
n isolation is therefore of no real clinical value.

5) Tympanic Membrane Perforation

Perforation of the tympanic membrane may occur naturally or may be
lone surgically as with the insertion of grommets during middle ear
surgery. The function of the grommet is to help ventilate the middle
ear cavity and prevent a recurrence of middle ear fluid. The impedance
bridge can help in identifying perforations and in assessing the function of grommets. If there is an open perforation, then of course no

Figure 2.32: Assessing the function of grommets.

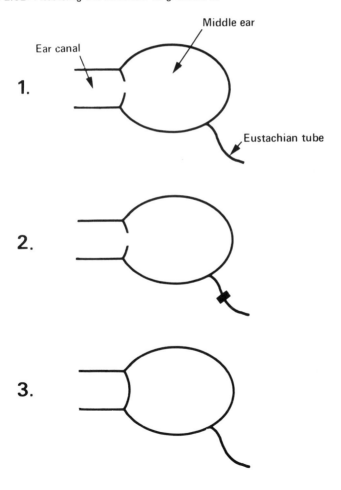

pressure differential can be applied across the tympanic membrane
In such a case, a straight line is normally obtained with attempted
variation of pressure (Figure 2.30).

However, variations upon this theme can occur and clinical obser
vations are useful in clarifying certain situations.

Figure 2.32 illustrates three possible situations that may arise with
grommets and in cases 1 and 2, drum perforations.

In case 1 the grommet is patent and the Eustachian tube is func
tioning normally. As a result it will not prove possible to maintain
a pressure greater than 100 mmH_2O because the Eustachian tube will
open and equalise pressure. Secondly, the compliance reading neces
sary to set the sound pressure in the cavity at the reference will be
very high, quite simply because the cavity will no longer comprise the
ear canal alone, but that plus the volume of the middle ear cavity
Therefore an abnormally high reading of ear canal volume C_1 is indica
tive of a perforation.

In case 2 the grommet is patent but Eustachian tube function
is abnormal. It will therefore prove possible to hold a pressure of
+200 mmH_2O. The compliance reading necessary to set the sound
level to the reference will be very high. The tympanogram will be a
straight line.

In case 3 the grommet is blocked. In this case it will be possible to
hold pressure at +200 mmH_2O. The compliance reading will now be
in accordance with normal when the sound pressure is set to reference
at +200 mmH_2O air pressure. The resultant tympanogram will be one
of those described earlier.

Gradient

The term gradient is sometimes used by clinicians as a means of quan
tifying the shape of the tympanogram. The gradient is defined as the
ratio of the change in compliance in going from middle ear pressure
(A) to ± 50 mmH_2O of middle ear pressure (B) to the compliance a
middle ear pressure (A), that is, gradient $= \dfrac{A - B}{A} \times 100$.

In normals this is 40 to 60 per cent while in cases of exudative
otitis media it is usually less than 10 per cent (Brooks, 1969) (see
Figure 2.33).

Measurement of middle ear function by means of the impedance
bridge is an extremely useful procedure. However, the measure provides
no information on hearing thresholds. Conductive hearing problems
rarely produce losses in excess of 70dBHL. Therefore, in cases where

Figure 2.33: Determination of the gradient of the tympanogram. (a) Normal; (b) middle ear fluid.

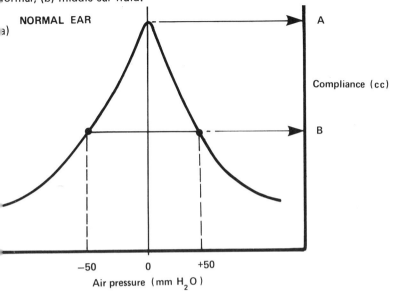

Gradient % = $\dfrac{A - B}{A}$ x 100

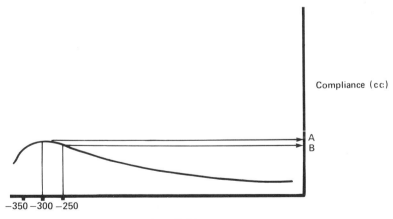

Gradient % = $\dfrac{A - B}{A}$ x 100

audiometric data indicate a more severe loss while impedance indicate a conductive problem, a mixed hearing loss would be concluded.

Tympanic Membrane Breaking Strain

Clinicians may be concerned at applying pressures to the tympani membrane using the impedance bridge equipment. However, Zalewsk (1906) cited by Peters Ltd, Sheffield, reported the breaking strain of th tympanic membrane for positive air pressure, in cadaver specimens as

Normal membranes — mean for 111 ears 160,000 mmH$_2$0
Thin membranes — mean for 12 ears 5000 mmH$_2$0
Scarred membranes — mean for 12 ears 3000 mmH$_2$0

The Stapedial Reflex — Acoustic Reflex

The middle ear includes two muscles — the tensor tympani and th stapedius. The latter is considered as responding to sound stimulation contraction occurring at levels of 70-90 dB above threshold in normal (Borg, 1972; Liden *et al*., 1970; Chiveralls and FitzSimons, 1973 Anderson *et al*., 1970). The muscle is attached to the posterior cru of the stapes and is innervated by the seventh cranial nerve (facia nerve). The reflex contraction occurs bilaterally and produces a increase in the stiffness of the middle ear.

It is possible for the acoustic reflex to be obscured from detection It has been found that it may be absent in many conductive disorder as well as in various types of sensori-neural loss. In fact the reflex i unlikely to be observed in an ear with anything but the slightest con ductive lesion apart from some cases of discontinuity (Chiveralls *et al*. 1976). Even normally hearing subjects can show an absence of th reflex — it has been suggested that this may be as high as 10 per cent.

It is unlikely that the reflex will be observed in the neonatal perio by means of a conventional impedance bridge. A probe tone of 800 H; or higher is needed to indicate its presence in such cases (Weatherby and Bennet, 1979).

It has been suggested that the reflex could be used as an estimate o hearing level. Various approaches to predicting an audiogram from reflex thresholds to pure tones and noise have been put forward (Popelka, 1981). Such methods tend to be prone to inaccuracy and while a recent method based on single frequencies seems to be more accurate it does appear to be impractical for general clinical application

(Sesterhenn and Brueninger, 1977).

It is generally accepted that it is the subjective loudness rather than the physical intensity of the stimulus which is the determining factor for innervation of the reflex. While the span between hearing threshold and reflex threshold is 70 to 90 dB in the normal, it can be as little as 5 dB in certain sensori-neural cases. This reduction in span is produced by an accelerated growth of loudness in relation to the norm and is indicative of recruitment (Liden, 1970). Use of the reflex as an objective measure of recruitment was suggested by Metz as early as 1952 (Metz, 1952). This can prove useful to the clinician, particularly in relation to hearing aid management.

Testing for the Reflex

The method of measuring threshold for the stapedial reflex may be described in the following way:

1. The tympanometric procedure is first applied. The headset should have been placed on the child — unless the machine comprised a hand-held probe and ipsilateral reflex function.
2. Once tympanometry has been carried out the applied pressure should be set to middle ear pressure, that is, set to the peak of the tympanogram.
3. The impedance bridge should then be set to be sensitive to small changes in compliance. This may involve selecting the measuring mode 'Reflex' on the modern bridges or selecting a sensitive compliance range on the older manual models.
4. The bridge should then be balanced so that the sound level in the cavity is at the balance level, for example, 65 dB SPL in many bridges, which is below reflex threshold for the probe tone frequency.
5. Two modes of stimulation may be applied to test for the presence of the reflex. In IPSILATERAL stimulation the signal is presented in the same ear as the probe via a miniature transducer. Test frequencies are usually restricted to 1000 and 2000 Hz.

In CONTRALATERAL stimulation the stimulus is presented in the opposite ear to the probe ear via a headphone. Therefore, in contralateral stimulation the probe ear acts as the indicator ear. Test frequencies are octave frequencies from 500 to 4000 Hz.

When a supra-threshold reflex stimulus is introduced into the headphone, the signal travels up (afferent pathway) the auditory nerve (eighth cranial nerve) to the reflex centre (superior olive) from there (efferent pathway) impulses travel down the facial nerves (seventh cranial nerve) to the stapedius muscles on both sides – bilateral contraction resulting. The stimulus mode should be selected.

6. The chart recorder should be set to ON. The pen will sweep across the paper at a steady level – equivalent to the cavity sound pressure level and hence compliance of the system.

7. To begin a signal of 1000Hz should be introduced at 80dBHL. The tone should last for about two seconds. The reflex is time locked being in evidence from onset to offset of stimulus. If the reflex is present it will produce a stiffening of the middle ear. This will result in a rise in cavity sound pressure level, equivalent to a decrease in middle ear compliance. A deflection of the pen in the direction of decreased compliance will occur (Figure 2.34).

Figure 2.34: Recording the stapedius muscle reflex.

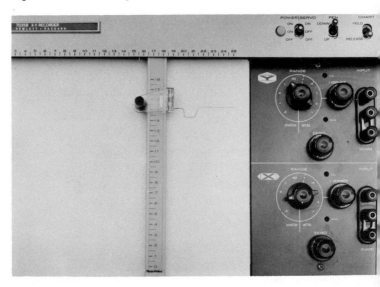

8. The signal level should be adjusted in 5dB steps until the reflex threshold is found.

9. The signal should then be changed to another test frequency the test then being repeated.

Stapedial reflex testing with young children can prove to be very difficult. Whereas it is possible to obtain tympanometric information on a crying or restless child, it is not so easy to observe reflex contraction in such children. A considerable amount of time, effort, patience and skill in handling young children will be needed if the measure is to be successful with many youngsters.

The presence or absence of the reflex is not indicative of anything when taken in isolation. However, when put together with other diagnostic findings it can prove to be useful. In particular, it can help to identify and pinpoint the location of an ossicular disruption. It can be taken as a very strong indicator, when present, of normal middle ear function (with the exception noted earlier). It can also help to draw attention to hearing-impaired children who may have tolerance problems. This is particularly important early on in life when standard 'upper tolerance' tests are difficult to apply. Reduced span does not necessarily mean that a child will have loudness discomfort problems using conventional linear response hearing aids. However, its presence should ensure that a close watch is kept on the child's use of hearing aids.

Speech Tests of Hearing

The tests of hearing that have been described thus far are all aimed at providing the clinician with information on the degree of loss and the functioning of the conductive mechanism of the hearing system. Another important measure that can be applied to children over the age of 2½ years is a speech test of hearing. Such tests provide the clinician with information on the child's ability to hear and comprehend speech and are clearly very useful since hearing speech is without doubt one of the most important functions of our auditory system. Furthermore, such tests provide the clinician with information on the overall reliability of the test battery, and when included in the ongoing management programme, on the child's potential for using his residual hearing.

The choice of speech test will be primarily a function of the child's language level rather than chronological age. This is of particular relevance when working with hearing-impaired children.

The early speech tests rely on the child's ability to demonstrate understanding of simple commands. This progresses to tests involving identification of familiar objects by pointing. Later the child's developing 'picture-vocabulary' skills are employed until at the age of approximately seven years 'speech repetition' is used as a means of quantifying 'hearing for speech'.

It is very important for the clinician to ensure before beginning a

speech test that the material reflects the child's receptive vocabular
level.

Tests with Children 2 to 2½ Years

Speech may be assessed in this age category by the co-operative tes
already described. The test demands understanding by the child an
therefore acts as a rudimentary speech test.

Alternatively, use may be made of the Doll Vocabulary List (Sher
dan, 1976) which involves the child in exploring a doll being aske
to 'show me her shoes', 'her hair', 'her nose', etc. This permits a rela
tively quick assessment of hearing for most of the common vowel
and consonants.

The 5-Sound Test (Ling and Ling, 1978) and the Auditory Number
Test (Erber, 1980) may also prove useful with this age group.

Obviously, such tests may prove useful with older hearing-impaire
children having delayed language development.

Children 2½ to 4 Years

The child's developing 'object-name' matching skills are used via th
Kendall Toy Test (KT) (Kendall, 1957). This test uses a selection o
toys, the names of which should be familiar to most normally hearin
children of this age. There are three sets of 15 toys in the test an
the usual procedure would be to choose one set of toys for a parti
cular child. Each set of 15 items comprises ten test items and fiv
distractors. The test should be applied in the following manner: first
each toy should be taken out and shown to the child. The clinicia
will probably ask the child to name the toy – 'What's this?' – jus
to check whether the child is familiar with it. 'Yes, it's a house isn'
it. Put it on the table.' Each item is placed on the table in front o
the child. The tester then moves out of vision at 1m from the chil
as shown in Figure 2.35 and asks the child to point to different item
on the table. The clinician should determine the level of voice require
by the child to identify the items accurately. Voice level will be mea
sured on a sound level indicator and the test repeated on the othe
ear.

The child is not required to give a verbal response and during th
build up to the test, the tester should provide plenty of reinforcemen
as to the name of each item regardless as to whether or not the chil
responds verbally. This type of test is very useful for children wit
limited or indistinct speech and has proved particularly effectiv
with mentally handicapped subjects (Nolan *et al.*, 1980).

Figure 2.35: Application of the Kendall Toy Test.

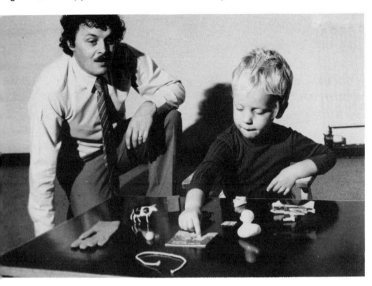

The items of the test are grouped according to vowel sounds as may be seen by reference to one of the test sets. For example:

TEST ITEMS: house, spoon, fish, duck, cow, shoe, brick, cup, gate, plate.
DISTRACTORS: mouse, book, string, glove, plane.

If a child requires a raised voice level in order to perform reliably the indication would be that a hearing impairment was present. However, no conclusion would be drawn until all test results were available.

Children 4 to 6 Years

The child's ability at picture-name matching would be used to evaluate hearing for speech in this age-group. The New Manchester Picture Test (Watson, 1957) and The Word Intelligibility by Picture Identification Test (WIPI) (Ross and Lerman, 1970) are employed with such children.

The New Manchester Picture Test, for example, comprises eight sets of 10 picture cards. Each card contains pictures of four objects, the child being asked to point to one specified object on each card. The test is designed to assess a child's ability to discriminate specific vowel and consonant sounds. Each set of 10 cards assesses the child's ability to hear five specific vowel and five specific consonant sounds. The distractors on each card contain sounds in common with the test item. For example:

test sound: vowel *e*
test item: a well
distractors: ball, wall, doll

The method of application is to show the practice card to the child who is asked to name the pictures. The child is then asked to show the tester one or two of the pictures on the card. This prepares the child to the task at hand. The tester then positions himself at 1m (as in the earlier described behavioural tests) and the child is asked to 'Show me the . . .' (see Figure 2.36). The card is then turned over and the next word presented. Voice level should be measured using a sound level meter. The test should be applied to each ear at a number of voice levels (one for each test set). The child's score as a percentage is calculated for each list and a speech audiogram — percentage score versus speech level should then be plotted. This is compared with the 'normal curve'.

Figure 2.36: Application of the New Manchester Picture Test.

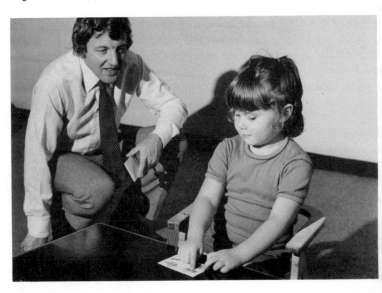

As children approach 6 years of age it is possible to use tests such as NU-CHIPS (Katz and Elliott (1978)) – which incorporates phonetically balanced lists of monosyllables and picture pointing response or the Manchester Junior Word Lists (Watson, 1957). This latter test involves the child in 'speech repetition', having to say back a word which is either presented live or via headphones from the cassette tape. The child's utterance is scored whole word and a percentage score is determined. A number of lists are applied over a range of signal presentation levels. A speech audiogram curve (percentage score versus signal level) is plotted and compared with the normal.

As with all diagnostic procedures no conclusions are drawn until every test has been completed.

Children 6 Years Plus

It is usual to assess such children by closed-circuit prerecorded word lists via headphones. The type of ear phone normally used is the TDH 39 in an MX41AR cushion. Various speech tests are available including the phonetically balanced lists (Fry, 1961), and the PBK-50 lists (Haskins, 1949) or the isophonemic AB lists (Boothroyd, 1968). The AB lists are very commonly used in the United Kingdom. The AB test comprises 15 word lists, each list containing 10 words (30 phonemes). The test format is that the child is fitted with headphones, each ear is assessed separately using a number of list-signal level configurations – the number of lists being sufficient to obtain a discrimination score range from maximum to less than 50 per cent. The child is expected to respond to each test word by repeating what he hears. The response is scored phonemically. For example:

test word:	house	
response:	house	3 points
response:	mouse	2 points
response:	cow	1 point
response:	five	0 points

It is important to encourage children during this type of test – 'have a guess if you're not sure', 'just say what you hear, it doesn't matter if it sounds silly'. The test should be applied at a reasonable speed but not too quickly in case the child misses out words and loses concentration. The clinician must not lose track of which test word it is that is being presented to a child; this can occur if the test is allowed to run without the clinician knowing when each word is presented.

Clinicians must therefore be able to hear the test words as they are presented (perhaps via a miniature earphone). Upon completion of the test a speech audiogram is plotted for each ear and compared with the normal ear response for the test equipment.

One may predict with a reasonable degree of accuracy the expected shift in a subject's speech audiogram relative to the normal curve on the basis of the pure tone audiogram. Although this is by no means absolute it has been found to be reliable, particularly for the most commonly occurring audiogram shapes. The relationship may be considerably different in unusual audiogram configurations such as U shapes, steeply sloping or rising ones. Various methods have been suggested, but the most appropriate for children using the speech material described is considered to be that of Markides (1980a).

Figure 2.37: The speech audiogram — normal and pathological result.

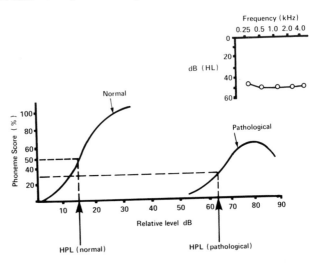

This involves the use of pure tone thresholds to predict the Half Peak Level Elevation (HPLE) of the child. HPLE is defined as the difference in decibels between the normal Half Peak Level (HPL) and the child's Half Peak Level. Half Peak Level is the speech level (dB) at which the child scores 50 per cent of his maximum discrimination score. For example, reference to Figure 2.37 shows hypothetical speech audiograms for a normal and a pathological subject. The normal HPL calculated at the 50 per cent discrimination score (that is 50 per cent of 100 per cent), was achieved at 15 dB reference level. The pathological HPL, calculated at the 30 per cent discrimination score (that is, 50 per cent of a maximum score of 60 per cent) was achieved at 65 dB reference level. The HPLE for the child was therefore 50 dB (65–15 dB).

It has been demonstrated that there is a good correlation for the commonest types of audiogram between the HPLE and the Best Two Average (BTA) hearing level in the frequencies 250-4000 Hz. The clinician simply identifies the two frequencies with the most sensitive air conduction hearing levels and averages these values. This average (dB) is a good guide as to the child's expected HPLE.

The clinician will compare the speech audiogram with the pure tone audiogram once all the diagnostic procedures have been completed. The information presented above can prove useful in checking for inter-test reliability bearing in mind the limitations of the procedure and the uncertain effects of some audiogram configurations. It is also very helpful when deciding upon the dB 'starting level' of the speech at the beginning of the test. The aim should be to present speech at a level where the child has considerable success (that is, 50 per cent).

Masking for Speech

It is important to realise that there is a possibility (as in pure tone audiometry) that the non-test ear can respond to speech during closed-circuit testing via headphones due to the cross-over of information. The speech discrimination score in the poor ear for a subject with asymmetry of loss may therefore be contaminated (improved) by the contribution of the non-test (better) ear. Masking may therefore be necessary in speech audiometric testing with children in the 6 plus category.

Speech is a wide band signal which contains many frequencies. It is unlike the pure tone which is one discrete frequency. When masking for speech it is necessary to shift sensitivity of the test ear over a wide range rather than a very narrow band of frequencies (as occurs in pure tone testing). Wide Band (WB) masking is therefore used for masking in speech testing. It has been shown that there is a linear 1 to 1 relation between threshold for speech and WB masking level Hawkins and Stevens, 1950). This means that above the minimum effective level of the masking each 1 dB increase in masking produces a 1 dB shift in threshold for speech.

The interaural attenuation for speech has been found to be approximately 50 dB (Liden *et al.*, 1959b; Smith and Markides, 1981). This means that when presenting speech via a TDH 39 headphone in an MX41 AR cushion, once the signal level is 50 dB above the bone conduction sensitivity of the non-test ear, the speech can cross over the skull via bone conduction and be heard in the cochlea in the non-test ear.

The clinician will be faced with three questions in relation to masking for speech. These are (1) What masking noise should be used? (2) When is masking required? and (3) How much masking will be required?

1. The answer to question 1 has already been given as wide band noise.

2. The answer to question 2 will be a function of:
   (a) Transcranial attenuation for speech.
   (b) Speech presentation level.
   (c) Bone conduction sensitivity in the non-test ear.

Transcranial attenuation for speech is taken at 50 dB.

In view of the fact that speech has a wide frequency range it is proposed that the bone conduction sensitivity in (c) be taken as the average of the thresholds for the test frequencies 500 Hz, 1000 Hz and 2000 Hz or alternatively in cases of steeply sloping or unusual shaped loss, the threshold at 500 Hz or 1000 Hz (whichever is the better). The decision as to when to mask is taken on the basis of whether the speech level in the test ear is 50 dB or more above the bone conduction sensitivity of the non-test ear then masking must be applied to the non-test ear.

3. The amount of masking used must be sufficient to prevent the non-test ear contributing to the results for test ear. It must not be unnecessarily high, however, as this can result in needless distraction or even discomfort for the child. A fixed level of masking should be presented to the child for a particular speech presentation level. This is determined by the formula:

Masking level (re masking threshold)	X	dB SL
Speech signal level	Y	dB SL
Bone conduction threshold non-test ear	Z	dB HL
Transcranial attenuation	50	dB
Correction factor	20	dB

$$X = Y - (50 + Z) + 20 \text{ dB SL}$$

The correction factor is applied so as to ensure that the masking is effective. The above assumes that the speech audiometry equipment is calibrated so that the normal threshold of detectability is at the OdB dial reading on the speech attenuator.

Decision Making

Once the diagnostic procedures have been completed the clinician will consider the results of all the tests. If, for instance, both the conventional hearing test and a speech test have been applied, the clinician will check for consistency. The impedance bridge measurements will aid in deciding on whether there are any conductive problems that should be dealt with before any sensori-neural ones are tackled. By this time the clinician should have a reasonably clear picture of both degree and nature of the loss. This information will be fundamental to the management programme.

If there is a conductive element in the hearing-impairment the first thing the clinician will do is arrange for an otologist to perform an Ear, Nose and Throat (ENT) examination. Children must be reviewed routinely following ENT treatment so as to determine whether improvement in hearing has taken place.

In cases where sensori-neural problems are indicated, the clinician will probably inform the parents of the position, discuss its implications and arrange for immediate help from the parent guidance service. During the short interim period between the diagnostic session and the first follow-up appointment, the clinician will be organising the hearing aid prescription and earmould provision and will be briefing the child guidance team, in particular the visiting teacher of the deaf, about the child.

The diagnostic tests should continue to be applied to a child as part of the management programme. This is crucial because more comprehensive information will be obtained as the child matures. Such information can have a critical effect on factors such as hearing aid prescription. Such prescription must therefore be very flexible and amenable to change – should change be indicated from information from the ongoing diagnostic tests.

The importance of applying routine checks on sensori-neural hearing-impaired children cannot be overemphasised. It has been reported that the incidence of middle ear effusion in childhood may be as high as 20 per cent at any one time. Children with sensori-neural impairments simply cannot afford to be 'carrying' an overlay conductive problem. For this reason regular checks, perhaps as part of the management sessions, should be carried out.

'Difficult to Test' Children

There will undoubtedly be a small number of children who for reasons such as developmental delay, mental and physical handicap, etc. prove to be 'difficult to test' by conventional procedures. The main point of note in relation to testing hearing in children is one must apply a test appropriate to the child's *level of development* and not *chronological age*. Skilled clinicians act quickly and decisively when working with children and are generally able to determine quickly which test is likely to be most appropriate for the child. The biggest problem for the inexperienced clinician is knowing how long to persevere on an 'age appropriate' test before moving back to another test appropriate for a younger age-group. Unnecessary time spent on an inappropriate test will often result in a totally unproductive session, the child being too tired or uninterested to continue when the decision is taken to 'break-down' to a less demanding test.

Mental Handicap

One group of children who are very prone to hearing-impairment and yet are often not assessed satisfactorily, audiologically speaking, are the mentally handicapped. All too often the lack of response to sound, speech in particular, is put down to the child's mental capacity rather than hearing integrity, this despite the fact that numerous studies (Nolan *et al.*, 1980; Lloyd, 1970; Cunningham and McArthur, 1981; Davies and Penniceard, 1980) have highlighted that the incidence of hearing loss in such groups is significantly higher than in the normal population. This is particularly so in the case of Down's syndrome. The comment that there is little point in assessing hearing in the mentally handicapped because they are usually untestable and have no problem with hearing anyway, is simply untrue and totally unacceptable. Hearing in such children can be successfully assessed by conventional procedures in the majority of cases and favourable results do occur as a result of treatment for conductive disorders and fitting of hearing aids (Balkany *et al.*, 1979).

Functional Hearing Loss

In routine audiological practice the clinician is generally required to advise on management of hearing disorders resulting from actual physical abnormalities of the auditory system. Such disorders are described as either conductive (related to diseases in the outer ear or middle ear) or sensori-neural (related to diseases of the cochlea or inner ear).

These disorders have an organic basis and may therefore be described in general terms as organic hearing losses.

Another category of patient may be seen where on conventional routine pure tone audiometric testing the results indicate a sensori-neural hearing-impairment. This may be bilateral or unilateral in nature. However, it may be subsequently shown that the patient is in fact simulating or exaggerating a hearing loss. Such losses are not therefore a result of pathology in the hearing system and are described as non-organic or functional in type.

Functional hearing loss in children has been recognised as a clinical entity for some considerable time. The studies carried out in this area are comprehensively described by Chaiklin and Ventry (1963), Martin (1978) and Nolan and Tucker (1981).

The importance of identifying such losses in children at the earliest moment has been emphasised by several authors (Ross, 1964; Miller *et al.*, 1968). Otherwise such children may be managed as hearing-impaired with all the unnecessary consequences resulting from misdiagnosis (otological referral, hearing aid fitting, peripatetic support). A study by Campanelli (1963) on school children who failed school screening tests emphasised the need for caution against preferential seating, special classes, hearing aid fitting and peripatetic back-up support until the organicity of the hearing problem is defined by proper audiological procedures. Inter-test inconsistencies, particularly between audiometry and speech testing, are often indicators of such problems.

Prevalence

The prevalence of functional hearing loss in children over the age of 7 years referred for audiological assessment was reported by Nolan and Tucker (1981) as 7.5 per cent (10 of 133 referrals) over a four-year period. This constitutes a significant proportion of referrals and emphasises the importance for clinicians to be aware of the existence of such children. Only four of the ten children who were found to have functional hearing loss in the study had aroused the suspicion of the referring party on the reliability of the pure tone audiogram they had obtained. The remaining six children had been pronounced hearing-impaired and had been referred for more detailed investigations into the cause and for advice on management.

It is of interest to note that all the children found to have functional hearing loss in the study had been assessed and referred to the clinic on the basis of one pure tone audiogram.

Sex Differential

An interesting finding that emerged from three clinical studies (Brockman and Hoversten, 1960; Dixon and Newby, 1959) was that functional hearing loss occurred three times more often in females than in males. No explanation for this sex differential has been provided. It is possible, however, that it is an artefact of numbers involved in the studies. The Nolan and Tucker (1981) study did not support a sex differential, there being no significant difference in incidence within male and female referrals (7·3 per cent in males, 7·8 per cent in females).

Identification

The identification of this type of problem usually results from gross inter-test inconsistencies. Included in the 'test battery' must be the initial interview with child and parents. One of the most important observations arising out of studies into functional hearing loss in children relates to the importance of the clinician interacting with the child. In the Nolan and Tucker (1981) study, it was readily apparent from the information gained in the initial interview that eight of the nine children with moderate to severe bilateral functional losses were able to converse without difficulty at normal conversational voice level. The subsequent audiometric results on these children were totally inconsistent with the interview observations. However such inconsistencies will not be apparent if clinicians direct all their questions to the parent and ignore interaction with the child. This observation is consistent with that reported by Barr (1960).

Clinicians must therefore make an effort at communication with the child – perhaps seeking information on sports, hobbies, television etc. The child's behaviour should be noted. Seek information on whether the child requires or indicates a need for lip-reading in the conversational situation. Sometimes children will claim that they are able to perform well in the interview situation provided they can see the speaker's lips, because of excellent lip-reading ability. This often accompanies a deafness of relatively recent onset. In the Nolan and Tucker (1981) study an example of one child who showed no response on audiometry and yet conversed freely provided the speaker's lips were visible was highlighted. This girl's lip-reading ability was found to be very poor on subsequent investigation, and indicated that she was 'hearing' conversation.

Lip-reading Test

A test of lip-reading ability may be applied to subjects who claim that lip-reading ability enables understanding of questions at normal conversational voice level, while audiometrically a significant hearing loss is observed. The material for the test may, for example, employ that described by Markides (1980b). This would be applied following the usual diagnostic procedures.

Test Approach Following Interview

The routine audiological diagnostic procedures of pure tone audiometry for air and bone conduction, impedance bridge measures, stapedial reflex studies and speech audiometry should all be applied.

Observations Relating to the Diagnostic Procedures

Performance on Pure Tone and Speech Audiometry. Chaiklin and Ventry (1963) and Coles and Priede (1971) have commented upon the inappropriate lateralisation of pure tone or speech stimuli in many cases of unilateral functional hearing loss. Such observations are clear signs of functionality.

In the Nolan and Tucker (1981) study it was noted that the one child with a unilateral functional loss failed to show a shadow curve response to pure tone stimuli presented in one ear while responses on the other ear were normal. A similar observation was made on speech audiometry. When testing for bone conduction without masking the child failed to respond with the vibrator on the functional mastoid but responded normally on the other ear.

Such observations may therefore prove useful in highlighting the functional behaviour of a child during routine audiometric assessment.

Audiogram Shape. It has been suggested by some writers (Barr, 1960; Dixon and Newby, 1959) that the pure tone thresholds in children with functional hearing loss have a characteristic shape and often lie between 40 and 70dBHL resembling equal loudness contours. The study of Nolan and Tucker (1981) supported this observation. Eight children showed such audiogram shapes for both ears. It therefore appears that many children with bilateral functional hearing loss do present with a characteristic audiogram shape. However, it must be remembered that such audiograms cannot be considered in isolation as proof of functionality (Chaiklin *et al.*, 1959).

It is of considerable interest to note the audiological findings relating to all of the children included in the Nolan and Tucker (1981) study. Sixteen cases of bilateral organic sensori-neural deafness were seen. It may be seen by reference to Table 2.5 that 14 of these children had mild losses of less than 35 dBHL in the poor ear. One child was found to have a loss of 45 dBHL and one child had a loss of 95 dBHL. (Loss classified as mean of 500, 1000, 2000 Hz test frequencies.) However, the child with the profound loss was a recent immigrant into the United Kingdom; the child with the 45 dB loss had been diagnosed as being hearing-impaired at the age of 2 years and had been referred for advice on an alternative hearing aid; seven of the children with mild losses had been diagnosed earlier in life elsewhere and were being seen for advice on management. Hence, only seven children over the age of 7 years were diagnosed as having bilateral sensori-neural deafness during the study period. This deafness was of a very mild nature.

Table 2.5: Distribution of degree of loss in children showing bilateral sensori-neural deafness on pure tone audiometry.

Classification	Mean Loss dB HL			
	≤35	36-55	56-75	75
Organic loss	14	1	0	1
Functional loss	0	3	5	1

In comparison, it may be seen from Table 2.5 that the children with bilateral functional hearing loss constituted 87 per cent of the children over the age of 7 years who were seen in the study and found to have a bilateral sensori-neural loss of greater than 35 dBHL on pure tone audiometry.

These results indicate that there is a high probability of functional hearing loss in children over the age of seven years who present with a moderate to severe (greater than 35 dBHL) bilateral sensori-neural hearing loss on pure tone audiometry, with no relevant medical history. This fact underlines the importance of clinicians being aware of such possibilities. Furthermore, it emphasises the need for implementation of other tests of hearing in addition to pure tone audiometry, before a decision is made on hearing levels in children in this age category.

This recommendation is supported by work of Beagley and Knight (1968) and Coles and Priede (1971).

Impedance Bridge Measurements — Stapedial Reflex Threshold. The impedance bridge measurements may prove useful in ruling out the possibility of any underlying conductive pathology.

The fact that stapedial reflex thresholds may be 'normal' for a child is of limited value. The reason for this results from the fact that the span between hearing threshold and stapedial reflex threshold may be as little as 5 dB in cochlea pathology. Chiveralls *et al.* (1976). Reflex information is of primary importance with reference to functional children (unilateral or bilateral) who show no response to sound. If these children display reflex thresholds below their admitted hearing levels then this is a clear indicator that functionality is present. Such observations have been reported by Feldman (1963), Lamb and Peterson (1967), Nolan and Tucker (1981).

Speech Audiometry. The most commonly reported indication of functional hearing loss in children relates to the discrepancy between pure tone audiometry (PTA) and speech reception threshold (SRT) (SRT being taken as the level for 50 per cent discrimination score). The SRT often approximates the patient's true hearing threshold (Brockman and Hoversten, 1960; Dixon and Newby, 1959). In the Nolan and Tucker (1981) study seven of the ten children's SRTs were consistent with a normal PTA. In addition, it was also noted that the seven children were also able to communicate without difficulty at normal conversational voice level. There is no doubt that speech audiometry does provide the clinician with much useful information on hearing although it must be remembered that the test may not be viewed as a strict quantitative measure of hearing threshold.

Speech testing with such children can prove very difficult. The children often need a great deal of encouragement and the clinician certainly requires a great deal of patience. It is useful to vary the signal level before settling on what the clinician can describe to the child as a nice 'loud' level which is in fact relatively quiet. Problems of children substituting a word rhyming with the test word or simply saying random jargon words do occur. However, by careful application, useful information may very often be obtained from speech testing.

Sound Localisation. The fact that asymmetry in hearing can lead to difficulty in localisation of sound led Azzi (1962) to the idea of suggesting the use of such a test as a means of identifying unilateral functional cases. However, such tests can only be scientifically applied on a standardised testing rig. This clearly limits the test's usefulness as such rigs are not available to many clinicians. The format and test procedure to be used in such a test are comprehensively described by Newton and Hickson (1981). While such results do not *prove* functionality, they are useful in the overall test battery.

Quantification of Organic Thresholds

A number of test procedures has been suggested as a means of estimating the true organic thresholds in suspected functional cases. Usually the clinician's suspicions will have been aroused by some inconsistency of the diagnostic procedure. The aim then would be to obtain an estimate of the true hearing levels. Such tests obviously also act to confirm the clinician's suspicions.

Child-oriented Play Tests

1. The Pointing Test. In this test the child is seated in the position adopted for pure tone audiometry. The child is then instructed:

> You are going to wear the headphones again. This time when the whistle comes I want you to point to the ear which you think it is in. If you are not sure make a guess. It doesn't matter if your guess is incorrect.

The child is then fitted with headphones, a suitable test frequency is selected and the signal is presented from the audiometer in a similar manner to that adopted in pure tone audiometry. The child is given no clue as to when a signal is presented and each ear is stimulated separately. The signal level is initially set 10dB above the admitted threshold level. It is important in the initial stages to encourage the child by reinforcing the point about guessing if there was uncertainty about which ear the signal is in. Once the child has been encouraged to listen and point in response to a stimulus, the signal level is slowly reduced in 10dB steps with alternation to the other ear, so that responses resulting from stimuli presented to both ears may be recorded. This procedure continues until the signal level reaches an accepted screening level or an intensity level below which the child does not respond. The frequency of the pure tone is changed and the test repeated.

The child's response is recorded as positive if pointing to either ear occurs in response to a tone. The fact that the correct ear is identified is of no consequence. The important point is that the child responds reliably to a stimulus without clues or prompting. It is important that the clinician varies the time interval between stimuli so as to check for random false positive responses. However, when clear consistent pointing responses are obtained it may be concluded that the stimulus is being perceived. It has previously been reported by Feldman (1963) and Chaiklin and Ventry (1963) that subjects with functional hearing loss rarely, if at all, give false positive responses during testing. This is contrary to the behaviour of many highly responsive co-operative subjects.

2. The Say Test. This test idea was originally suggested by Miller *et al*. (1968) and was adopted for evaluation by Nolan and Tucker (1981). In that study the form of the test employed the format of the pointing test in that the child was seated in the position normally adopted for pure tone audiometry and instructed:

> You are going to wear headphones again. This time when the whistle comes I would like you to say yes when you hear it, no when you don't.

The child was then fitted with the headphones. A suitable test frequency was selected on the audiometer and the intensity level set at 10 dB above the admitted threshold. The child was then instructed to listen carefully and the procedure then followed that of pure tone audiometry. The child was given no clue as to when the signal was to be introduced. At the beginning of the test the child was encouraged to listen and respond. If, when the signal was presented, the child responded by saying 'yes, I heard that' or 'no, I couldn't hear that one', then the response was a positive one and the signal intensity was reduced as in the pointing test. Once consistent responses had been obtained for a particular frequency the frequency was changed and the test repeated. This test was devised following the observation that some children with functional hearing loss had shown evidence of hearing below their admitted thresholds on pure tone audiometry. Their behaviour was one of headshaking or saying, 'no, I didn't hear that one' at the instance a test tone was presented to them. These subjects were observed as being quiet and unresponsive during the interim periods between stimuli. The only time such behaviour was observed was whenever the stimulus was present. It was therefore considered that this behaviour was evidence of hearing the stimulus and could be used both as an indicator of functional hearing loss and true organic hearing thresholds.

3. The Counting Test. In this test the child is instructed in the following manner:

> You will be fitted with headphones. This time you will hear a series of several whistles, rather than just one whistle. I would like you to count the whistles out as they occur. There will be one, two, three, or four of them.

The child is then fitted with headphones and the method of signal presentation is the same as that used for pure tone audiometry. No clues as to when the tones are presented is given. The signal level is initially set 10dB above the admitted threshold and the child is encouraged to listen and count out loud. If positive responses are elicited, in that the child begins to count when the signals are presented, then the response is scored positively and the signal level reduced as in the previous tests.

The above three tests may be used with children showing bilateral or unilateral functional losses.

Effectiveness of Tests Designed for Identification of Functional Hearing Loss

It was reported by Nolan and Tucker (1981) that the pointing test was extremely effective. In all ten cases of functional hearing loss it proved possible to demonstrate consistent pointing responses at a level of 15dBHL. Included in the group were two children, one with no response unilaterally and one with no response bilaterally to conventional audiometry.

The 'Say Test' was effective in 50 per cent of the children, enabling the clinician to demonstrate reliable responses at 15dBHL. The children in whom this test failed only co-operated at the level shown in audiometry.

The counting test proved to be the least effective, only working with one child.

One of the major advantages of such tests relates to the fact that no specialised equipment is required. Furthermore, the tests are simple to apply and do not demand too much of children in terms of maturational level required to complete the test.

Such tests may prove useful in verifying normality of hearing, or in uncovering an underlying pathology which is resulting in a milder degree of hearing loss than indicated.

Unilateral Functional Loss

The Stenger Test. This test is useful with unilateral functional cases. It may be applied using pure tones or speech. However for normal clinical practice pure tone Stenger is most suitable (Newby, 1964). The Stenger principle states that when two tones of the same frequency are introduced simultaneously into both ears, only the louder tone will be preceived. This test is performed by introducing a tone of a particular frequency into the good ear at a level of 10dB above threshold and into the 'bad' ear at a level of 10dB below admitted threshold. If the loss in the 'bad' ear is genuine the patient will respond to the tone in his good ear since it is 10dB above threshold. If the patient does not respond this is a positive Stenger. This indicates that the tone in the 'bad' ear is precluding hearing of the tone in the good ear. Since the patient does not want to admit hearing in the bad ear, he fails to respond.

It is possible to quantify hearing levels using a pure tone Stenger. Clinically this may be achieved by use of a twin channel audiometer. Normal interrupted pure tones are employed. Having set the signals as instructed and obtained a positive Stenger the signal in the 'bad' ear is reduced until the patient begins to respond again. At this level the patient is hearing the tone in the good ear and therefore responds. This level is noted. The signal level is then slowly increased in 5dB steps in the 'bad' ear until the patient ceases to respond. This is recorded. At this level the patient is only perceiving the signal in the bad ear and is unaware of the signal in the good ear. Threshold may be assumed to lie between the recorded levels.

Electric Response Audiometry

Electric Response Audiometry is another useful component in the identification of functional hearing loss. The test applied needs to be relatively quick and non-invasive. BSER is considered to be most appropriate and when put together with other test results should enable the clinician to have a very comprehensive picture of the child's hearing capacity.

Causes and Management. The causes of this problem are generally considered to be of a psychogenic basis (Beagley and Knight, 1968). The fact of the matter is that while the child may not have a significant hearing problem, he certainly has a problem which will probably require the skills of a child care team comprising psychologist, otologist, psychiatrist and audiologist. It is vital for clinicians to ensure that parents understand the situation very clearly and are not simply informed that the child's hearing is satisfactory. This may be interpreted by the parents as 'child wasting everyone's time'. It should be pointed out that while hearing is not a significant problem as such, the child is having difficulties which require investigation and help. The parents should be advised very carefully on what they should do – this depending upon the prevailing situation with reference to the child.

Final Comments

Diagnostic Management Model

The point was made at the beginning of the chapter that early diagnosis is something that all clinicians should be working towards for every hearing-impaired child. It is fundamental to any effective audiological service that staff are well-trained and, in relation to screening in particular, that they receive regular refresher courses where their testing procedures are reassessed.

The role of parents in early diagnosis cannot be overemphasised. We propose that all parents should be asked when the baby reaches 4-6 months of age either by official letter or as part of a visit by the health visitor, whether they have any doubts about the child's hearing. The child should be thoroughly assessed at once by the diagnostic team in cases where concern is expressed. If a child at any time from birth onwards gives concern to parents with reference to hearing, then that child should be automatically referred by the person responsible for the medical care to the diagnostic team, this regardless of whether the baby has passed screening. All too often parents are fobbed off with comments such as 'don't worry he's just a little slow', 'it will only be wax', 'his father was slow to talk', when they suspect a hearing problem early in life. Such parents eventually obtain a diagnostic assessment for their child perhaps 18 to 24 months later. But by this time their child has failed to develop language, a disaster for the child and the family which ought not to be allowed to happen. Parents' assessments of their children are usually very accurate – take notice of them!

References

Anderson, H. Barr, B. and Wedenberg, E. (1970) 'The early detection of acoustic tumours by the stapedial reflex test' in G.E.W. Wolstenholme and J. Knight (eds.), *Sensori-neural Hearing Loss*, Ciba Foundation Symposium, J. & A. Churchill, London

Azzi, A.A. (1962) 'Hearing tests in simulation', *International Audiology*, *1*, 134

Balkany, T.J., Downs, M.P., Jafek, B.W. and Kragicek, M.J. (1979) *Clinical Pediatrics, 18*, 116

Barr, B. (1960) 'Non-organic hearing problems in school children. Functional Deafness', *Acta Otolaryngology, 52*, 337

Barratt, H. (1980) 'Electric response audiometry and its application to the assessment of hearing in children', *Journal British Association Teachers of the Deaf, 4 (4)*, 116

Barratt, H. and Rowson, V.J. (1982) 'Normal variation in the masking effectiveness of the narrow band noises of one audiometer', *British Journal of Audiology*, *16*, 159

Barry, S.J. and Resnick, S.B. (1978) 'Absolute thresholds for frequency modulated signals: effects of rate, pattern and percentage modulation', *Journal of Speech and Hearing Disorders*, *43*, 192

Bayne, S.M. (1968) 'Vibrotactile thresholds in air and bone conduction audiometry'. Dissertation submitted for the Diploma in Audiology, Department of Audiology, University of Manchester, Manchester

Beagley, H.A. and Knight, J.J. (1968) 'The evaluation of suspected non-organic hearing loss', *Journal of Laryngology, 82*, 693

Bench, R.J. and Boscak, N. (1970) 'Some applications of signal detection theory to paedo-audiology', *Sound*, *4*, 58

Bench, J. (1978) 'Why early diagnosis?' in S.E. Gerber and G.T. Mencher (eds.), *The Early Diagnosis of Hearing Loss*, Grune and Stratton, New York

Bennet, M.J. (1979) 'Trials with the auditory response cradle: I neonatal responses to auditory stimuli', *British Journal of Audiology*, *13*, 125

Bennet, M.J. and Wade, H.K. (1980) 'Automated newborn hearing screening using the auditory response cradle' in I.G. Taylor and A. Markides (eds.), *Disorders of Auditory Function III*, Academic Press, London

Blair-Simmons, F., McFarland, W.H. and Jones, F.R. (1979) 'An automated hearing screening technique for newborns', *Acta Otolaryngology*, *87*, 1

Boothroyd, A. (1968) 'Developments in speech audiometry', *Sound*, *2*, 3

Borg, E. (1972) 'On the change in the acoustic impedance of the ear as a measure of middle ear muscle reflex activity', *Acta Otolaryngology*, *74*, 163

Brasier, V.J. (1974) 'Pitfalls in audiometry', *Public Health*, *89*, 31

British Society of Audiology (1981) 'Recommended procedures for pure tone audiometry using a manually operated instrument', *British Journal of Audiology*, *15*, 213

British Standard Institution (1969) 'Reference zero for calibration of pure tone audiometers', B.S. 2497 pt. 2

Brockman, S.J. and Hoversten, G.H. (1960) 'Pseudo Neural Hypacusis in Children', *Trans. Amer. Larng. Rhinol. Otol. Soc.*, 603

Brooks, D.N. (1967) 'An objective method of detecting fluid in the middle ear', *International Audiology*, 7, 280

Brooks, D.N. (1968) 'Clinicial use of the acoustic impedance meter', *Sound, 2*, 40

Brooks, D.N. (1969) 'The use of the electro-acoustic impedance bridge in the assessment of middle ear function', *International Audiology*, 8, 568

Campanelli, P.A. (1963) 'Simulated hearing losses in school children following identification audiometry', *Journal Auditory Research*, 3, 91

Chaiklin, J.B., Ventry, I.M., Barrett, L.S. and Skalbeck, G.S. (1959) 'Pure tone threshold patterns observed in functional hearing loss', *Laryngoscope, 69*, 1165

Chaiklin, J.B. and Ventry, I.M. (1963) 'Functional hearing loss' in J. Jerger (ed.), *Modern Developments in Audiology*, Academic Press, New York, p. 76

Chalmers, P., Mentz, L. and Bench, J. (1974) 'On the acquisition of skills in judging infants auditory behaviour: knowledge of peers' assessment', *British Journal of Audiology*, 8, 89

Chiveralls, K. and FitzSimons, R. (1973) 'Stapedial reflex action in normal subjects', *British Journal of Audiology*, 7, 105

Chiveralls, K., FitzSimons, R., Beck, G.B. and Kernohan, H. (1976) 'The diagnostic significance of the stapedius reflex', *British Journal of Audiology, 10*, 122

Coles, R.R.A. and Priede, V.M. (1971) 'Non-organic overlay in noise induced hearing loss', *Proceedings of the Royal Society of Medicine, 64*, 194

Cunningham, C. and McArthur, K. (1981) 'Hearing loss and treatment in young Down's syndrome children', *Child: Care, Health and Development, 7*, 357

Davies, B. and Penniceard, R.M. (1980) 'Auditory function and receptive vocabulary in Down's syndrome children' in I.G. Taylor and A. Markides (eds.), *Disorders of Auditory Function III*, Academic Press, London

Denes, P. and Naunton, R.F. (1952) 'Masking in pure tone audiometry', *Proceedings of the Royal Society of Medicine, 45,* 790

Dillon, H. and Walker, G. (1982) 'Comparison of stimuli used in sound field audiometric testing', *Journal of the Acoustical Society of America, 71*, 161

Dixon, R.F. and Newby, H.A. (1959) 'Children with non-organic hearing problems', *AMA Archives Otolaryngology, 70*, 619

Dockum, G.D. and Robinson, D.O. (1975) 'Warble tone as an audiometric stimulus', *Journal of Speech and Hearing Disorders, 40*, 351

Downs, M.J. and Silver, H. (1972) 'The A.B.C.D.'s to H.E.A.R.', *Clinical Paediatrics, 11*, 563

DeSouza, S.W., McCartney, E., Nolan, M. and Taylor, I.G. (1981) 'Hearing, speech and language in survivors of severe perinatal asphyxia', *Archives of Disease in Childhood, 56*, 333

Erber, N. (1980) 'Use of the auditory numbers test to evaluate speech perception abilities of hearing-impaired children', *Journal of Speech and Hearing Disorders, 45*, 527

Ewing, A.W.G. (1957) *Educational Guidance and the Deaf Child*, Manchester University Press, Manchester

Feldman, A.S. (1963) 'Impedance Measurement at the eardrum as an aid to diagnosis', *Sound of Speech and Hearing Research, 6*, 815

Fletcher, H. (1940) 'Auditory patterns', *Review of Modern Physics, 12*, 47

Flood, L.M., Fraser, J.G., Conway, M.J. and Stewart, A. (1982) 'The assessment of hearing in infancy using the post auricular myogenic response', *British Journal of Audiology, 16*, 211

Forse, A. (1980) 'Interaural intensity differences in the free field'. Unpublished MSc dissertation, Department of Audiology, University of Manchester, Manchester

Fraser, J.C.L. (1971) 'Validation of the new Manchester picture test'. Unpublished dissertation for the Diploma in Audiology, University of Manchester, Manchester

Froding, C.A. (1960) 'Acoustic investigation of newborn infants', *Acta Otolaryngology* (Stockholm), *52*, 31

Fry, D.B. (1961) 'Word and sentence tests for use in speech audiometry', *Lancet*, ii, 197

Gatehouse, S. and Browning G.G. (1982) 'A re-examination of the Carhart effect', *British Journal of Audiology*, *16*, 215

Gibson, W.P.R. (1978) 'Essentials of clinicial electric response audiometry', Churchill Livingstone, Edinburgh

Haskins, H. (1949) 'A phonetically balanced test of speech discrimination for children'. Unpublished master's thesis, Northwestern University, Evanston, Illinois

Hawkins, J.E. and Stevens, S.S. (1950) 'Masking of pure tones and of speech by white noise', *Journal of the Acoustical Society of America*, *22*, 6

Health Visitors' Association (1977) 'Survey on hearing testing – summary of findings'. *Talk* (September), 19

Hood, J.D. (1957) 'Measurement of noise', *Proceedings of the Royal Society of Medicine*, *50*, 689

John, J.E.J. (1957) 'Acoustics and efficiency in the use of hearing aids' in A.W.G. Ewing (ed.), *Educational Guidance and the Deaf Child*, Manchester University Press, Manchester

Katz, D. and Elliott, L. (1978) 'Development of a new children's speech discrimination test'. Paper presented at the American Speech and Hearing Association Convention, San Francisco, California

Kendall, D.C. (1957) 'Mental development of young children' in A.W.G. Ewing (ed.), *Educational Guidance and the Deaf Child*, Manchester University Press, Manchester

Kiang, N.Y.S., Christ, A.H., French, M.A. and Edwards, A.G. (1964) 'Quarterly Progress Report', Laboratory of Electronics, Massachusetts Institute of Technology, *28*, 218, Mass.

Lamb, L.E. and Peterson, J.L. (1967) 'Middle ear reflex measurements in Pseudohypacusis', *Journal of Speech and Hearing Disorders*, *32*, 46

Langford, C. and Bench, J. (1973) 'Neonatal auditory responses assessed by trained and untrained observers: A preliminary study', *British Journal of Audiology*, *7*, 29

Liden, G., Nilsson, G. and Anderson, H. (1959a) 'Narrow-band masking with white noise', *Acta Otolaryngology* (Stockholm) *50*, 116

Liden, G., Nilsson, G. and Anderson, H. (1959b) 'Masking in clinical audiometry', *Acta Otolaryngology* (Stockholm), *50*, 125

Liden, G. (1970) 'The stapedius muscle reflex used as an objective recruitment test: A clinical and experimental study' in G.E.W. Wolstenholme and J. Knight (eds.), *Ciba Foundation Symposium on Sensori-neural Hearing Loss*, J. & A. Churchill, London

Liden, G., Peterson, J.L. and Hartford, E.R. (1970) 'Simultaneous recording of changes in relative impedance and air pressure during acoustic and non-acoustic elicitation of the middle-ear reflexes', *Acta Otolaryngology*, *263*, 208

Ling, D. and Ling, A. (1978) *Aural Rehabilitation*, Ch. 6, A.G. Bell Association for the Deaf, Washington, DC

Lloyd, L.L. (1970) 'Audiologic aspects of mental retardation' in N.R. Ellis (ed.), *International Review of Research in Mental Retardation*, Academic Press, London

McDermott, J.C. and Hodgson, W.R. (1982) 'Auditory thresholds in children for narrow-band noise and warble tones in sound field', *British Journal of Audiology, 16*, 221

McFarland, W.H., Blair-Simmons, F. and Jones, F.R. (1980) 'An automated hearing screening technique for newborns', *Journal of Speech and Hearing Disorders, 45*, 495

Martin, F.W. (1978) 'Evaluation of pseudohypauisis' in J. Katz (ed.), *Handbook of Clinical Audiology*, 2nd edn, Williams & Wilkins, Baltimore, p. 276

Martin, J.A.M., Bentzen, O., Colley, J.R.T., Hennebart, D., Holm, C., Iurato, S., de Jonge, G.A., McCullen, O., Meyer, M.L., Moore, W.J. and Morgon, A. (1981) 'Childhood deafness in the European Community', *Scandanavian Audiology, 10*, 165

Markides, A. (1980a) 'The relation between hearing loss for pure tones and hearing loss for speech among hearing-impaired children', *British Journal of Audiology, 14*, 115

Markides, A. (1980b) 'The Manchester speechreading (lipreading) test' in I.G. Taylor and A. Markides (eds.), *Disorders of Auditory Function III*, Academic Press, London

Mecox, K. and Galambos, P. (1974) 'Brainstem auditory evoked responses in human infants and adults', *Archives of Otolaryngology, 99*, 30

Metz, O. (1952) 'Threshold of reflex contractions of muscles of the middle ear and recruitment of loudness', *Archives of Otolaryngology, 55*, 536

Miller, A.L., Fox, M.S. and Chan, G. (1968) 'Pure tone assessments as an aid in detecting suspected non-organic hearing disorders in children', *Laryngoscope, 78*, 2170

Mokotoff, B., Schulmann-Galambos, C. and Galambos, R. (1977) 'Brain stem auditory evoked responses in children', *Archives of Otolaryngology, 103*, 38

Moncur, J.P. (1964) 'Videotape analysis of hearing responses in children', Progress Report, USPHS, NB4019, June

Moncur, J.P. (1968) 'Judge reliability in infant testing', *Journal of Speech and Hearing Research, 11*, 348

Moore, J.M., Thompson, G. and Thompson, M. (1975) 'Auditory localisation of infants as a function of reinforcement conditions', *Journal of Speech and Hearing Disorders, 40*, 29

Moore, J.M., Wilson, W.R. and Thompson, G. (1977) 'Visual reinforcement of headturn responses in infants under 12 months of age', *Journal of Speech and Hearing, 42*, 328

Morgan, D.E., Dirks, D. and Bower, D.R. (1979) 'Suggested threshold sound pressure levels for frequency-modulated (warble) tones in the sound field', *Journal of Speech and Hearing Disorders, 44*, 37

Newton, V.E. and Hickson, F.S. (1981) 'Sound localisation: A clinical procedure', *Journal of Laryngology, 95*, 41

Newby, H.A. (1964) *Audiology*, 2nd edn, Appleton-Century-Crofts, New York, p. 157

Nolan, M., McCartney, E., McArthur, K. and Rowson, V.J. (1980) 'A study of the hearing and receptive vocabulary of the trainees of an adult training centre', *Journal of Mental Deficiency Research, 24*, 271

Nolan, M. and Tucker, I.G. (1981) 'Functional hearing loss in children', *Journal British Assoc. Teachers of the Deaf, 5*, 2-10

Nueva Espana, E.A. (1979) 'Diagnostic significance of otoadmittance measurements in the middle ear pathologies'. Unpublished MSc dissertation, Dept. audiology, University of Manchester, Manchester

Popelka, G.R. (1981) *Hearing Assessment with the Acoustic Reflex*, Grune and Stratton, New York

Porter, T. (1974) 'Otoadmittance measurements', *American Annals of the Deaf*, *119*, 47

Rainville, M.J. (1959) 'New method of masking for the determination of bone conduction curves', *Trans. Beltone Institute Hearing Research*, no. 11

Redell, R.C. and Calvert, D.R. (1969) 'Factors in screening hearing of the newborn', *Journal of Auditory Research*, *3*, 278

Reilly, N. (1958) 'Frequency and amplitude modulation audiometry', *Archives of Otolayrngology*, *68*, 363

Robinson, D.W. and Vaughn, C.R. (1976) 'Relative efficiency of warble tone and conventional pure tone testing with children, *Journal of the American Audiology Society*, *1*, 253

Robson, J. (1970) 'Screening techniques in babies', *Sound*, *4*, 91

Ross, M. (1964) 'The variable intensity pulse count method (VIPCM) for the detection and measurement of pure tone threshold of children with functional hearing loss', *Journal of Speech and Hearing Disorders*, *29*, 477

Ross, M. and Lerman, J. (1970) 'A picture identification test for hearing-impaired children', *Journal of Speech and Hearing Research*, *13*, 44

Ruben, R.J. (1972) 'The ear' in H.L. Barnett and A.H. Einhorn (eds.) *Paediatrics*, Ch. 21, Butterworths, London, p. 959

Ryerson, S.G. and Beagley, H.A. (1981) 'Brainstem electric responses and electrocochleography: a comparison of threshold sensitivities in children', *British Journal of Audiology*, *15*, 41

Sanders, J.W. and Rintelmann, W.F. (1964) 'Masking in audiometry: A clinical evaluation of the methods', *Archives of Otolaryngology* (Chicago), *80*, 541

Sanders, J.W. and Josey, A.F. (1970) 'Narrow-band noise audiometry for hard to test patients', *Journal of Speech and Hearing Research*, *13*, 74

Sesterhenn, G. and Brueninger, H. (1977) 'Determination of hearing threshold for single frequencies from the acoustic reflex', *Audiology*, *16(3)*, 201

Shallop, J.K., Tubergen, L.B. and Jones, J.K. (1982) *Clinical Applications of Tympanometry and Acoustic Reflexes*, Indiana University School of Medicine, Madsen Electronics Publication, Indiana

Sheridan, M.D. (1976) *Manual for the STYCAR Hearing Tests*, NFER Publishing Company Ltd, London

Smith, B.L. and Markides, A. (1981) 'Interaural attenuation for pure tones and speech', *British Journal of Audiology*, *15*, 49

Staab, W.J. and Rintelmann, W.F. (1972) 'Status of warble-tone in audiometers', *Audiology*, *11*, 244

Studebaker, G.A. (1962) 'On masking in bone-conduction testing', *Journal of Speech and Hearing Research*, *5*, 215

Studebaker, G.A. (1964) 'Clinical masking of air and bone conducted stimuli', *Journal of Speech and Hearing Disorders*, *29*, 23

Suzuki, T. and Ogiba, Y. (1960) 'A technique of pure tone audiometry for children under 3 years of age. Conditioned orientation reflex (COR) audiometry', *Rev. Laryngology* (Bordeaux), *81*, 33

Taylor, I.G. (1964) *Neurological Mechanisms of Hearing and Speech in Children*, Manchester University Press, Manchester

Taylor, I.G. (1980) 'Medicine and Education', *Proceedings of Conference for Heads of Schools and Services for Hearing-impaired Children*, University of Manchester, Manchester

Telesensory Systems Inc. (1982) *Crib-o-gram Validation Study. A Summary of Results*, Telesen Inc., Palo Alto, California

Thomsen, K.A. (1955) 'Eustachian tube function tested by employment impedance measuring', *Acta Otolaryngology*, *45*, 252

Walker, G. and Dillon, H. (1983) 'The selection of modulation rates for fⁱ quency modulated sound field stimuli', *Scandinavian Audiology*, *12(⸴* 151

Wallace, G. (1973) *Canadian Study of Hard of Hearing and Deaf*, Canadiₐ Rehabilitation Council for the Disabled, Ottawa

Watson, T.J. (1957) 'Speech audiometry' in A.W.G. Ewing (ed.), *Educationₐ Guidance and the Deaf Child*, Manchester University Press, Manchester

Weatherby, L.A. and Bennet, M.J. (1979) 'The neonatal acoustic reflex', *Scₐ dinavian Audiology*, *8(4)*, 233

Wedenberg, E. (1956) 'Auditory tests on new born infants', *Acta Otolaryngoloₐ* (Stockholm), *46*, 446

Zalewski, T. (1906) 'Experimentelle Untersuchungen uber die Resistenzfahigkₐ des Trommelfells', *Zeits. f. Chrenheik.*, *52*, 109

Zwislocki, J. (1953) 'Acoustic attenuation between the ears', *Journal of tₐ Acoustical Society of America*, *25*, 752

3 PARENT GUIDANCE AND COUNSELLING

The Educational Audiologist may be directly involved in both counselling and guidance — the area related to the emotional reactions to handicap and the area related to the management of deafness. This is frequently the case in the United Kingdom, where Educational Audiologists receive special training in these areas, but even where direct involvement with the counselling aspect is not the audiologist's role, everything he does with hearing aids will largely depend for its success on the family of the hearing-impaired child. Child acceptance of the aids depends on parental acceptance and the child's linguistic experience through his aids will depend on many parental factors, which in turn relate to the counselling area. The Educational Audiologist should be very familiar with common reactions to having handicapped children and what steps the professionals involved will be taking to support the family. He cannot isolate himself from the human factors, concentrating solely on the application of technology to the hearing problem.

There is a danger, in this area of interest, of making statements which only refer to a small minority of the parents of handicapped children and the basis of little experience some workers are apt to generalise *vis-à-vis* the whole population of handicapped children and their families. There would seem, however, to be a good deal of support for the suggestion that there are a variety of very common reactions to having a hearing handicapped child and it would be useful to highlight a number of them.

Some Common Initial Reactions to Hearing-impairment

The reported reactions of parents range from shock, guilt, embarrassment, inadequacy and on occasions even relief, relief that it is deafness and not something else that they fear even more. Many parents feel a great sense of isolation and inadequacy. They feel entirely alone in having to solve what, for them, must seem an enormous, perhaps insoluble problem. They have gone through all of the stages of expectation of having a normal healthy child and now they have a child with a permanent disability. How much that disability becomes a handicap will depend on many things including how they are managed, both in

terms of the child's amplification requirements and educational stim\
lation and in terms of the support available to overcome the earl\
emotional reactions to the discovery of the disability.

The first step of any support programme is to convince the famil\
that they are not *alone* with their problems, that there is someon\
who cares about them and their child. Telling them that support \
available is one thing, but actually being supportive when they nee\
it is what really counts. A counsellor being outgoing to the baby itse\
can be an early positive step. Some mothers feel that no one will regar\
them or the baby as 'normal' again and when the counsellor picks u\
the baby, or plays with the toddler this sense of isolation can start t\
fade. Undoubtedly the early stages of counselling are more atuned t\
the emotional needs of the parents than the practical and specifi\
aspects of the child's development.

The scene is set in the clinic where the diagnosis is carried out. Ho\
parents are told of the outcome of the testing requires a great deal o\
tact and skill. As Thomas (1978) has suggested 'this period calls fo\
intensive support, not only in practical day to day child care, bu\
also in working through emotions aroused'. He also suggests a relation\
ship between parental attitudes and subsequent adjustment and progres\
of the child. Any contribution the counsellor can make to gettin\
'attitudes' right will be valuable indeed for the long-term developmen\
of the child.

Neuhaus (1969) examined the social and emotional adjustment o\
84 hearing-impaired children. All of the children he studied were o\
average or near-average intelligence, had no secondary handicap an\
came from complete families. Maternal and paternal attitudes wer\
rated independently and teachers used a scale to assess the child'\
adjustment. Neuhaus compared adjustment levels with parental atti\
tudes and found a close correspondence between maternal attitude\
and child adjustment level. Positive attitudes produced emotional an\
social stability (paternal attitudes correlated more highly with the olde\
age group of children).

Why Did it Happen?

This is a very common early reaction and a typical question asked o\
the counsellor.

Parent of M.S. — diagnosed at 14 months with average hearing los\
of 100 dB HL. Cause of deafness not discovered but sensori-neura\
in nature. He expressed his feelings after the diagnosis as follows:

Empty really. My wife just broke down. I would have liked to as well, but it would have looked stupid both of us walking through Manchester like that. One of us had to be normal you know. Times are when things are quiet and you think why? why? and no reason.

Following on from diagnosis every possible medical test should be carried out to ascertain the cause of deafness.

In about half of sensori-neurally impaired patients these tests will reveal no obvious causative agent and in these cases there is high risk that the impairment is of a recessive genetic causation, where mother and father carry a gene for deafness. In these cases the risk of producing further hearing-impaired children will be about one in four at each subsequent pregnancy. Obviously genetic counselling is vital here. The tests are needed not just to satisfy the parents' question 'why' but also to provide a bank of information which will help to let the child himself know if he also will risk hearing-impaired children when he marries. Many of the tests must be done early if they are to be of any value.

However, the parent quoted above was not just saying 'why' in the sense of 'why did it happen?' He is saying why out of all the people who have lovely normal babies have we been so cruelly selected to have a child with such a serious disability. In other words, whatever the cause, why did it happen to us? The world seems a harsh place indeed for parents with shattered expectations.

Shock and Sorrow

Thurston (1960) has suggested that grief was one of the main initial reactions of parents. Solnit and Stark (1961) have asserted that the birth of a handicapped child was seen by the parents as an 'object loss', that is, the loss of the expected healthy child at a time of regression, great stress and physiological and psychological depletion. The parents may grieve, the course of this grief being dependent on such factors as the abruptness of loss and the preparation for it. It is further suggested that there may be two further extreme reactions resultant upon feelings of guilt and depression. On the one hand guilt can lead to an absolute dedication to the welfare of the handicapped child, on the other the parents feel intolerance of the defect and an almost irresistible impulse to deny their relationship to the child. Where parents are poorly handled or given inadequate counselling they may become fixated between recognition and denial and chronic mourning may result. It was Olshansky (1965) who suggested that most parents who

have a mentally handicapped child suffer from a reaction he identi
fies as 'chronic sorrow' particularly if the child is severely impaired.

> Mother of M.M. — diagnosed at 11 months. M.M. was severely
> impaired with an average hearing loss of 100dB. 'When M. was
> diagnosed ... it was a terrible shock ... and the shock lasts for
> years really and all the time you're trying to cope with the child
> You gradually become adjusted, but it's not easy.'
>
> The above mother's face was clearly anguished as she recalled
> the early days after her daughter was diagnosed several years pre
> viously.

There are similarities in the responses of some parents of hearing
impaired children, particularly those with severe additional handicaps
One of the problems as the present authors see it is that in our culture
sorrow is concealed. That is the socially accepted practice, so comment
like 'She's bearing up very well' may be said of a recently bereaved
wife. On occasions professionals mistake this concealment of sorrow
for a pathological symptom. Workers say then that the parents are
denying the reality of the child's handicap, when in fact what may be
happening is that parents are denying their sorrow. Rather than a
neurotic manifestation, sorrow should be seen as an understandable
response to what is indeed at the start a family tragedy. Olshansky
too, reminds us that very few parents, after the initial shock, do not
recover enough to mobilise their efforts on behalf of their child. Tumim
(1977), a parent of two hearing-impaired children, has suggested that
there is great danger in professionals assuming that having a deaf child
brings about a sort of 'pathological metamorphosis' in the family.

> Julius and Martha Allen from the United States (Allen and Allen
> 1979) are parents of a profoundly hearing-impaired mainstreamed
> son and they have revealed their reactions through their advice to
> other parents of hearing-impaired children:

> When we meet parents of a newly diagnosed deaf child we find
> ourselves remembering all too well the inner turmoil of those early
> weeks and months after our first child was diagnosed profoundly
> deaf. We find ourselves looking into their eyes and seeing the naked
> pain, or perhaps we see a mask wherein the eyes are vague and
> unemotional. At the beginning, we usually say, 'Believe it or not,
> you will laugh again.' Often that brings tears, tears for everything

that is gone, for everything that will never be the same. We tell them to cry and usually we cry with them. We say it is normal to cry and to hurt, but it can't be for too long. Then we tell them how it was when our world seemed to come to an end and that it is possible to reconstruct a new one; not the same as before, but certainly an acceptable one. Since the scheme of things has changed, there will be new problems, new goals and new expectations. There will be much pain and much frustration, as well as guilt and anger. Life a series of adjustments and compromises at best, now demands critical adjustment. We tell parents that they'd better get on with it because if they don't this child will not make it alone. Finally we try to tell them what to expect in the next few weeks and months, both from their child and from themselves. We talk to them only from our own experience and hope that their progress in adjusting to this devastating blow will be faster than our own.

The present authors certainly do not believe that many families with hearing-impaired children present as 'psychiatric cases'. There are reactions such as those described, and others, but the underlying fact from our experience of seeing many families with young hearing-impaired children is that within the family unit is the inner resource, the strength to face up to the problem of hearing-impairment and with the help of caring, sensitive professionals, the ability to overcome their grief and their fears. As the Allens say, 'The child cannot make it on his own, the parents have to help.'

Relief

Inexperienced workers may be unaware that a frequent reaction to diagnosis of hearing-impairment is relief. This often stems from the fact that parents have suspected deafness long before the diagnosis is made. Those involved in carrying out diagnostic procedures would do well to take great note of what the family say about the child. If they think he has a hearing problem, in our experience he almost always has. We strongly advise parents not to be put off by *any* professional until they have achieved a full audiological assessment at a specialist audiology centre. Too many people, who know nothing about testing the hearing of young children, are too ready to give an opinion about his hearing status.

J.H. was victim of professional muddle and not diagnosed with his 90 dB HL sensori-neural hearing loss until he was nearly four years old.

His mother expressed her feelings as follows:

> We were convinced that he had a hearing problem long before h
> was diagnosed. I felt when he diagnosed — well thank God some
> body has finally appreciated the problem. I felt very concerne
> about it obviously, but the main thing was that at least now i
> was diagnosed something can be done about treating it.
>
> I began to feel that people, I mean my own mother and di
> ferent people, were saying I was stupid to be thinking there wa
> something wrong with him, he was perfectly normal and I reall
> began to think that there was something other than a hearing prob
> lem and that it was a mental thing with him — I am sure I wa
> relieved that it was what we had suspected and nothing more
> There was a sort of resistance from our parents to the fact tha
> there was anything wrong with him. We felt we were battling, not onl
> against the first doctor who said his hearing was normal, but it wa
> also our own families who said 'Oh no he's just a slow talker.' S
> you see we met resistance all the way along.

This parent was not only relieved that she had finally convinced some
one that her child was hearing-impaired, she was relieved that it wa
deafness and not something, in her view, far worse. This is not a
infrequent comment, parents being much happier to accept hearing
impairment than say mental handicap, or 'brain damage'.

> A.J.'s parents were convinced she had a problem but no profes
> sional diagnosed it until Mrs J., when A. was nearly two and a half
> finally realised what it was. A.J. has an average hearing loss o
> 90 dB HL, sensori-neural in nature.

> Relief really — that's the only way I can describe it because we'
> been warned, but it was up to us to find out what was wrong wit
> her. We were told that she might be brain damaged and that was it
> There was nothing after that. She was two and a half by the tim
> I finally put my finger on it, that it was deafness. Some people migh
> think it is a silly thing to say, but as opposed to being brain damage
> I'd prefer that she was deaf because you can do a lot whereas wit
> brain damage there's not a lot you can do — not as much anyhow
> Our reaction was relief.

The above 'bright' child progressed very well after a late diagnosis an vas placed in a partially hearing unit in an ordinary school. Much of he research into reactions to handicap has been carried out on families where the child is very handicapped, both physically and mentally and t is advisable therefore for the workers with families of hearing-impaired hildren to bear in mind the possible differences in reaction and acceptance of sensori-handicapped as opposed to more globally handicapped hildren.

Stress

Tumin (1977) highlights the *external* stresses the family face rather han the more usual (professional) model of the *internally* stressed handicapped family'. She points out the paradox of the educational, medical and social services, etc., which are supposed to help handicapped children and their families, but may actually make them more wretched — in some cases even more so than the problems they are designed to alleviate. She cites examples of teachers giving parents unrealistic tasks, that make them feel guilty, inadequate or anxious and she calls this 'pedagogenically induced stress'. She extends her criticisms to doctors, psychologists and education authority bureaucrats because they frequently fail to give parents enough information, or give it in an unintelligible way, and make decisions about handicapped children without giving the parents any semblance of 'partnership'.

There are indeed many things both within and outside the family which can lead to stress and anxiety for the parents. As already mentioned many parents are forced to battle through a series of obstacles to get their child diagnosed. There are the doctors who say 'parents worry too much' or that 'it will just be a wax build-up or catarrh'. All this is very stressful to a parent who is convinced that the child's problem is more serious than this. Some workers have referred to the process of getting the child diagnosed as getting through the *minefield* or the *obstacle* course. Even when they get to the audiology clinic it is not always incident-free, with reports of casual or hasty diagnosis, with the clinician showing little interest in the family, talking to colleagues about the diagnosis whilst ignoring the family, and reports of families being given a totally unintelligible account of the child's problems. If the clinic is slow to fit the hearing aids, or if the earmoulds do not allow the appropriate volume control setting to be used, then this too is likely to add to the family's already high state of anxiety. Poor diagnostic work, where the family are not convinced of the findings, leads to stress and often induces the response some clinicians call *diagnosis shopping* where the parents take the child from clinic to clinic, from specialist to specialist. It is part of the clinician' job, in our view, to demonstrate his findings to the parents so that they are convinced. This can be followed up later in more detail, using demonstration tapes, etc. but the clinician must show the parents that the level of hearing loss is as he says it is. It is also true that one of the reactions to diagnosis of hearing-impairment is to search for a specialist not so much to get a better diagnosis, but in the hope that he will say that the loss is not there, or that if present it can easily be cured. Parents must be told the truth and convinced that it is the truth.

In any event diagnosis shopping would be much reduced if audio logists ascertained the extent of the problem and then got on with positive features of stressing the child's abilities in other aspects of his development, and positive effects of the use of amplification. I is most helpful if the professionals involved get together and provide a united approach to the family. This was a positive recommendation of the Warnock Report (HMSO, 1978) and co-operation in the way information is collated about a handicapped child is embodied in the United Kingdom Education Act 1981. In the United States similar prin ciples now apply following recent legislation. Teamwork is crucial since i is most stressful for the family if there are big differences on major issues from members of the support team. There are always shade of opinion about issues, but our partners in the venture of helping the hearing-impaired child (the parents) often start with little or no knowledge of the subject and are only made anxious by professional wrangling over methodology.

Within the family, maternal or paternal differences can cause stress and it would seem a wise plan to advise parents to discuss and devise agreed procedures for handling the hearing-impaired child. This is appropriate for such issues as discipline, table manners, etc. where it can be stressful for one partner to be insisting on certain responses and the other to be accepting inappropriate behaviour. It could easily be argued that this applies equally to the treatment of normally hearing children and we would agree, but parents of normally hearing children are much more relaxed about their children achieving skills and th reduction of handling conflicts in the family with a hearing-impaired child may enable them too to adopt a more relaxed approach. Add on top the worries of school placement, the fears for the future, the stress of a multitude of clinic appointments and one might wonder how they cope, but cope they do and most of them very well.

The parents seem to be in a double bind. On the one hand they are eing encouraged to be less anxious because anxiety can affect the elationship they have with their baby. On the other hand, they cannot void feeling anxious about many things. The advice of the mother of everely hearing-impaired twins is, we feel, a contribution that some arents could accept from another parent, that perhaps they could not ccept from professionals. The twins had just started at a school for partially hearing children, although their hearing losses are both in xcess of 100 dB HL, so we asked their mother if, with the benefit of hindsight, there was anything in the way she had handled or managed he children that she would have changed, if she could. She replied hat had she known how well they would grow up she would have done ll the same things, but she would have been far more relaxed and ess anxious about doing them.

Guilt

A very commonly reported reaction to hearing-impairment is guilt. The parents are reported as seeking someone to blame for the child's disability or blame themselves. This can be particularly true where the known cause is rubella in pregnancy. If the child is deafened because of the rubella virus and the mother had not had the rubella vaccine his can be particularly stressful. Of course there is a small percentage of women who have the vaccine and do not build up antibodies to the disease. There is also a problem related to the whole question of vacination in the United Kingdom. Vaccination is given to teenage girls whose parents sign a form saying they agree to this procedure, yet often the disastrous effects of rubella to the foetus have not been sufficiently emphasised. We are sure that many parents see the disease as the mildly irritating rash they had as a child. A vigorous parent education programme is required. There are also those who would argue that the vaccination programme should include all teenage girls unless their parents opt out, rather than parents having to sign a form to opt in. Sanctions against unvaccinated persons are used in the USA and this could well be followed in Britain. The aim should be to vaccinate every girl who does not already have antibodies to the disease. This is said advisedly since many parents, who produce a rubella child, believe they already had the disease. The test should be, does the patient *have* the antibodies to rubella, NOT does the patient think she had the disease as a child.

There is no doubt that there is a possibility of parents experiencing guilt feelings throughout the child's life. They feel guilty about not being able to get Bill to wear his aids all day when they see Mary wearing hers happily. They feel guilty when you, the audiologist, tell them to set the aid at volume setting five and they cannot because the earmoulds are a poor fit as the child is in a growth spurt. They must be encouraged to seek support when these problems, over which the parents have little control, arise. Improvement of the aid fitting in the latter instance would remove the cause of the guilt and appropriate advice on tactics for encouraging the wearing of the aids would offset the former problem.

Guilt can spread to attempts to blame others. In one example of a family known to us, the mother had been married before and had produced two normally hearing children. The implication of her comments were that she felt her second husband was somehow to blame for the third child being hearing-impaired. There was little doubt that her attitude had put severe strain on the marriage. All the possible medical tests were carried out on the child and both families were investigated with no dominant line of genetic inheritance being found. The conclusion was that there was a strong possibility that the deafness was genetic, but of a recessive nature, where both mother and father must carry a gene for deafness. An appointment with a genetic counsellor greatly helped in resolving this conflict.

Guilt can also arise in communication situations with the child. One aim is to encourage parents of hearing-impaired children to provide as many situations and activities as possible where communication can and needs to take place. Some parents, however, adopt this attitude to such an extent that they feel guilty if they are doing something and *not* involving the child. They need to be encouraged to treat communication in as relaxed a manner as possible and to enjoy the child as a child. There is a real danger of too much attention being focused on the 'problem' and not enough on the child himself. Parents should be advised that there is no doubt that the child will make communication attempts both in the vocalisations he makes and in other non verbal ways. Parents should watch for these attempts (and there is growing body of evidence that they can and do) learn to read them and to respond with appropriate linguistic stimulation. Giving the child his 'turn' in communication must start early and certainly mother/child turntaking will be well established long before the child speaks his first words.

One of the problems with guilt as a concept is its deeper meaning for psycho-pathologists. This can in our view obscure the fact that practical responses often remove its basis for parents of hearing-impaired children. In fact quite a lot of what is written about guilt in relation to andicap is not helpful − either to the parents or to those who are rying to help them. Roith (1963), a consultant psychiatrist writing bout the parents of mentally handicapped children and the question f guilt, suggests that there is a lot of woolly thinking and false reasoning on this issue. Some experts allege that the guilt is based on the lack f knowledge of causation. Parents believe that the problem is caused y heredity, the child must have inherited it from them, so they feel uilty. On the other hand some experts suggest that if the parents new that the cause was heredity-based, they would *not* feel guilty ecause they would realise there was no way they could have done nything about it. This variety of expert suggests the causation of uilt is external and the parents see it as being caused by their drinking habits or some other such thing. Some say parents are guilty because they love and overprotect the child, others say that these expressions mask an impulse to reject the child. Parents are guilty, if they ressurise the support services, being accused of *projecting* their guilt n to these services, they are guilty if they do *not* pressurise the support services, because they are *repressing* their feelings. It seems that hatever they do they are guilty. Above we have tried to briefly escribe guilt, although we are not at all sure that it is a useful concept nd in our contact with families parental reactions are treated pragmatically, placing emphasis on an attempt to sort out areas of lack of nowledge, of fear, of confusion, and then guilt takes care of itself. ractically oriented support, in a guidance sense, often takes the pressure off the parents and allows them time to sort out for themselves he intra-family emotional difficulties and problems of personal relationship.

The parents often fear that what they do will not work so it is rucial to monitor progress carefully. We find video records very useul from this point of view as they can enable parents to see that their fforts with the child are having positive practical results.

rogress in Adapting to Having a Hearing-impaired Child

ost writers have suggested that if parents ever do adjust to the impact f having a handicapped child they do so in orderly stages. Readers ill recall the parent who said 'it was a terrible shock and the shock sts for years'. Some authors suggest that in the initial stages the arents endulge in 'self pity' asking the question 'Why did it happen o me?' At this stage the concern is for oneself, one's own feelings.

Later the parents move to concern to help the child overcome his problems and finally the concern broadens to include the spouse and others. Boyd (1951) suggested that only a few parents reach the third stage. Rosen (1955) suggested a five stage adaptation to handicap: (1) awareness of the problem; (2) recognition of the nature of the handicap; (3) search for a cause; (4) search for a solution; and (5) acceptance of the problem. The latter may never be attained fully.

Luterman (1973) suggested that in order for parents to deal positively with their child's needs, they must be allowed the luxury of working through their own feelings of guilt, fear and confusion. Shontz (1965), in an article about parental reaction to crises, suggested a five stage schema. He hoped that this would be useful in describing adjustment to having a handicapped child. He listed: (1) Shock (2) Recognition (3) Defence (4) Retreat (5) Acknowledgement and Constructive Action. Sensitivity and patience he regarded as counsellor requirements. The present authors accept that several of the responses mentioned and probably others too are noticeable in the families of hearing-impaired children, but we are not at all sure that adaptation follows a predictable line as would be the case if it were a stage-by-stage response. There is movement towards greater understanding and perhaps what some authors call 'acceptance' of the handicap, but there are setbacks for some and not all parents take the same route.

Acceptance itself is methodologically very difficult since it is almost always used without clear definition. There is a great danger in our view of defining acceptance of the handicap as seeing it as we professionals see it and reacting and treating the child as we would want them to. It is possible that knowledge of the handicap induces a high drive state in the parents which can be channelled to productive ends. In the early stages of guidance workers should be most careful to present any information in a way that will be meaningful to parents, since there is little doubt that descriptions that are 'over the heads' of parents produce marked feelings of inadequacy. Nowhere must we be more careful than in our interaction with the handicapped child. The professional's experience of child development and coping with young children may mean more skilful handling of the child, say in a play situation, than the parents would manage — where it is their first child, for example, but they should avoid this as it only serves to drive a further wedge between family and child. The aim should be to encourage parental growth, fostering and encouraging the parents handling skills. This will reduce the risk of parental feelings of inadequacy.

One wonders if the view of Adamson *et al.* (1964) that the entire ssue of acceptance is 'wasted' and 'overstated'. If workers accept a model of fairly firm stages in adaptation to having a handicapped child then the danger is that they will try to fit parents to stages rather than try to understand their individual needs.

The Professional Response – Theory

This is clearly a difficult area and traditionally, in the United Kingdom, teachers of the deaf have provided basic support in terms of counselling and guidance, often without special additional training. Some teachers are good at this work, realising at once that the skills of advising and counselling adults are very different from their classroom teaching experience. Others become good at the work after time and practice. The pity is that they get their practice and learn their skills at the expense of the families of hearing-impaired children, the ones on whom they make their mistakes! More recently, educational audiologists with special training in this field have become more involved with young hearing-impaired children and their families. The parents have counselling needs to help offset their reactions to handicap and they have guidance needs related to the practical steps they can take to help their child benefit from amplification and benefit educationally and socially. As mentioned above, this chapter is focusing on the counselling need and many aspects of guidance will be covered in the chapters on hearing aids, language development, etc. The great diversity of reactions and family situations requires a worker who is knowledgeable in many fields with a flexible outlook and capable of a variety of responses.

This adult-oriented approach stresses the working with parents to help the child. As an example, in guidance areas relating to language development it is regarded as far more important to get the ideas over to the parents who will then apply them daily with the child than to spend half an hour teaching the child. The counseller/guider is not a child teacher; he would hope that his hours spent with the parents would mushroom into activities with the child the whole week through.

Counselling

Theories of counselling are usually insight or action-oriented and the present authors believe that families of hearing-impaired children, in general, do not require a highly psychiatric action-oriented approach. Recent studies have shown that psychotherapeutic technique is not as important as the counsellor's general style of social behaviour and the type of relationship he develops with his client. Recovery rate in anxiety type cases is reported as faster where the counsellor is warm, permissive, is interested in and likes the client, and is able to empathise with him. Particular techniques are not the major criteria for success with parents of hearing-impaired children, this relying more on the personality and attitudes of the counsellor.

One insight approach, that of Carl Rogers (1942) — Client Centred Therapy — seems to be a useful approach in the context of the above comments. Rogers reacted to the highly diagnostically oriented probing, and interpretive methods which he felt were not very effective. Such insight theories imply that the primary objective of counselling is to help the client to gain insight into his own thoughts, feelings and behaviour. The responsibility for the counselling processes rests with the client whilst the counsellor facilitates rather than directs his efforts at insight. The efforts and decisions regarding change of behaviour after counselling also remain the responsibility of the client. The action theorists on the other hand are much more problem-oriented and would try to find the problem, then using various techniques try to change behaviour in the hope that the problem would thus be alleviated.

The Client Centred Approach in More Detail

One view of human beings is that they are by nature irrational, unsocialised, and destructive of themselves and others. The client centred point of view is the reverse of this, the client being seen as basically rational, socialised, forward-moving and realistic. When human beings are free of defensiveness their reactions are positive, forward moving and constructive. The process from maladjustment to adjustment is a self-regulatory one.

The basic philosophy of the counsellor is represented by the attitude of respect for the individual, for the individuals capacity and right to self-direction and for the worth and significance of each individual. The theory suggests that for therapy to occur the following conditions must be present:

1. Two people are in contact.
2. One person, the client, is in a state of incongruence, being vulnerable or anxious.
3. The other person, the counsellor, is congruent in the relationship.
4. The counsellor experiences unconditional positive regard toward the client.

5. The counsellor has an empathic understanding of the client's internal frame of reference.
6. The client perceives at least to a minimal degree conditions 4 and 5 above.

The above results in a process with the following characteristics:

1. The client feels more able to express his feelings.
2. This expression of feelings increasingly has reference to the self.
3. The client becomes more able to differentiate and accurately symbolise his experiences.
4. He experiences fully, in awareness, feelings which have in the past been denied to awareness or have been distorted.
5. There is reorganisation of the self-structure, his concept of self becoming increasingly congruent with his experiences with the result that defensiveness is decreased.
6. He becomes increasingly able to experience the counsellor's positive regard without feeling threatened and feels positive self-regard.

There is the basic assumption in the theory that the individual is capable of changing by himself or herself, in ways they choose, without the direction or manipulation of the therapist. The counsellor should be accepting of the client as an individual with all his conflicts and inconsistencies, good and bad points. The ideal counsellor is thus a unified, integrated and consistent person with no inherent contradiction between what he is and what he says. The counsellor must seek to develop an understanding of his client's world as seen from the inside, as if it were his own, but without losing the 'as if' quality. This is the basis of *empathy* which seems essential to counselling — feeling 'with' rather than 'for' the client. It is most important that the client sees the counsellor as accepting, congruent and understanding. If he has these attitudes he will express them in many ways both verbally and non-verbally. The counsellor-client relationship will then be seen by the client as safe, secure, free from threat and supporting but not supportive.

The worker in the role of counsellor as opposed to guider is not strictly helping the client by his knowledge. The relationship helps the client to discover within himself the capacity to use that relationship to change and grow and is not a cognitive or intellectual one.

The Professional Response – Practice

There is much in the literature about poor practice in diagnosis and early follow-up work, perhaps the harshest criticism being reserved for doctors. We are very keen in this text to stress positive features of the work, but educational audiologists should be aware that they may come into contact with parents who have, or believe they have, been treated very shabbily, with a casual and hasty diagnosis, not being given any information regarding cause, extent or possible effects of the disability. The severest criticism which is commonly reported is that of abruptness and lack of interest. A greater awareness through changes in training, of the extent and nature of reactions to handicap should help to offset this criticism. Of course it is medical people who are often the first and most frequent contacts of the family in the time around diagnosis so logically they would be more 'prone' to criticism as being in contact at a time of great trauma for the family. One of the problems may be that medical people are usually heavily trained to an action-oriented approach and when the disability is permanent (is inoperable or will not respond to medical intervention) they lack skills in the then essential areas of information, explanation, counselling and support.

In the United States an attempt to answer this problem has been the setting up of government-subsidised speciality clinics. The response in the United Kingdom has in some ways been similar in that there has been a gradual build-up of regional audiology centres and, significantly, the formation of a new medical speciality, the Audiological Physician, with special training and the availability of consultancy posts in the National Health Service. In the USA the speciality clinics have led to greater satisfaction with diagnostic procedures, but less so with subsequent guidance and counselling function. The clinics seem to have avoided getting involved with long-term management. In the United Kingdom visiting teachers of the hearing-impaired are closely involved in follow-up counselling work. It is vital that there is a close link between diagnosis, aid fitting and subsequent guidance and counselling. There is a great need for courses of additional training for teachers involved in this specialised work.

Counsellor Qualifications

The relationship which the counsellor has with the family can have the profoundest effect on the stability and well-being of the family group and also on the future possibilities of the hearing-impaired child. Thi work with adults and their children is more straining than any class-room teaching and must be approached very carefully and circum-spectly, so that the advice given is the most appropriate available. The strain is increased by the fact that mistakes can have visibly adverse effects. Inappropriate comments like 'everything's all right' when parents give tearful pleas for reassurance, or make anxious comments about the child's future only serve to make the situation worse.

It is our view that the counsellor's professional background is largely irrelevant — neither possession of a medical degree nor a teach-ing qualification qualifies or disqualifies anyone from counselling and managing parents of hearing-impaired children. There are a number of professional backgrounds which lend themselves basically to the work and those mentioned above are only two of several which are possible. The essential is the follow-on training in counselling and audiology which the person undertakes and the attitudes and person-ality he brings to that training. As an example Social Workers, who may have substantial counselling training would not be regarded as suitable without further training in audiology and the educational aspects of guidance. In a British report by the Paediatric Society it is stated that whoever counsels the parents must be exceedingly well informed about all facets of the situation. It must be our aim that counsellor guiders become experts in their chosen specialism, experts in counselling, experts in the handicapping effects of deafness in children and how they may be overcome.

Summary of Skill Areas Required

1. Knowledge of paediatric audiology especially the use of ampli-fication with young children.
2. Counselling skills.
3. Knowledge of child development in its widest sense.
4. Broad knowledge of pre-school and school resources, including other agencies.
5. Freedom from stereotypes about deafness and its results.
6. Possession of positive attitudes.
7. Knowledge of current trends in educational philosophy and practice.
8. Sensitivity to the needs of the family of the hearing handicapped child.
9. A willingness to go further than traditional approaches to help parents.

10.   A measure of patience but also a keenness to 'get things done'.

Workers need to keep clear of the view that the parents are patients and also to be sure of what their own views about the handicap of deafness really are. They may even hold, perhaps unawares, the same sort of attitudes as those of the community at large and harbour conscious or unconscious antipathy towards the handicapped and their problems. With some workers it has been suggested that they surround themselves with non-directive, redirective and reflective techniques and obscure vocabulary which are not allied to any theoretical strategy for counselling, but are merely means of maintaining distance yet seeming to be involved.

If the counsellor is truly to work with the parents then the traditional professional client distance must be narrowed and this can only be done by the professional in how he presents himself and interacts with the family.

Some Do's and Don'ts of Parent Counselling

1.   Become competent in the counselling area of the work — it is vital that you do.
2.   Always be honest, with yourself and the parent.
3.   Prepare for the meeting particularly if you propose to provide information.
4.   Aim to involve both parents since if you don't it can lead to marital friction later. It also puts an unfair burden on one partner as the 'carrier' of all the information. When you involve both parents you help them to focus on the mutual nature of their responsibility for the hearing-impaired child and also the mutual nature of their feelings. This is an aid to marital integration.
5.   Remember that diagnosis is the beginning of professional involvement, not the end of it.
6.   Written information is under-used, but it must be appropriate and written in language that the parents can understand.
7.   Professionals should aim for a continuous relationship with the family and not pass the family around a number of different professionals.
8.   Outdated and ambiguous terminology should be avoided.
9.   The counsellor should be cautious when talking about prognosis particularly in relation to the very young child.

10. Be empathetic (feel with) rather than sympathetic (feel for).
11. Always allow the family sufficient time, that is, do not book so many appointments that each family only has a very limited time with you.
12. Be aware of the 'doorstop syndrome' where the parents save their major worry for when they are going out of the door. Allow plenty of time for this.
13. Be outgoing to the child since you may be the first outside the family to play in a normal way since the child's diagnosis. This will give the parents a welcome boost.
14. Keep records of each meeting and record the information as soon as possible after the meeting. Indicate any preparation needed before the next meeting.
15. Be willing to *not* do what you had planned for a particular meeting and to focus on what the parents need at that time. In other words, *be flexible*.
16. Reward and encourage what parents say to you since they may find it difficult to talk at all.
17. Be prepared for a variety of reactions from parents from hostility and anger to warmth and friendship.
18. Gradually aim to develop a relationship with the family such that they grow in confidence and knowledge, thus being in a position to make the important decisions for their child.
19. Build up an armoury of practical suggestions for parents. They want things they can *do* to make a positive contribution to their childs progress.

Interpersonal Skills

Effective listening is a key area for the counsellor and Argyle (1972) has provided some useful tips on listening skills, together with ways of encouraging a person to talk more. Firstly it is not only polite but encouraging if the counsellor shows a keen interest and gives the person his full attention. Doodling, writing up case notes and not making appropriate eye contact is what we would see as a discouraging environment. It is most helpful if the counsellor meets the parent on his own grounds by adopting his terminology and conventions where necessary. In order to encourage a parent to talk more there is the natural corollary that we should talk less. It is also helpful if open ended questions are asked rather than those just requiring a yes/no answer or other single word answer. Concentration on what is of interest to the family on that day is particularly important, as are rewards for what is said. The counsellor should search for the main point of the problem at that time and not just sit back and think he has heard it all before. To this we might add the practical details that workers should see that families are not kept waiting for long periods and that the meeting is not frequently interrupted. Krasner (1958) showed that non-verbal signals such as head nods as well as their verbal equivalents can make a person say more and that the absence of these can make him say less.

Self-assessment is a useful exercise following a session with the family and thinking about areas such as the following could be valuable:

1. Did I put the parents at ease?
2. Did I cope with anxiety, hostility, etc?
3. Did I listen well?
4. Did I begin to see the problem from the parents point of view?
5. Did I clarify confused ideas?
6. Did I go at the parents' speed?
7. Did I provide relevant factual information when required?
8. What skill did I need to develop most?

Logically an educational audiologist involved in this work would need to add to the above list such things as:

1. Were the aids the correct type appropriately fitted?
2. Were the aids operating at the correct settings for the child's hearing loss?
3. Are the parents capable yet of handling the aid and making routine daily checks?
4. Are attempts being made to provide a good language base for the child? etc, etc.

The present authors would place very high on their list of priorities the *individual* nature of the work with families. Indeed the great majority of contacts with families in the clinics at Manchester University are on this basis. Group meetings also take place but they have guidance aims rather than counselling aims. Parents have personal problems, they have personal needs and any guidance and counselling programme should reflect this fact. Efficiency might lead us to consider a system where group guidance/counselling was the major way of helping families, but in this way we feel that parents are rapidly reduced to membership of a category and lose their individuality and any counsellor understanding of their personal needs. General principles do not help us to know what situation parents are in, only personal knowledge. We also cannot assume that the needs of one family are much the same as another simply because they seem to have much the same problem. We must get to know families individually if we are to be effective counsellors.

It is difficult to describe the level of involvement required, but it must be deeper than most professional client relationships. We must respond warmly, show empathy, understand the unspoken as well as the spoken feelings, but workers would be wise to remember that the relationship itself is controlled and is not analogous to friendship. The counsellor respects the parent for what he is, not for what he would like him to be. They are not there to sit in judgment on families, but to help them make progress in their own emotional status and in the guidance role to support the family to help their child make progress on all fronts, cognitive, social and emotional.

Finally in this chapter it is worth stressing again the need for parents to be treated as partners in respect of what happens to their child. This in our view does not mean *informing* them, it does not mean just *consulting* them, it means *sharing* with them all the important decisions which will be made about their child.

References

Adamson, W.C., Ohrenstein, D.F., Lake, D. and Hersh, A. (1964) 'Separation used to help parents promote the growth of their retarded child', *Soc. Wk.*, *9(4)*, 60-7

Allen, J. and Allen, M. (1979) 'Discovering and accepting hearing-impairment: Initial reactions of parents', *Volta Review*, *81*, 5

Argyle, M. (1972) *The Psychology of Interpersonal Behaviour*, Penguin, London

Boyd, D. (1951) 'The three stages in the growth of the parent of a mentally retarded child', *Amer. J. Ment. Deficiency*, *55*, 608-11

HMSO (1978) *Report of the Committee of Enquiry into the Education of Handicapped Children and Young People*, Cmnd no. 7212, Special Educational Needs – The Warnock Report

Krasner, L. (1958) 'Studies of the conditioning of verbal behaviour', *Psychological Bulletin*, *55*, 148-70

Luterman, D. (1973) 'On parent education', *Volta Review*, *75(8)*, 504-8

Neuhaus, M. (1969) 'Parental attitudes and the emotional adjustment of deaf children', *Exceptional Children*, *35*, 721-7

Olshansky, S. (1965) 'Chronic sorrow: A response to having a mentally defective child' in E. Younghusband (ed.), *Readings in Social Work*, vol. I, Allen and Unwin, London

Rogers, C. (1942) *Counselling and Psychotherapy*, Houghton Miflin, Boston

Roith, A.I. (1963) 'The myth of parental attitudes', *Journal of Mental Subnormality, 9*, 51-4

Rosen, L. (1955) 'Selected aspects in the development of the mothers understanding of her mentally retarded child', *Amer. J. Ment. Deficiency, 59*, 522-8

Shontz, F.C. (1965) 'Reaction to crisis', *Volta Review, 67*, 364-70

Solnit, A.J. and Stark, M.H. (1961) Mourning and the birth of a defective child', *Studies in Childhood, 16*, 523-37

Thomas, D. (1978) *The Social Psychology of Childhood Disability*, Methuen, London

Thurston, J.R. (1960) 'Counselling the parents of the severely handicapped', *Exceptional Children, 26*, 351-4

Tumin, W. (1977) 'Parents of Deaf Children', in *Report of the Proceedings of the Conference on the Diagnosis and Early Management of the Deaf Child*, University of Manchester, Manchester

4 THE HEARING AID AS A SYSTEM

The Hearing Aid

At the present time there are four main types of hearing aid systems in use with hearing-impaired children. These are:

(1) Body worn or pocket aid (Figure 4.1).
(2) Post-auricular or behind the ear aid (Figure 4.1).
(3) Radio hearing aid of the pocket type (Figure 4.2).
(4) Radio hearing aid of personal type which links up with the conventional aid of category (1) or (2) via direct connection or by loop induction (Figure 4.2).

In addition, an increasing but very small number of children use 'in the ear' or modular aids. Certain groups of hearing-impaired children also have access to amplification systems specific to education. The Group Hearing Aid, which is a hard-wire system, is perhaps the most familiar member of this category.

A system which uses infra-red light is finding more widespread use particularly in special schools for the deaf. The auditory training unit (in effect a 'single module' of a group aid), which finds application particularly with pre-school hearing-impaired children, is not specifically an educational aid, but rather an extension of the child's personal hearing aid, to be used for short sessions such as an interactive play situation with mother, these sessions being aimed at fostering development of the child's linguistic skills.

The Role of the Hearing Aid

All of these amplification systems are designed to improve the auditory experience of the hearing-impaired child. The quality of this hearing experience is of paramount importance, because without effective experiences of the sounds of speech, hearing-impaired children will have little or no chance of developing spoken language. A child's language development proceeds most rapidly in the early years of life. If a child's hearing is such that some or all of the sounds of everyday conversational speech are inaudible, then that child's speech and language will be severely restricted.

131

Figure 4.1: (a) The pocket aid. (b) The post-aural aid.

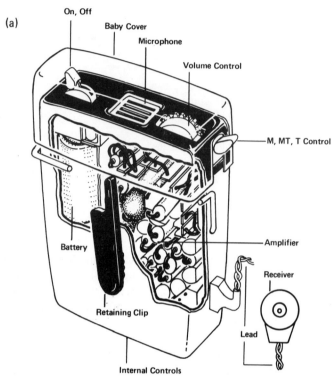

(a)

On, Off

Baby Cover

Microphone

Volume Control

M, MT, T Control

Amplifier

Receiver

Battery

Retaining Clip

Lead

Internal Controls

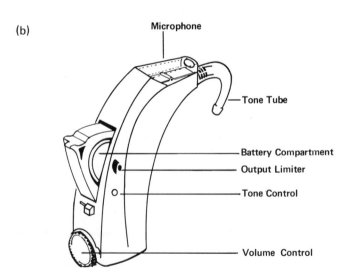

(b)

Microphone

Tone Tube

Battery Compartment

Output Limiter

Tone Control

Volume Control

Figure 4.2: (a) Radio microphone hearing aid (type 1) configuration (Phonic Ear 431 system). (b) Personal radio microphone hearing aid (type 2) configuration connected to a post-aural aid via direct input (Phonic Ear 44 system with a Phonak PPCL).

(a)

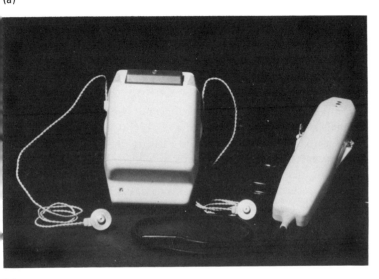

(b)

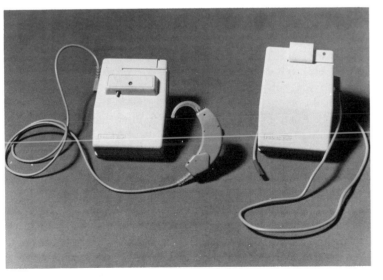

A child's ability to make use of his residual hearing depends to some degree on the severity of the hearing loss. It is vitally important to appreciate the potentially devastating effect that hearing-impairment can have on a child's linguistic attainments. While a hearing aid will not restore a child's hearing to normal, it will provide experiences of sound that would be otherwise unheard. It therefore plays a vital role in the child's sensory stimulation and contributes enormously to subsequent linguistic development.

Effective Hearing Aid Management

The effective management of hearing-impaired children requires a comprehensive child-oriented service. Professionals have to deal with a completely different population (having child-specific problems) to that encountered by those working with the adult deaf. It is a fact of life that young hearing aid users rely heavily on their parents and later, teachers to ensure that their aids are used efficiently. Generally speaking, young children are not able to set their own aids or even fit them. Furthermore, they rarely indicate when a fault arises, even when it results in reduced, distorted or total lack of output. Parents and teachers therefore have the responsibility of ensuring that hearing aids are well maintained and used to maximum effect.

The fundamental point of note at the onset of a management programme is that one is not simply dealing with a handicapped child — one is dealing with a family with a handicap. Families have a very important role to play in the utilisation of the child's residual hearing via a hearing aid fitting. They must therefore be carefully counselled, advised and supported, not only early on immediately following the traumatic time of diagnosis, but throughout the child's pre-school years and during the school years where necessary.

Hearing handicap in a young child is often unrecognised by the public at large — that is until people see the child wearing hearing aids. This concept of 'total child' being child plus hearing aids is one which parents may need time to come to terms with and fully accept. Parental acceptance of the hearing aid and an understanding of the importance of its continued efficient use is without doubt the primary aim of the early habilitative programme. This programme should provide a saturation service for the family, whereby guidance sessions, both in the home and perhaps on occasions at the resource centre, are organised on a regular basis, but with a built-in flexibility of support and help on demand.

Parents initially find it difficult to absorb information so the sessions should be spaced over time and new information only introduced gradually. This will include aspects of hearing aid management and day-to-day fitting procedures. Obviously, in the initial stages following diagnosis the *care* of the aids will be the sole responsibility of the professional, but gradually parents must be encouraged to develop their own hearing aid management skills. The eventual aim should be that the parents are competent hearing aid handlers (*but* not technicians or electronics experts). They should be able to fit aids, routinely check them prior to fitting and be able to spot faults and remedy the commonly occurring ones without recourse to the hearing aid clinic.

Concept of the Hearing Aid

It is important for everyone concerned with the day-to-day management of hearing-impaired children to conceptualise the hearing aid not from their own 'adult' or 'audiological specialist' viewpoint, but through the eyes of the child. Only in this way is it possible to begin to appreciate those child-specific problems which if left unchecked can spell disaster for effective auditory stimulation. Furthermore, such an approach also enables the 'professional advisor', who may have studied hearing aids over many years, to appreciate the difficulty that those 'new' to hearing aids (that is, parents and teachers alike) face in understanding just what kind of device is the hearing aid, how it works, what can go wrong, and what potentially it has to offer to the future of a hearing-impaired child. It is all too easy for familiarity to breed a 'too technically offputting' explanation on what is a vital piece of equipment that must become an integral part of the child.

The hearing aid is best seen as an interactive system, a system comprising a number of building blocks or components, that is, a chain of building blocks. If a single component is weak or faulty, the overall performance of the system will be INEFFICIENT – putting at risk the child's reception of auditory information. It is the job of parents, teachers and professional advisors to maintain this interactive system in as efficient a condition as possible. The aid is only as effective as the weakest link in the chain of building blocks.

Many of the problems influencing the efficient day-to-day use of hearing aids by children relate to the ergonomic design of the hearing aid (Powell, 1975) – the vast majority of hearing aids being designed for the adult user. These design features produce weak spots on the hearing aid, resulting in a risk of inefficient or totally ineffective amplification.

What is a Hearing Aid?

While hearing aids come in various shapes and sizes they all basically perform the same function — that of providing the hearing-impaired with experiences of sound which would otherwise go unheard. The interactive system comprising a conventional hearing aid is shown in Figure 4.3. All hearing aids whether pocket, post-auricular or 'in the ear' comprise this system of units. The only difference between these 'conventional' systems and other alternatives (for example, radio hearing aids, group aids, infra-red, etc.) is simply that the alternatives have extra components 'added on', some of these being worn or used by others. This is why such systems are known by the term 'hearing aids not entirely worn on the listener' (IEC, 1979). However, as will be described later, they too are equally vulnerable to 'component faults' the majority of which are common to the conventional systems.

Figure 4.3: The building blocks comprising a hearing aid.

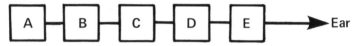

The units comprising a conventional wearable hearing aid.

A — Microphone, amplifier, other controls i.e. the 'hearing aid' box of either body or post aural type.

B — Battery

C — Lead

D — Receiver

E — Earmould

The Earmould

It may be seen by reference to Figure 4.3 that the earmould is seen as an integral part of the wearable hearing aid. This is an important point because all too often little or no attention is paid to this particular component, with the result that amplification is totally unsatisfactory. While the subject of earmoulds is seen as sufficiently important to warrant its own chapter, it is pertinent to make a number of comments at this juncture.

1. The ear impression should be taken in 'addition cured' silicone.

2. The injection or syringing procedure of impression taking should be employed.

3. Earmoulds should be made in soft acrylic, vinyl or silicone rubber.

4. Earmoulds should be issued with as wide a bore as possible (for the majority of children) and with a meatal projection which does not reach past the junction of the cartilaginous and bony canal.

5. Shell, not skeleton, moulds should be issued to children.

6. Thick walled tubing (1mm wall thickness) should be employed with high power post-aural instruments — to help reduce the problem of acoustic feedback.

7. Guidance staff must fully appreciate the impact that the earmould can have on the overall performance of the hearing aid. Parents must be advised along the following lines.

  (a) Not to accept an inadequate ear mould. They must return to the supply centre and continue to do so until a satisfactory product is made available. Parents should draw the attention of the support service and their own national body (National Deaf Children's Society) where earmould provision is unsatisfactory.

  (b) Earmoulds must be replaced whenever necessary regardless of the time interval since the previous fitting. If the child is unable to use his hearing aid efficiently and effectively because of the earmould then that mould must be replaced. No rigid earmould replacement programme should apply. There is no way of predicting when a child will require new earmoulds, other than to test whether it delivers the required gain.

  (c) A child must be encouraged to take responsibility for the aftercare of the earmoulds. Routine nightly cleaning of earmoulds should be part and parcel of getting ready for bed — this regardless of whether the child goes to sleep with his aids on.

  (d) Children should be trained to put in and remove their earmoulds. They should be encouraged to blow out the perspiration that can accumulate in sound tubes of shell moulds.

  (e) Regular attention should be paid to earmould plumbing — a good supply of tubing being made available so that the problem of cracked or 'dried out' tubing can be avoided. Parents must be instructed on how to retube an earmould. Alternatively, this retubing may be done by a member of the support service. If the earmould's potential for destroying the effectiveness of a hearing fitting is to be minimised then a stringent ear mould management programme must be applied.

The Battery

Two distinct categories of battery are used with hearing aids. The PRIMARY or disposable cell which is employed in all conventional pocket and post-auricular hearing aids is used until its energy is drained whereupon it is replaced with a new cell. The exhausted cell is thrown away or safely stored for return to the issuing centre for disposal. On no account should any attempt be made to recharge primary cells.

The SECONDARY or rechargeable battery which finds particular use with radio hearing aids can by definition be recharged to full capacity when exhausted. Such cells may be recharged hundreds or even thousands of times. Recharging is achieved by use of special battery chargers which obtain power from the mains supply.

The nominal voltage of these batteries lies between 1.3 and 1.5 volts. The actual value for a particular battery is a function of cell chemistry (see Table 4.1).

Figure 4.4: Maximum dimensions as established by the IEC for the penlite R6 and the pellet R44 and R48 cell.

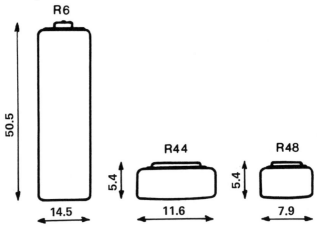

Source: after Philips, 1982b.

In terms of dimensions, there are three primary batteries employed in conventional hearing aids. The pocket aid uses the large cylindrical penlite cell which is commercially identified by IEC regulations as the R6 cell (Figure 4.4). The majority of post-aural aids use the pellet or button cell having an IEC code of R44. This is probably more familiarly known as the '675' cell (Figure 4.4). The miniature pellet cell with IEC code R48 is employed in the smaller post-aural aids and 'in the ear' systems. It is probably more familiarly known as the '13' cell (Figure 4.4).

The rechargeable batteries are produced in the primary size format and also in power pack configurations. For example, certain radio aid systems (for example, Phonic Ear Personal and Connevans systems) employ the PP3 power pack format, while others (for example, Phonic Ear Stereo and Mono, Cubex Radio Link) use the cylindrical penlite format. The application of rechargeable batteries to conventional hearing aids is not recommended on account of service life and financial factors.

Battery Chemistry. The penlite cell is available in either carbon-zinc (Leclanche) or manganese alkaline configuration (Ever Ready, 1980). The carbon-zinc cell has been effectively replaced by the manganese alkaline cell, carbon-zinc cells now having very limited application for hearing aid use.

The pellet or button cells that are employed in hearing aids come in mercury-oxide and zinc-air configuration. Both cells have widespread use in hearing aids and are available in both R44 and R48 format.

The rechargeable batteries are all of one type — nickel-cadmium.

Battery Properties. All batteries have certain characteristics or behaviour properties. A knowledge of these properties is valuable in relation to an effective battery management programme.

The CAPACITY of a battery relates to the current the cell can deliver over time. It is equal to the product of current and time. It is expressed in milliampere hours (that is, mAh). If, for example, a battery has a capacity of 100 mAh this indicates that the battery can provide a constant 1 mA current for 100 hours, or 2 mA current for 50 hours, etc. before exhaustion. This parameter can prove useful in estimating battery life in an aid (Pollack, 1980).

The NOMINAL VOLTAGE is an expression of the 'driving force' of the cell. It is the difference between the electrode potentials of the cell. As mentioned earlier, the voltage of primary cells lies between 1.3 and 1.5 volts when cells are new. This voltage declines during use — decline being characteristic of a particular cell chemistry (Ever Ready, 1980). The declining voltage is accompanied by a reduction in cell capacity which can influence the effectiveness of the hearing aid.

It is therefore of particular importance to those responsible for hearing aid management.

The VOLTAGE DISCHARGE PROFILE is a graph or curve which shows the above behaviour of change in nominal voltage with time while the battery is being used in the hearing aid.

The INTERNAL RESISTANCE of a cell is an expression of the cells' 'built in' hindrance to the flow of electrical current. This is usually of the order of two or three ohms. However, rechargeable and manganese alkaline cells have lower resistances. Dangerously high currents may therefore result in the case of a short circuit.

The SHELF LIFE is a term that is used to express the period over which a battery may be safely stored prior to issue without significant loss in capacity. This figure, particularly for child usage, should be based on a maximum loss of capacity of 10 per cent.

Penlite Batteries. The properties of the zinc-carbon and manganese alkaline cells are summarised in Table 4.1 and Figure 4.5. Manganese alkaline cells have distinct advantages over zinc-carbon ones. While both have a nominal voltage of 1.5V, the voltage discharge profile of the manganese alkaline is far more gradual. The capacity of the manganese alkaline cell is such that under similar load conditions, service life will be enhanced by a factor of 1.6 to 2 in relation to zinc-carbon (Ever Ready, 1980). The shelf life of the manganese alkaline cell is significantly better than that of zinc-carbon — for example, the zinc-carbon cell is often completely flat (that is, total discharge) after two years of storage while the manganese alkaline cell would still have at least 90 per cent of its original capacity.

Table 4.1: Properties of primary cells.

Dimensions	Type	Nominal voltage (volts)	Capacity (mAh)	Shelf life (months)
R6	zinc-carbon	1.5	1500	6
R6	manganese-alkaline	1.5	2500	24
R44	mercuric oxide	1.35	220	18
R44	zinc-air	1.35	350	24[+]
R48	mercuric oxide	1.35	95	18
R48	zinc-air	1.35	160	24[+]

Source: after Philips, 1982b.

Figure 4.5: Average discharge curve for discharge in hearing aids: (a) carbon-zinc (Leclanche); (b) manganese alkaline; (c) silver oxide; (d) zinc-air; (e) mercury; (f) nickel-cadmium (rechargeable).

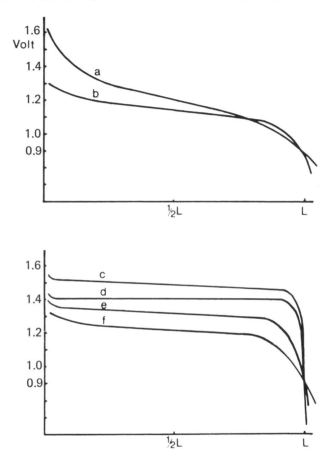

Source: after Philips, 1982b.

The Pellet Batteries. The properties of mercuric oxide and zinc air batteries are summarised in Table 4.1 and Figure 4.5. Both cells have a characteristic voltage discharge profile of a slight initial reduction in voltage followed by a long period when voltage is virtually constant. This latter factor is particularly so in the zinc-air cell. The voltage then decays very rapidly when the end point is reached. Cell capacity is greater in the zinc-air system being increased by a factor of approximately 1.6. However, this factor may vary as a function of load conditions and shouldn't be assumed to apply to all conditions of use. The shelf life of both cells is good in relation to an effective battery stock rotation and issuing service. The zinc-air cell does not function until the adhesive seal is removed thus allowing for a supply of air to enter through the small holes in the base of the battery. It is important that this seal is not removed until the cell is required, otherwise the useful life of the battery will be reduced.

The current drawn from a zinc-air battery is limited by the rate at which the air can diffuse into the case. There is a possible risk that the current drain demanded by a high power post-aural aid (for example, BE51, Oticon E28P, Phonak PPCL) may be too much for the cell with the aid on high gain setting. This would result in a small but significant reduction in hearing aid performance (~2 dB). If this does occur and causes problems for the user, then it would be necessary to replace with a mercuric oxide cell. Where children are concerned it is recommended that zinc-air cells are employed whenever possible because such cells have a particularly flat discharge profile that is ideal for child users.

A word of caution is warranted at this point with reference to the day-to-day use of the pellet cells. These cells are easily mistaken for a sweet by a child and swallowed (Reilly, 1979). The *mercuric oxide* cell presents as a source of potentially lethal poisoning for a child, should the cell rupture following ingestion into the stomach. It is imperative that medical advice be sought should ingestion occur. Corrosion occurs while the cell is in the acidic environment of the stomach — not because of the corrosive effects of the gastric juices but electrochemical polarisation of the battery canister (Nolan and Tucker, 1981). Once a cell passes out of the stomach into the small intestine corrosion will cease and the cell should then pass freely out of the system. The major problem associated with ingestion of cells of this type occurs when the cell remains in the stomach for a considerable time (greater than two hours). On occasions it has been found necessary to perform surgical procedures to remove heavily corroded cells so as to avoid harm to the child (Reilly, 1979; Barwick, 1983).

The zinc-air cells do not present as significant a risk to health primarily because of their chemistry and the fact that they show no significant corrosion when swallowed (Nolan and Tucker, 1981). Clearly, however, ingestion of any pellet cell regardless of type demands the advice of a medical practitioner.

Steps must be taken to 'child proof' the battery compartment of post-aural aids of *all* young children. This can be achieved at the present time by the use of surgical tape. Ideally battery compartments should be made child-proof by means of locking 'shoes' (as are used for direct input connection with radio aids) or snap-fit protective 'caps'. Perhaps future generations of post-aural aids will have such facilities built into their design. At present the design of the battery compartment is a typical example of the 'designed for adult' syndrome.

Storage of Batteries. It is strongly recommended that parents and teachers are advised to store batteries in a safe place out of reach of children. Older hearing aid users such as grandparents should be similarly advised. Batteries should be stored in dry, cool conditions. They must not be stored in direct sunlight, nor near sources of heat, for example, radiators. If possible a temperature below $15°C$ is desirable. In schools it is important not to stockpile too many cells with the danger of post shelf-life cells being issued. A policy of effective stock rotation must apply. Parents of pre-school children must be provided with a stock of batteries that will cover them for one month's use at any one time. It is important to note that mercuric oxide pellet cells are not to be discarded in dustbins as they present as a source of pollution to the environment (DHSS, 1982). They must be stored in the issuing dispenser pack when exhausted (marked with felt tip pen so that old and new cells do not become mixed up) and returned to the visiting teacher or hearing aid centre for safe disposal. The DHSS applies a policy of insisting that all mercury, zinc-air and manganese alkaline cells be returned to the issuing centre where they are exchanged for new cells.

Batteries should not be left in hearing aids that are not in regular use. They may leak corrosive substances that can permanently damage the aid.

The Rechargeable Battery. The discharge profile of a nickel-cadmium battery is shown in Figure 4.5. It may be seen that the picture is somewhat similar to that of the pellet cells, the voltage remaining fairly steady during the effective lifetime of the battery. The main point of note in relation to rechargeable batteries is that of the relatively short lifetime before the end point of the cell is reached. This is a function of the particular cell configuration and hearing aid system in use.

The Battery and its Relation To Hearing Aid Performance

It should be clear that the greater the CAPACITY of a battery the longer the hearing aid will operate without the battery having to be changed.

The voltage of the battery has a direct influence on the performance of the hearing aid — the higher the voltage the greater the maximum sound intensity and maximum amplification. The performance of a hearing aid during the operative life of a battery is also connected with prevailing battery voltage. It has already been shown (Figure 4.5) that the voltage discharge profiles for different batteries have characteristic shapes — the manganese alkaline battery, for example, shows a steady gradual decay in voltage over time to the end point. This is accompanied by a corresponding decay in amplification from the hearing aid (Figure 4.6) such that the user would notice a reduction in loudness of the amplified signal and would in the case of an adult, turn up the volume control to compensate for this decline. The amount of reduction in amplification varies between hearing aids and is therefore specific to a particular aid (Philips, 1982a).

Figure 4.6: The change in gain for a fixed volume setting of a pocket aid powered by a penlite battery. A loss of gain of 5dB occurred after 28 hours of use.

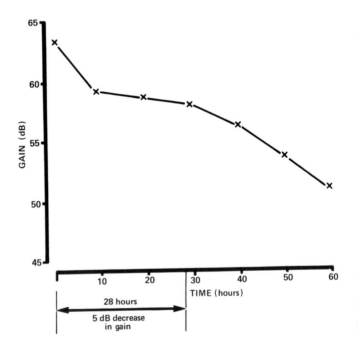

The zinc-air cell, on the other hand, shows a very steady voltage over a considerable time with a corresponding steady amplification performance. This is followed by a sudden and effectively 'without warning' rapid decay in voltage and amplification which warrants battery replacement. Hence, while the penlite battery with its gradual decay of voltage and accompanying hearing aid performance 'gives notice' to the adult user that the battery is becoming run down, the pellet battery gives no warning at all — the cell suddenly ceases to operate over a very short time indeed. Another consequence of a decaying battery voltage is that distortion of the processed sound signal increases with a consequent deterioration in sound quality. Most of us have experienced this ourselves when persevering with batteries in a transistor radio when they really ought to be replaced. This problem of distortion is particularly noticeable with penlite cells.

The Battery — Its Effective Management

It is of interest to note that the majority of comments, pertaining to hearing aid performance above, were made in relation to the 'adult user'. This was done deliberately because it helps to emphasise the 'child-oriented' problems that must be overcome in order to achieve a continuity of efficient amplification.

The most important comment relating to battery use in a hearing aid is that the battery has the potential for causing greater periods of inefficient amplification than any other component of the hearing aid system. Unlike other components, batteries must be changed regularly, otherwise the amplification delivered by the hearing aid will become ineffective and the child's linguistic progress will be impaired.

The battery should be seen as 'the heart' of the hearing aid — in this way it should be obvious that a poorly conditioned battery will result in an inefficient amplification system. Effective management of a hearing aid involves a routine management programme for the battery. It is therefore necessary for the professional adviser to provide battery changing guidelines and also to encourage parents and teachers to carry out routine checks on 'battery condition' in the interim period between battery changes.

Battery Management — A Summary

Battery management is achieved by a 'two-prong' approach:

1. Routine daily checks of the aid. To check the battery the procedure is as follows:

(a) Switch aid on.

(b) (i) For a pocket aid, turn the volume to full and hold the receiver a lead length from the microphone. The aid should produce a characteristic squeal. (ii) For a post-aural aid − turn on the aid to full volume and direct the plastic elbow towards the ear canal − the aid should squeal.

(c) If the expected result in (b)(i) or (ii) does not occur then the battery should be replaced and the procedure repeated.

(d) Parents and teachers should be provided with a stetoclip. They should become accustomed to the power of the child's aid and know the volume setting which they themselves find comfortable. They should listen through the aid and check for low or distorted output and replace the battery should they suspect a fault with this component. The audiologist should ensure that:

(i)   Parents and teachers have a months supply of batteries.
(ii) A stetoclip is made available for each family and class teacher.
(iii) Parents and teachers know how to change the battery (that is which way the battery fits and how to gain access to the battery compartment).

2. The second prong of the attack is to apply battery changing guidelines. The audiologist should therefore advise on the appropriate routine for a particular child's hearing aids.

Battery changing guidelines for a range of commonly used hearing aids are shown in Table 4.2. It may be seen that they are presented in a weekly format. This was considered to be the only practical mode of application particularly for school use. The service life of hours in each aid-cell combination is also given so that if necessary a more flexible changing approach can be applied perhaps with individual pre-school children. The guidelines are empirically based and are routinely applied in our parent guidance programme (Shaw, 1983).

The Microphone

A hearing aid is designed to pick up sounds of everyday life and reproduce them at the ear at a raised level. The microphone is that first link between the sound-wave travelling through the air and the AMPLIFIER

Table 4.2: Battery changing routines.

Make and Model	CP1	CP101	CP6
BE10 Series (11, 12, 14 & 16)	Every two weeks (165h)	Every four weeks (347h)	—
BE30 Series (31 & 32)	Every week (estimated)	Every two weeks (178h)	—
BE50 Series (51)	Twice a week (40h)	Twice a week (66h)	—
Danavox 775PP	Twice a week (62h)	Once a week (84h)	—
Oticon E22P	Twice a week (47h)	Twice a week (69h)	—
Phonak PPCL	Twice a week (47h)	Twice a week (71h)	—
Philips 8276	Twice a week (51h)	Once a week (89h)	—
Unitron E1P	Twice a week (estimated)	Once a week (96h)	—
BW61	—	—	Once a week (129h)
BW81	—	—	Twice a week (71h)
Philips 8146	—	—	Twice a week (55h)
Windsor	—	—	Twice a week (52h)

Source: after Shaw, 1983.

which is going to boost the signal and make it audible to the hearing-impaired child. A microphone is a transducer, that is, a device that converts energy from one form to another. In the case of the hearing aid microphone, sound energy is converted into electrical impulses which are then processed by the 'electronics' of the hearing aid (Figure 4.7). We want to provide a hearing-impaired child with as wide an experience of the sounds of speech as possible. It is therefore desirable for the microphone to be sensitive to a wide range of frequencies, this sensitivity being equal across frequency, if practically possible.

Nowadays, with the pure transistorised circuitry of hearing aids, one particular type of microphone, the ELECTRET microphone, has been established as an effective 'standard'. The electret or condenser microphone has very desirable properties for hearing aid application.

Figure 4.7: The basic mode of operation of a hearing aid.

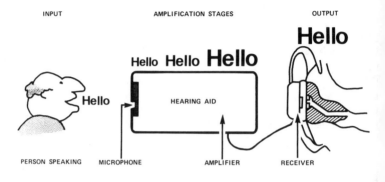

It has a wide flat frequency response, high sensitivity and a low noise level. It is also quite resilient to the everyday bumps and bangs of the child user.

The electret microphone consists of a membrane (an electret) made of a plastic foil with a high insulating characteristic. This has the ability of permanently retaining an electric charge which it is given during manufacture. This membrane is situated at a small distance from a fixed counter electrode. A voltage between foil and counter electrode accompanies vibration of the foil in response to an impinging sound wave. These voltages are amplified by a field effect transistor (FET) which is normally located inside the microphone housing and then led to the input terminals of the hearing aid amplifier (Niemoeller, 1978). This transduction of sound energy first into mechanical vibration of the membrane and then into electrical impulses is achieved by the microphone — the 'signal source' for the amplifier.

It is important to note that the quality of the incoming electrical signal from the microphone is crucial for achieving good sound quality at the ear. The amplified signal is no better in quality terms than that received from the 'signal source' — the microphone. This is analogous to the ear impression/earmould relationship, whereby the quality of the final earmould is determined by the accuracy of the initial impression.

One major advantage of the electret microphone for child users relates to the fact that it only produces a small electrical output when vibrated. This reduces the problems of clothes' rub noise and mechanical feedback which were significant with the earlier types of microphone (Hueber, 1972). The incorporation of electret microphone into hearing aids is seen as a very important and beneficial develop ıent for hearing-impaired children.

Microphone Configuration

The majority of hearing aids are fitted with what are technically described as omnidirectional microphones. The microphone housing is constructed in such a way that the sound energy enters through one portal and is directed on to the foil membrane. The term omnidirectional implies that the sensitivity of the microphone is equal for all angles of incidence of the sound waves.

An alternative microphone format that is available on certain postural hearing aids is the directional microphone. This microphone configuration differs from the omnidirectional in that the microphone housing is designed with two portals through which sound may enter (Lentz, 1975). The microphone is purposely designed to be more sensitive to sound originating from in front of the hearing aid user. The job of the two portals is to deliver sound energy to opposite sides of the microphone diaphragm. Sound entering the front portal acts on the superior diaphragm surface, while that entering via the rear portal acts on the inferior diaphragm surface.

The manner by which the directional microphone achieves its purpose may be best understood from the following description.

When a sound-wave originates from a source placed behind the hearing aid, the time of arrival at the rear microphone portal is earlier than that at the front microphone portal. The directional microphone is designed to be less sensitive to sound from the rear. This is accomplished by delaying the sound-wave which enters the rear portal so that it arrives at the inferior surface of the diaphragm at the same time as the sound-wave entering by the front portal arrives at the superior diaphragm surface. The two sound-waves attempt to displace the diaphragm in opposite directions and some cancellation occurs. A reduction in the degree of amplification therefore results. This delay of the sound-wave via the rear portal is achieved by incorporation of a damping resistive element into the portal. This together with the 'sponginess' of the air in the rear portal act to delay the sound-wave via the rear portal so that its time of arrival at the diaphragm coincides with that for the sound-wave coming via the front portal.

Sounds originating from in front of the hearing aid are amplified in a normal manner without attenuation. This is due to the fact that when the source is in front of the hearing aid the signal will arrive at the front portal first. This signal meets no significant delay when entering the front portal (unlike that entering the rear portal) and proceeds normally to the diaphragm. It reaches it well in advance of the signal via the rear portal and the temporal advantage of the initial input prevents the occurrence of cancellation.

Comments Relating to Microphone Configuration

If a hearing aid is fitted with a one portal microphone housing it is usually described in the technical literature as omnidirectional in nature. A truly omnidirectional aid may be considered as undesirable for hearing-impaired youngsters because by being equally sensitive regardless of source location, it is going to pick up and amplify 'unwanted sound' (for example, noise from behind the user) equally as well as the 'wanted sound' (for example, speech from the front of the user). This unwanted noise will act to mask out the speech and reduce the effectiveness of the hearing aid.

Reasoning that hearing aid users would orient their heads towards the sound source, design engineers saw the potential of a directional microphone for hearing aid application. By having a reduced sensitivity to sound from the rear, such a microphone should in theory furnish the hearing aid user with a more favourable signal to noise ratio.

It is important to realise that all of the above comments relating to the two microphone configurations are theoretically based. Significant changes in the behaviour of these microphones occur immediately they are taken out of the 'laboratory' and put into use in the 'real world' (that is, on people's heads) (Kasten *et al.*, 1967; Olsen and Carhart, 1975). The first significant point of note is that when a hearing aid with an omnidirectional microphone is mounted on a person that aid becomes a directional instrument. It is not possible to state just 'how directional' a particular aid will become because many factors influence this matter. Microphone placement, size of child, listening environment and frequency of sound are all significant in this respect. The only way of knowing this is to make measures on the aid.

With reference to the so-called directional microphone it is important to note that directional aids have been shown to vary widely in their directionality (Sung *et al.*, 1975). Furthermore, the directionality is a function of the listening environment — research having shown that such aids become functionally non-directional in more reverberant environments such as mainstream classrooms, where the reverberation time is in excess of 0·8 seconds (Studebaker *et al.*, 1980).

In practice therefore, the actual subjective differences between the two configurations may not be as great as may be implied in the technical iterature. The technical information on such aids is normally produced rom tests carried out in an anechoic room with the aid freely suspended n space. Alternatively, the aid may be mounted on a mannequin (for xample, KEMAR — Knowles Electronics Mannequin for Acoustic Research) but again situated in an anechoic room. Such test set-ups nay be far and away removed from the situations in which a child nay be using an aid.

To conclude this section it may be stated that two microphone onfigurations are in use with hearing aids. The directional microphone s designed to be more sensitive to sounds coming from one direction han from other directions. By the user orienting his head towards he sound it has been suggested that the wanted sound will be amplied more favourably than the unwanted, thus improving the signal-o-noise (S/N) ratio relative to that provided by an omnidirectional mit. This must be interpreted with caution. Research findings to date uggest that:

1) All microphones (as is the unaided ear) are directional to some degree.
2) In conditions of relative quiet there are no significant differences between children's speech discrimination abilities using either microphone configuration (Chan, 1980; Nielsen, 1974).
3) When listening conditions are poor (S/N ratio low) the directional instrument may provide a significant improvement in discrimination ability. However, this benefit is significantly influenced by room acoustics and may be entirely negated in the more reverberant mainstream classroom. Sound treated rooms with reverberation times of less than 0.6 seconds appear desirable (Nielsen and Ludvigsen, 1978).

At the present time most hearing-impaired children are fitted with he conventional one portal aids. It may prove beneficial for certain hildren to be fitted with a directional facility. Perhaps the most ignificant objection to such provision may come from the child himelf, who having become accustomed to the 'less pronounced' directionality of the 'omnidirectional unit' may dislike the change in emhasis of the directional unit. On no account should the directional nicrophone be considered as a satisfactory substitute for a specific mplification system for education such as the radio hearing aid. uch microphones are vulnerable to poor acoustic conditions and otally inadequate for overcoming the problems of 'communication at a distance' as often occurs in the classroom. They are, howeve fittings which may prove beneficial to certain individual childre in certain listening situations.

The Microphone and the Child User

The hearing aid microphone is a fairly resilient component particularl in the electret format. However, it is not immune to the everyda bumps and bangs of child usage and any steps that can be taken t protect it helps to ensure a continuity of efficient performance. one examines the pocket aid (Figure 4.1a) it quickly becomes clea that the appropriate placement of the microphone from an acousti viewpoint is probably the most inappropriate practically speakin; The acoustic placement demands a good ear-voice link for the chil and the aids should therefore be worn high up on the chest. Howeve this placement is directly below the chin and is therefore perfectl placed to catch the dribbles of food and drink from the mouth an chin. This problem is one which must be tackled — otherwise th microphone portal and all controls on top of the aid will becom clogged with debris. The use of a baby cover — a plastic cover whic is custom-made for a particular aid is necessary. This cover clips ove the top of the aid and protects the microphone — without significantl influencing the performance of the hearing aid. One major criticis: of certain manufacturer's baby covers is that they appear to be co: structed from 'rice paper' thin plastic. Their usable life may be sho — some youngsters delighting in removing and snapping them. Paren should always be provided with spare covers and asked to discourag their children from such behaviour. It is possible in an emergenc to child-proof an aid by use of cling film sandwich wrap. This shou be wrapped tightly around the aid — the aid then being totally pr tected from child debris. Cling film is reported as having no significar effect on the frequency response of a hearing aid (Powell, 1975). Hov ever, it is advisable to check this as a matter of routine on each mod of pocket aid in service by means of a hearing aid test box. Certai recently introduced pocket aids do show a change in performanc (for example, characteristic 'dip' of $\sim$5-8dB in gain 500-1000H: which would contra-indicate long-term use of cling film. By chec ing each model of aid with and without cling film it soon becom apparent on which aids this child proofing measure can be used o longer than an emergency basis. Overall, a good stock of baby cove s essential in ensuring that effective amplification is maintained.

The pocket aid has one major fitting advantage for use with young-ters and this is that it can be well secured to the child by means of a etaining clip and harness. This ensures that the aid does not fall on to he floor when the child is involved in play situations. The harness nust be comfortable and well fitting. It must be designed to provide he child with a good ear-voice link and not a good ear-tummy link is is sometimes noted. The harness must be worn on top of clothing o that the hearing aids are not buried under layers of jumpers, shirts ind even vests. This only acts to muffle the sound and at the same ime generate unnecessary noise due to clothes rub. A little thought n harness design can make a considerable difference to the impact ind effectiveness of hearing aids of this type. The aids should not be overed by a flap of material when in a harness nor should an elastic trip cover the microphone inlet. If elastic is to be used to secure the id it should be sited towards the ends of the aid away from the micro-hone. The depth of harness pocket is also important and should be uch that the top of the aid is 'proud' of the pocket so that sound an pass freely into the microphone.

All children who use pocket aids should have a selection of harnes-es — perhaps to match the outfits they usually wear. The harness nust be clean when fitted — tatty, food-stained harnesses only act to leter from the importance of the hearing aid fitting, this being parti-ularly so when seen through the eyes of the lay person. One important oint to remember with respect to the fitting of binaural pocket aids s that the signals delivered to each ear should be presented homolater-lly. The technique of criss-cross or contralateral routing of the signal o avoid acoustic feedback should not be employed because of its nown deleterious effects on a child's localisation ability (Markides, 981).

Clearly problems of food spillage and clothes' rub do not arise with ost-aural aids — the aid being worn behind the ear. However, there is much higher risk of damage or loss of the aid from falling from the ar because it is more difficult to secure to a young child. This is rimarily a result of the fact that young children's ears are soft and mall and often have difficulty in supporting the weight of a relatively arge, adult oriented instrument, particularly during the rough and umble of play. There are now a range of smaller post-aural aids avail-ble (these use the R48 button cell) which are more oriented to the hild user (Figure 4.8). Such aids should be considered if a post-aural tting is contemplated. However, the performance of these instruments,

Figure 4.8: The normal (a) and miniature (b) size post-aural aid; (c) unfitted.

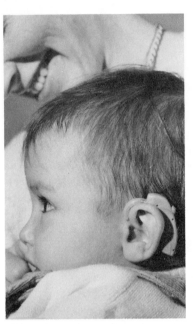 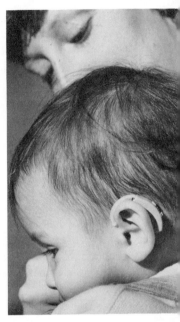

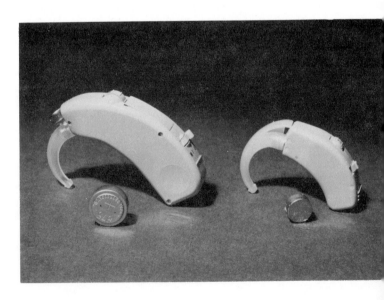

particularly for severe and profoundly deaf children is lacking in relation to that of the conventional size post-aural unit.

The microphone is located in one of two positions on post-auricular hearing aids: either at the top of the aid close to the acoustic elbow or at the bottom of the casing, the microphone entrance being behind the ear when the aid is worn. It is important to note that microphone placement may influence the performance of a hearing aid when worn on the head. This means that if two hearing aids (one with a top front microphone, the other a bottom mounted microphone) have equivalent performance when evaluated in a test box (that is, not on the head) their performance may be different when worn on the head. In particular it has been reported that an enhancement (8-10dB) in the frequency response from about 1 to 3kHz occurs for the top front microphone (Pollack, 1980). It has therefore been suggested that the optimal placement for the microphone on post-aural aids is just in front and above the ear, that is, the top front location. Interestingly, work done by Chan (1980) failed to demonstrate any statistical difference between children's speech discrimination scores when using equivalent top and bottom mounted microphones on post-aural hearing aids in the presence of background noise. This may have been a function of test set-up as speech was from directly in front of the children. The only meaningful way of determining whether this factor is significant for a particular child is to carry out an evaluation programme, using varying azimuth locations for the speech source.

Children sometimes complain about the 'noise' generated by post-aural aids due to air flow across the microphone inlet. This can be a real problem when hearing aids are used outdoors. Attempts should be made to resolve it. The problem is particularly noticeable on top front microphone fittings but is not specific to this fitting. One way of reducing the problem is to use a hearing aid with a wind protector. This protector is fitted as standard to certain hearing aids. Alternatively, as with baby covers, it may be obtained as a special accessory. The effectiveness of these protectors varies and it may well prove necessary to try the child on a bottom mounted microphone in cases where the problem proves difficult to resolve. Whilst this is no guarantee of success it has been found on occasions to be effective in our own clinical experience.

The Amplifier

The relatively small electrical signals that are generated by the microphone are directed to the amplifier whereupon they are increased in strength (amplified). Amplifiers are obviously small packages particularly in post-aural and 'in the ear' hearing aids. Prior to the 'silicone chip revolution' all amplifiers comprised separate components of resistors, capacitors and transistors which were assembled 'by hand'. Nowadays an increasing number of amplifiers comprise integrated circuits where the components have been deposited by a special photochemical process on to silicone chips. This has led to a reduction in the size of the hearing aid.

The amplifier circuit contains a number of amplifying 'stages' which boost the small microphone signals, and a power stage which is capable of handling sufficient power to drive the earphone receiver. The amount of gain or amplification available from modern hearing aids can be as much as 80 dB. This means that the voltage gain (input to output) is increased by a factor of 10,000 (each 20 dB increase in equivalent to a real change of voltage of $\times$ 10). The number of stages involved in an amplifier is a function of the amount of gain required.

Two types of amplifier are employed in hearing aids. The low and moderate power aids with gains of less than 45 dB use a class A or single ended amplifier. This comprises three to five amplifier stages, and means that the small incoming microphone signal receives a series of boosts (three to five) before the signal is directed to the power or output amplifier stage ready for feeding into the earphone receiver. This power stage comprises one transistor in class A – hence the name single ended amplifier. It ensures that the processed signal has sufficient strength to drive the earphone receiver.

The class B or 'push-pull' amplifier is used in the higher power aids (maximum gain greater than 45 dB). In this amplifier the signal is fed not into a single transistor power stage, but a power stage comprising two transistors connected in balance so that one acts to 'push', the other to 'pull' the receiver. Each output stage therefore only effectively operates during one half of the signal cycle.

Apart from their amplifying task, many hearing aid amplifiers contain special adjustments which can be used for more accurate compensation of various hearing deficits. These adjustments are controlled by small potentiometers or variable resistors which may be adjusted by a small screw drive or via a finger operated wheel. The volume control is one facility that is common to all aids. This is normally set by the user, or in the case of young children, by the parent or teacher on the advice of the audiologist. In addition to the volume control, hearing aids may also have tone controls and facilities for limiting the maximum output of the hearing aid (peak clipping or compression) incorporated into the amplifier circuits.

Volume Control

The volume control of a hearing aid enables the user to alter the sound intensity delivered to the ear. It is usually built into the aid in the form of a dial or serrated wheel. Some aids have numbers on the dial while others are unmarked. The volume control is in fact a potentiometer (a variable resistor) which controls the flow of the current between the output of one transistor and the input of another in the amplifier. One point of particular importance to teachers and parents is the fact that the volume control is not necessarily linear in nature. Research (Kasten and Lotteman, 1969) has revealed a wide range of taper characteristics, that is, volume control rotation and amount of signal increase. Some hearing aids, for example, may attain their maximum gain when the volume control reaches 50 per cent of its total range. Above this setting no further increase in gain occurs. It is important for the audiologist to know about the taper characteristics of a child's hearing aid and the range over which the volume control operates. This information is rarely given by manufacturers, and must therefore be obtained by the audiologist using a hearing aid test box.

Parents and teachers must be informed of the volume setting at which the child should wear a hearing aid. It is advisable, particularly where settings are different for the two ears, to place a sticky label inside the casing or on the back of the case with the required setting and the ear into which the aid is to be fitted. Some hearing aids do not have a labelled volume control. In such cases it is necessary to carefully mark the control with quick drying paint at the setting required by the child. This must be done when the aids are issued, the parents being advised as to the appropriate setting.

Tone Control

The tone control provides a means of manipulating the frequency response of a hearing aid. Usually three tone control settings are available, these being labelled L, N and H. The N setting is the normal 'reference' response of the hearing aid. The L and H settings alter the shape of the N response. The L setting is not (as may be implied) a base boost or low frequency emphasis (LFE), rather a high frequency de-emphasis or treble cut; and H setting is not (as may also be implied) a treble boost or high frequency emphasis, but rather, a low frequency de-emphasis or base cut.

The electronic tone control is usually built 'into' the amplifier and comprises capacitors and resistors. Tone controls are really filter networks, the L setting being a low pass filter the H setting a high pass filter. Tone controls may be situated externally and operated by a lever or internally and operated by a screwdriver. Recall too that manipulation of a hearing aids' frequency response may be achieved non-electrically by attention to the earmould and associated plumbing (Chapter 5).

Gain Control

Certain models of hearing aid have, in addition to the volume control, a pre-set gain control (GC) which can be adjusted by means of a screw pot. This control acts to reduce the gain of the aid − possibly by up to 10dB. It can be particularly useful for older people because the effect of altering this control is that greater rotation of the volume control is necessary to produce a particular sound intensity. For old people with arthritic fingers (where it may be difficult to make small adjustments to the volume control), it protects them from sudden large increases in sound input into their ears as a result of their unsuccessful attempts at a small adjustment of the volume control. The gain control is situated within the amplification stages and is simply a variable resistor. It does not effect the maximum output of the aid − the input simply has to be greater in order to reach maximum output when the GC control is reduced.

Output Limitation

The majority of pocket aids and some post-aural hearing aids have a screw adjustment (usually internally situated on the pocket aid) to reduce the maximum intensity of sound that the aid can generate. This facility ensures that a child is not subjected to intolerably loud sounds such as a door banging or traffic noise, while at the same time receiving speech optimally amplified.

Peak Clipping

This is commonly used in many hearing aids as a means of limiting the maximum output. There is a limit to the amount of current a transistor can handle. When this limit is reached, further increases in input produce no further increase in output. The output plateaus and the amplifier is said to be in saturation. The process may be best understood by reference to Figure 4.9. In the top diagram the amplifier is working in its 'linear' mode in that there is a 1 to 1 relation between

Figure 4.9: Input-output function in a linear 1:1 (a) and a non-linear peak clipped (b) system.

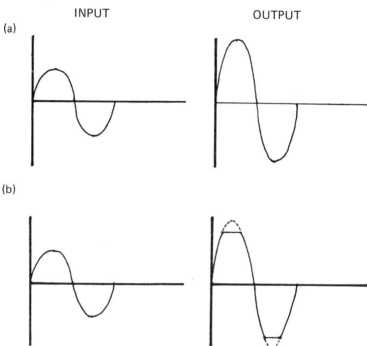

increase in input and increase in output. The amplifier is not driven into saturation and the output waveform is simply an increased or amplified version of the input. In the lower example the situation is different. In this case the input-output relationship is no longer 1 to 1. The transistor in the amplifier attempts to follow the input signal as long as it can. However, beyond a certain point it cannot deliver any greater signal and the peaks of the input signal are chopped off or clipped. The maximum output is therefore limited — the term peak clipping being used to describe this limiting process. It may be seen by reference to Figure 4.9 that the relationship between input and output (I-O function) is linear 1:1 until the saturation level is reached when peak clipping prevents any further increase in output. The aid therefore goes into a non-linear mode. The limitation of current-flow usually takes place in the output stage transistor leading to the earphone. All hearing aids therefore have an 'inbuilt' output limiter which is a function of the power handling capability of the output stage of the amplifier. The peak clipping level can be fixed or adjusted by means of a screw pot. Peak clipping may be seen as simply a characteristic of the amplifier which prevents the output from exceeding a certain (usually adjustable) value. Peak clipping only operates on the powerful sounds which are picked up by the aid and are capable of driving the aid into the non-linear mode. The act of clipping the signal, which is instantaneous, causes distortion in that there will be a change in the relative intensities of the processed signals (that is, these powerful components receive less amplification than the weaker ones). Further, the act of clipping introduces 'new sounds' (distortion products) into the output signal because as may be seen by reference to Figure 4.9 the output is no longer a sinusoid but more a 'square' wave. Harmonics and intermodulation products appear in the output (Hodgson and Skinner, 1981). This will be considered in more detail shortly. There is no standard convention for labelling of the peak clipping control. On certain hearing aids it is labelled as PC; on other hearing aids it is labelled as power control and there is no difference in the action of these controls. It should be noted that peak clipping acts to limit the maximum output of the aid. It does not affect the gain of the hearing aid unless the input signals put the aid in saturation.

Automatic Gain Control (AGC)

An alternative method of limiting hearing aid output is by use of a system known as automatic gain control (AGC). This acts to decrease the gain of the aid so as to prevent the output from exceeding the child's upper tolerance limit. This approach usually prevents the output signal from reaching saturation when the aid is confronted with high inputs. This prevents the occurrence of significant distortion as does occur when output limitation is facilitated by peak clipping. AGC utilises the electronic feedback principle for self-regulation. In AGC circuitry part of the electrical signal at a certain stage of the amplifier network is fed back to an earlier stage. This is done in such a way as to oppose the regular current flow through the amplifier and results in a reduction of amplifier gain and therefore a limitation of signal output level. When sound input to the microphone is weak and the corresponding electrical signals passing through the amplifier are small, the feedback signal is so small as to have no significant influence on the amplification performance. However, if the input signal is strong with a consequent large electrical signal at the feedback site then the amplification will be reduced and the output from the hearing aid is therefore limited. This type of circuit is often described by the term compression amplification, because it acts to compress the dynamic range of the input signal without producing significant distortion at the output.

A number of labels have been used in describing compression circuits (AGC, DRC dynamic range compression, AVC automatic volume control, ALC automatic loudness control, LDC linear dynamic compression) but the differences are often in name only (Philips, 1982a). The term AGC will be used in this discussion. There are two main types of AGC circuit both of which by definition act to reduce gain of the hearing aid. One circuit produces a pattern of a gradually decreasing gain which starts at an input of around 60 dB ('compressor' compression). The other circuit acts as an effective 'limiter' and starts to operate close to the predetermined maximum output and prevents the output from being increased further ('limiter' compression, Figure 4.10). It may be seen that the 'limiter' compression circuit maintains a 1 to 1 input-output function until the limiting level is reached. The 'compressor' does not show this 1 to 1 relationship. In effect the only basic difference between these circuits relates to the input level at which the compression comes into action and the resultant input-output function. This level is known as the lower AGC limit (or knee point) as may be seen by reference to Figure 4.11. Both circuits limit the maximum output without introducing significant distortion. This means that the intended signal is reproduced more accurately than occurs with peak clipping.

AGC circuits may be distinguished in another way. This distinction is a function of whether the AGC circuit is reacting to the incoming signal early on in the amplification stages, or to the signal from the output stage of the amplifier going to the earphone.

AGC circuitry that works on input is known as input dependent compression (IDC). In such hearing aids a portion of the output from an early stage of the amplifier is fed back to preceding stages. The signal level arriving at the microphone therefore determines when the compressor will come into action. The feedback takes place prior to the volume control and as a result compressor action is totally independent of volume control setting. The effect of this is that the AGC system operates for all positions of volume control. The child can therefore adjust the maximum sound level by manipulation of the volume control. Output dependent compression (ODC) by definition operates on the output signal going from the amplifier to the receiver. In this case the volume control is situated within the feedback loop

Figure 4.10: Input-output curves of hearing aids with peak clipping, 'limiter' AGC and 'compressor' AGC output limitation facility.

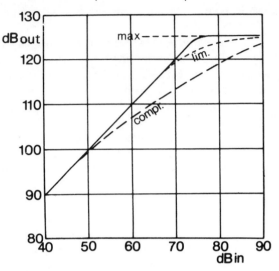

Figure 4.11: Example of a steady state AGC input/output graph.

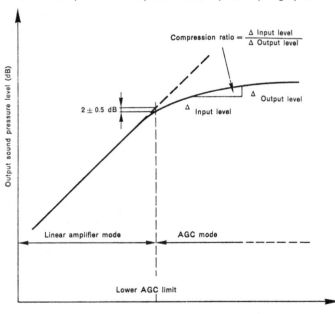

Source: IEC, 1979, with permission.

and its setting therefore influences the action of the compressor. When the volume control is situated within the AGC system the child cannot manipulate the maximum acoustic output. This output is fixed to some predetermined level by the AGC circuit and the child can only alter the gain of the hearing aid by adjustment of the volume control (Figure 4.12). The AGC level will be set in such cases by the audiologist.

Figure 4.12: The input/output relationship as a function of gain control position in (a) output dependent compression and (b) input dependent compression.

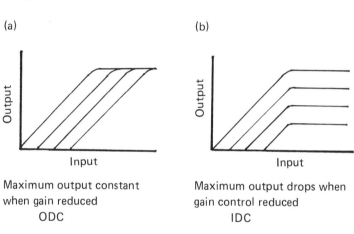

(a)   (b)

Maximum output constant   Maximum output drops when
when gain reduced   gain control reduced
         ODC   IDC

One potential advantage of input dependent compression over the output dependent type is that there is likely to be less distortion produced because of the fact that the compression occurs prior to rather than after the amplification stage. It is important to note that AGC circuits do take a finite time to operate. The term 'attack time' refers to the length of time required for the controlling action to take effect. Recovery or release time is defined as the time taken for the amplification stages to return to 'normal' amplification after a strong signal is no longer present. These parameters are important in relation to effective use of amplification (Johansson, 1973). Values of the order 18 msec for attack and 180 msec for recovery times are common in hearing aids.

The point was made earlier that AGC causes gain reduction and prevents output saturation when the input signal is high. There is, however, on linear compressors, a compression ratio (see Figure 4.11). It is therefore important to realise that for high input the output level may exceed the child's upper tolerance limit. This is why many hearing aids with AGC also have an adjustable maximum power control (Philips, 1982a).

The Hearing Aid Lead

The hearing aid lead carries the electrical signal from the output stage of the amplifier to the receiver. In pocket aids this is an insulated wire which plugs into the output socket of the hearing aid at one end and the earphone receiver at the other end. It is imperative that this lead is kept in first class working order. It has known weak spots at the two ends where the adaptors are attached. Day-to-day wear and tear eventually results in broken or intermittent leads with a resultant unacceptable hearing aid performance. One reason why faults develop on leads is that people coil the lead inappropriately during periods of non use. This produces unnecessary stress on the lead connector and perhaps more importantly on the socket of the hearing aid and results in the danger of intermittent performance. The most appropriate way to store the aid, for example overnight, is to disconnect the lead and coil it carefully. Child length (45cm) leads must be obtained for youngsters. It is not acceptable to fit children with leads of adult length — to conceal long lengths of lead under children's clothing is difficult and often causes discomfort and distraction to the child. The leads should be concealed as much as possible, for example, into the straps of the harness. Every effort should be made to prevent trailing leads which can otherwise result in problems of the moulds being pulled out of the ears during play, children chewing their leads, a greater risk of lead faults and of course aids looking less attractive particularly from the parents viewpoint.

The parents and teachers must apply a management programme that is effective in identifying lead faults. This is most easily done by use of a stetoclip — lead checking being another component of the daily checking routine. The hearing aid should be set to a comfortable level via the stetoclip. The condition of the lead and incidentally the output socket of the aid is checked by talking into the aid and wiggling the lead at the two noted weak spots. If intermittency or total lack of output is apparent (having replaced the battery), then a faulty lead should be suspected. If an intermittent fault is noted which persists with a new lead then a faulty socket should be suspected. Parents and class teachers must have a supply of spare leads. These leads as well as being of child length must also be specific to the child's hearing aid. If the aid has a side entry socket for the lead, then the lead must be fitted with a right-angle connector. If the socket is on top of the aid then the lead must have a straight connector. The lead socket on some hearing aids is polarised, that is, one pin is wider than the other while on others it is non-polarised, that is, two holes of the same size. The lead must have the correct connector. A polarised lead must not be fitted to a non-polarised socket because intermittent contact may result.

The lead on a post-aural hearing aid is simply a short connector from the amplifier to the internal receiver. However, this receiver has to convey the amplified signals to the ear. A plastic elbow, tubing and an earmould are usually employed in this respect. Interestingly 'lead-like' faults can arise on post-aural aids due to problems arising in the above-mentioned plumbing. The most commonly occurring problem is that of condensation in the elbow or tubing. Dried out and cracked tubing, strangled tubing and the problem of wax in the sound tube can also contribute to an inefficient system. Management of these factors is described in the earmould chapter.

On-off Switch

The on-off switch by definition switches the power supply in and out of the system. This switch may be separate from or incorporated into the volume control of the aid. On certain models of post-aural aids there is no 'switch' as such, the power to the aid being switched on and off by manipulation of the battery compartment. Obviously, parents and teachers must be shown how to switch the aid on and off and they must be made aware of the need to switch the aid off when not in use. Otherwise the capacity of the battery will be significantly reduced.

The Telecoil (T)

Many hearing aids are equipped with a magnetic induction pick-up which is mounted vertically in the aid casing. This coil is simply a conductor wound in a tight spiral which allows a high concentration of conductor material in a small space. The hearing aid is normally equipped with a switch labelled M-MT-T or M-T-O. This switches the microphone in and out of the system and obviously also energises the coil. When the switch is set to the M position the microphone will be sensitive to the sound-waves impinging on the diaphragm and will direct electrical signals to the amplifier. When this setting is at T, the microphone is no longer sensitive to sound and the aid will only function if used in an induction loop system.

Originally the T mode was known as the 'telephone coil' and was intended to allow individuals to use their hearing aids with the telephone. The basic principle involved is that of electromagnetic induction (Halliday and Resnick, 1962). Briefly when a conductor (a wire) is carrying current, that current sets up a magnetic field around the wire. If another conductor is situated in the vicinity of the first then a current will be induced into this conductor whenever a change occurs in the strength of the current through the first conductor. Now recall that the telecoil is simply a high concentration of conducting material (rather than one wire) which permits a more effective induced current flow to occur when a changing magnetic field is introduced in its vicinity. The telecoil passes on this induced current to the amplifier in a similar manner to the microphone.

When telecoils were first introduced into hearing aids the electrical energy at the output of the telephone produced a magnetic field which induced current into the hearing aid coil. As the coil is not sensitive to acoustic signals the aid simply amplified the telephone message and not the competing noise around the telephone. Unfortunately, the modern generation of telephones such as the push button and trim phone use a microphone-receiver system that allows only a tiny magnetic field which is totally inadequate for the telecoil to operate effectively. There are ways of overcoming this problem. These will be discussed later under the section dealing with auxiliary aids.

The main use of the teleloop with children is via classroom loop or FM induction systems. These will be also discussed later in the chapter under 'Educational Amplification Systems'.

It should be remembered that when the aid is set to T it will be insensitive to acoustic energy arriving at the microphone. The MT setting allows the child to pick up both acoustic signals and signals from the loop induction system. It should be noted that the gain of an aid is very likely to be less with the aid on MT rather than M. Parents and teachers must be advised of this fact and the audiologist must determine just what effect the switch from M to MT has on the performance of the aid. The volume setting of the aid may require adjustment in going from M to MT to ensure optimal use of the aid. If this is so parents and teachers must be notified of the appropriate settings for young children. A simple guideline relating to everyday use of a hearing aid is that it should be set to the M position, unless there is a loop induction or other system in use with the child (for example, direct input radio hearing aid — see the section on 'Radio Hearing Aids').

While all pocket aids have the M-MT-T settings the same cannot always be said of post-aural systems. Some post-aural aids have only M and T settings. This is not desirable for child usage and such aids should be avoided if at all possible. Children must be able to hear their own voices at all times particularly in educational settings. They must be able to hear the contributions of other children too. This will be impossible with the hearing aid on the T setting in a classroom loop with the loop microphone close to the teacher.

The Receiver

The receiver, like the microphone, is a transducer. In effect the receiver is a microphone in reverse, converting electrical energy into sound energy ready for delivery to the ear.

In the pocket aid the receiver is a button-shaped unit with a small nub on one side that clips into the earmould. When a child is fitted with a pocket aid a specific receiver will also be chosen for the child to use. This is because a particular pocket aid may be used with a range of receivers which have differing sensitivities to the speech frequencies and therefore allow manipulation of the hearing aid's frequency response. Parents must be made aware of the type of receiver that has been selected for their child. They must also appreciate the detrimental effect that an inappropriate receiver can have on the effectiveness of the hearing aid fitting. This is best achieved by playing them a cassette tape of speech through an aid with an appropriate receiver and a totally inappropriate mismatched receiver (available from authors if required). Parents and teachers should know where the identifying code is stamped on the receiver. They should be encouraged as part of their daily aid checking routine to check that the correct receiver is being used (has not been swopped at school as does occur) and that the quality of sound (this is something they 'tune' into after a time) from the hearing aid is satisfactory. If it is not they should try replacing the receiver to see whether this improves the quality. Clearly a supply of appropriate spare receivers should be available to parents and teachers.

The majority of modern pocket aids may be used with subminiature receivers. These are desirable for the child user because of the problems that children's small soft ears have in supporting standard 'adult' size receivers. Typical problems of moulds continually falling out of the ears and acoustic feedback were very apparent when the standard size receiver was the order of the day. Although in theory it is possible to obtain more power from the standard PP receiver relative to the subminiature power unit, in practice it often turns out that this power cannot be used because of the above mentioned problems. As a rule therefore, subminiature receivers should be employed with young children. The problems of acoustic feedback are discussed in Chapter 5. It is important to recall that the receiver can contribute to this problem and that steps can be taken to reduce its contribution significantly.

The receiver in the post-aural aid is internally situated and directs sound energy into the acoustic elbow at the top of the aid. Being internally situated it is less prone to many of the button receiver child-oriented problems. Its main weakness basically relates to its integrity under child usage. It is clearly 'at risk' if the aid is persistently falling from the ear and steps must obviously be taken to prevent this. All of the receivers that are used in hearing aids are electromagnetic in type.

Usually the receiver is of an air conduction type whereby the sound energy is presented to the earmould and directed down the ear canal to the eardrum. An alternative is the bone conduction receiver which is sometimes used with children suffering chronic ear discharge or deformity of the external ear. This works just like the bone oscillator in audiometry and sets up skull bone vibration when coupled to the mastoid bone via a headband. Bone conduction receivers may be used with pocket and spectacle aids. Post-aural aids may also be adapted if required. It is possible to use such systems with FM aids as well. The major drawback of this type of receiver relates to the importance of good contact between mastoid and receiver for efficient performance of the aid. This can lead to discomfort for the user from prolonged wearing sessions. It is vitally important for the audiologist to produce as effective and comfortable a fitting as possible in cases where bone conduction is employed. Attention to the design and size of headband is particularly important. Nowadays, it is fair to say that the receiver may be rightly seen as the most influential component of the 'electronic package' in relation to high-fidelity performance of the hearing aid. Recall that the electret microphone has an extremely wide flat frequency response. However, electromagnetic hearing aid receivers do not. They have a much narrower 'peaky' response which severely restricts the range of speech frequencies that are 'effectively' handled y the hearing aid and experienced by the child.

The button receivers have a good low frequency response, their main limitation being in the higher frequencies above 3 kHz. The overall shape of frequency response can obviously be manipulated, but it is important to note that one cannot obtain both very high power and a wide band 'smooth' response. High power (~130 dB) necessitates a reduction in the band width of the processed signal (that is, a narrower range of frequencies).

The air conduction receivers in post-aural aids are by definition miniature and as a result haven't the same capacity of output in the low frequencies. Nevertheless, progress is being made here with the development, for example, of improved low frequency performance VLF aids. Post-aural receivers do provide better high frequency performance in relation to the button receiver. The weakness of many post-aural receivers relates to the marked peaks in their frequency response (resonances, for example, around 1 kHz) with, in certain cases, quite significant 'troughs' in the frequency region 1-2 kHz. It is possible to smooth out and extend the response as described in Chapter 5. This smoothing is often done in manufacture and built into the post-aural instrument – for example, 'etymotic response' (Philips, 1982a). This 'peaky response' characteristic is something that audiologists should pay attention to, particularly during hearing aid evaluation. Attempts should be made to assess the real ear performance of the aid on the child, because of the fact that a considerable amount of 'language information' lies in the 1-2 kHz region. Tests at more than octave frequencies are necessary to identify such troughs which cannot be tolerated with hearing-impaired children. (See section on aid evaluation for further comments.)

The bone conduction receiver requires considerably more power than the button receiver. It has a very limited low and high frequency response with little output below 500 Hz or above 4000 Hz.

It is of interest to note that the other type of receiver that is used with hearing-impaired children is the large circumaural or supra-aural earphone of the group aid or auditory training unit. This receiver can deliver high power wide range output and is particularly suited to the needs of profoundly deaf children. This is one reason why such systems are often seen as 'extending' a child's linguistic experience, particularly when one considers the 'filtering' effects of children's earmoulds on top of the frequency 'narrowing' effect of the hearing aid receiver. There is no doubt in our minds that use of headphones is still a very valuable exercise for hearing-impaired children.

References

Barwick, S. (1983) 'Beware the panic button', *Daily Mail*, 2 July 1983

Chan, T.M.Y. (1980) 'A comparison of speech discrimination in partially hear ing children'. Unpublished MEd dissertation, University of Manchester, Man chester

Department of Health and Social Security (1982) 'Primary batteries – Appli cations', *Services for Hearing-Impaired People – Information Sheet, B051* DHSS, London

Ever Ready (1980) *Modern Portable Electricity*, Ever Ready Company, London

Halliday, D. and Resnick, R. (1962) *Physics for Students of Science and Engineer ing*, Part II, 2nd edn, John Wiley, New York

Hodgson, W.R. and Skinner, P.H. (1981) *Hearing Aid Assessment and Use i. Audiologic Habilitation*, 2nd edn, Williams and Wilkins, Baltimore

Hueber, F. (1972) 'The hearing-aid microphone – past and future', *Journal o. Audiological Technique*, *11*, 46

International Electrotechnical Commission (1979) 'Hearing aid equipment no entirely worn on the listener', *International Electrotechnical Commission* IEC 118-3, Geneva

Johansson, B. (1973) 'The hearing aid as a technical-audiological problem' *Scandinavian Audiology*, *3*, 55

Kasten, R.N., Lotteman, S.H. and Hinchman, M.J. (1967) 'Head shadow and head baffle effects in ear level hearing aids', *Acoustica*, *19*, 154

Kasten, R.N. and Lotteman, S.H. (1969) 'Influence of hearing aid gain rotatio on acoustic gain', *Journal of Auditory Research*, *9*, 35

Lentz, W.E. (1975) 'An introduction to directional hearing aids', *ORL Digest 37(4)*, 12

Markides, A. (1981) 'Effect of homolateral and contralateral routing of signal through body worn hearing aids on the localisation ability of hearing-impaire people', *Journal of the British Assoc. Teachers of the Deaf*, *5(3)*, 63

Nielsen, T.E. (1974) *Hearing Aid Characteristics and Fitting Techniques fo Improving Speech Intelligibility in Noise*, Oticon Technical Library Series Oticon, Denmark

Nielsen, H.B. and Ludvigsen, C. (1978) 'Effects of hearing aids with directiona microphone in different acoustic environments', *Scandinavian Audiology* *7*, 217

Niemoeller, A.F. (1978) 'Hearing aids' in H. Davis and S.R. Silverman (eds.) *Hearing and Deafness*, Holt, Rinehart and Winston, New York

Nolan, M. and Tucker, I.G. (1981) 'Health risks following ingestion of mercury and zinc air batteries', *Scandinavian Audiology*, *10*, 189

Olsen, W. and Carhart, R. (1975) 'Head diffraction effects on ear level hearing aids', *Audiology*, *14*, 244

Philips (1982a) *Basics of Audiology*, 6th edn, Philips Audiological Equipmen Division, Eindhoven

Philips (1982b) *Batteries in Hearing Aids*, Product Information Services Hearing Aids, Philips, Eindhoven

Pollack, M.C. (1980) *Amplification for the Hearing Impaired*, 2nd edn, Grun and Stratton, New York

Powell, C.A. (1975) 'The ergonomic design of hearing aids for children', *Pro ceedings of the Congress on Education of The Deaf*, Tokyo

Reilly, D.T. (1979) 'Mercury battery ingestion', *British Medical Journal*, *1* 859

Shaw, D.A.J. (1983) 'Battery usage in hearing aids'. Unpublished MEd disserta tion, University of Manchester, Manchester

Studebaker, G.A., Cox, R.M. and Formby, C. (1980) 'The effect of the environment on the directional performance of head-worn hearing aids' in G.A. Studebaker and I. Hochberg (eds.), *Acoustical Factors Affecting Hearing Aid Performance*, University Park Press, Baltimore

Sung, G.S., Sung, R.J. and Angelelli, R.M. (1975) 'Directional microphone in hearing aids; effects on speech discrimination in noise', *Archives of Otolaryngology*, *101*, 316

5 THE EARMOULD

The earmould plays a very important role as a constituent part of wearable hearing aid. Its role may be summarised as:

(i) linking the hearing aid to the patient;
(ii) conveyor of sound from the output transducer of the hearing aid (the receiver) to the external auditory meatus.

The earmould can and does have a very significant influence on the *frequency response* of a hearing aid (Lybarger, 1967; Curran, 1978; Corell, 1978; Ewertsen *et al.*, 1957). It is often considered the 'weak link' in the amplification chain because of the fact that the 'quality of fit' of the mould in a child's ear may give rise to the problem of acoustic feedback (Nolan *et al.*, 1978). The 'quality of fit' – particularly with young hearing-impaired children, often determines the usable gain of the hearing aid. Under such circumstances the clinician may be unable to set the aid at the 'desired' gain level because of feedback howl.

The Requirements of an Earmould

The earmould has to satisfy the demands of both the patient (the user) and the professional (the provider). Patient wants may be summarised as:

(i) good cosmetic appearance
(ii) comfort
(iii) good acoustic fit
(iv) ease of insertion and removal
(v) simple to clean.

The professional 'wants' in addition to the above are:

(i) reliable product
(ii) no shrinkage
(iii) ease of working

(iv) quick processing time
(v) compatible with commercial hearing aids
(vi) instant (= ideal condition).

Types of Earmould

There are two distinct types of earmould in use. The INSTANT or DIRECT mould has particular advantages for the child user because of speed of replacement. The manufacturing process for this category of mould may be summarised as:

$$EAR\ IMPRESSION \rightarrow PROCESS \rightarrow FIT$$

The ear impression acts as the final mould, the only work necessary being the provision of sound tube, lock spring (pocket aids), venting tube (if required) and varnishing before fitting can take place (Nolan et al., 1979). This process has three important advantages over the INDIRECT or TWO STAGE earmould process:

. It minimises delay in the making and fitting the earmould, which is particularly important to children where 'turn over' is high, the moulds having relatively short life span because of child growth.
. It enables the technician to repeat a fitting without delay should the mould prove to be unsatisfactory.
. It reduces inaccuracies which are intrinsic to a two stage process.

If a one stage earmould is to be acceptable for use it must have certain characteristics or properties. Resilience is an obviously desirable property both for comfort, safety and a good fit. A flexible earmould will maintain close contact with the contours of the ear under working conditions and provide a better acoustic seal with less irritation than a hard mould. A good acoustically fitting earmould is an obvious requisite for the severe and profoundly deaf.

The most common one stage earmould used up to the mid-1970s was an acrylic cold curing material (ADI, 1967). This material is not acceptable for general use today because of its intrinsic properties. It shrinks considerably on curing ($\sim$6 per cent) and is hence unstable and dimensionally poor. It cures by an exothermic procedure which is not acceptable for use particularly with children. It can be unstable in its curing reaction being particularly influenced by age, quantities of mix and room temperature. The final product is hard and inflexible. Modern day instant earmoulds are silicone based. Their dimensional stabilit is far superior to the acrylic, the material is flexible and curing occu without exotherm. While such materials have clear advantages ove acrylic, they too have intrinsic characteristics which are not ideal fo earmould use. Relatively low shear strength (a weakness to tearing an inability to support a conventional lock spring for body aids an a well-known non-stick characteristic being of particular relevance It has been possible to minimise these drawbacks and produce mould which, while having a relatively short lifetime in comparison to two stage materials, have still proved to be reliable and adequate for th needs of children where turnover of moulds is quite high (Insta Mould 1979; Tucker *et al.*, 1978; Sneyd, 1979). This has been achieved b use of composite structures (acrylic backplate, silicone interior) speci wire lock springs and lock springs with collars. Such moulds shoul prove useful, particularly for short-term fitting while a two-stage moul is in preparation. These moulds are far superior to ear-pips or tempo ary moulds and will have great value in an earmould service.

The alternative category of earmould is the INDIRECT or TW(STAGE. In this approach the final mould results from a procedure of:

EAR IMPRESSION → PLASTER CAST → MOULD CAST →
PROCESS → FIT

The approach accounts for the vast majority of children's earmould The fundamental difference between this and the ONE STAGE proces is that the ear impression does not act as the final earmould. The ear mould is made in a special laboratory often some distance from wher the impression is taken. This means that the impression has to be sen by post to the laboratory. This and the 'turn round' time of the labor atory add delay to the fitting or continued efficient use of a hearing ai by a child. 'Turn round' time from taking of an impression to fittin, of the final mould should be seven to ten days and certainly no longe than fourteen days.

The TWO STAGE process follows along well-defined lines onc the impression reaches the laboratory. This may be summarised as:

   (i)   impression numbered
  (ii)   trimmed and possibly wax dipped
 (iii)   invested in plaster
 (iv)   plaster model filled with ear mould material
  (v)   heat cured under pressure
 (vi)   processed (drilled, polished)

vii) returned to clinic
iii) fitted.

Table 5.1 summarises the currently used range of earmould materials.

Table 5.1: Earmould materials

Materials in which earmoulds are commonly fabricated
   Hard acrylic
   Soft tip acrylic
   All soft acrylic
   Vinyl
   Silicone rubber
   Polymethyl methacrylate

Good Fitting Earmoulds

Good fitting earmoulds are a vital component of a successful hearing aid programme. The good fitting mould minimises the likelihood of acoustic feedback — a factor that can both limit the usable gain of the aid and significantly influence both parent and child *attitudes* to the hearing aid. The good fitting mould reduces the risk of the aid slipping from the ear and possibly being lost. Furthermore, unsightliness or discomfort resulting from an earmould may lead to rejection of the aid by the child or parent. The importance of the good fitting mould is again seen to be crucial to efficient effective amplification. Parents and children must develop good positive attitudes to amplification systems and professionals must do everything in their power to prevent those attitudes being tarnished by inefficiency in technical parts of the habilitative programme.

Those professionals who are involved in the management of hearing-impaired children will be faced with four major earmould problem areas which they must resolve if a good and acceptable earmould is to be provided for the child. These may be summarised as:

1. Texture of earmould material — soft or hard?
2. Type of earmould material?
3. Comfort and cosmetic aspect.
4. Acoustic fit.

The four factors obviously interact. The results of various studies into the provision and use of earmoulds by children indicate that soft textured

materials are a primary requisite (Nolan *et al*., 1978; Dawson, 1977
Furthermore, in the light of present technological developments th
most appropriate earmould materials are considered to be silicon
rubber, vinyl and soft acrylic.

The factors that can have a significant influence on the acoustic f
and comfort are:

(a) impression material;
(b) impression maker;
(c) impression technique;
(d) earmould material;
(e) earmould maker;
(f) earmould manufacturing technique.

A primary requisite for a good comfortable earmould is *an accurat
ear impression*. The earmould manufacturer can only provide a fin
product to the quality level of the initial impression. Whilst man
clinicians have little or no involvement in the manufacture of the ea
mould at the earmould laboratory, they can have a direct influenc
on the earmould quality as a result of the accuracy of their ear impre
sion.

Getting An Accurate Ear Impression

There is a simple practical process involved in obtaining an accurat
impression of a child's ear. The process is based on: a fundament
knowledge on the part of the clinician of the anatomical landmark
of the external ear relevant to the earmould; an ability to interac
positively with the child and parent; a knowledge of the techniqu
to use in obtaining an accurate impression of the ear; an awarenes
of the importance of using the most appropriate ear impressio
material.

The Anatomical Landmarks (Figure 5.1)

The most important anatomical landmark is that of the junction of th
cartilaginous and bony canal. It is very important to ensure that the ti
of the earmould does not reach into the bony part of the ear cana
Otherwise, discomfort and pain may result with jaw movement. Furthe
more, long tip earmoulds attenuate the higher speech frequencies whic
are vital for good speech intelligibility (Nueva Espania, 1980). There i
therefore nothing to be gained from provision of long tipped earmould
— in fact for the vast majority of children they are disadvantageous.

Figure 5.1: (a) The external ear showing site for tamp. (b) 1 Helix, 2 tragus, 3 lobe, 4 concha.

(a)   (b)

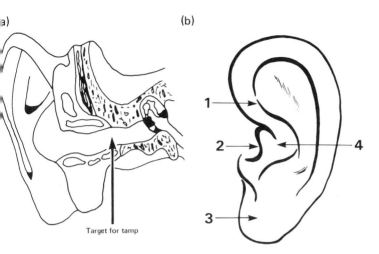

Figure 5.2: Correct (a) and incorrect (b) fitting of a child's earmould.

(a)   (b)

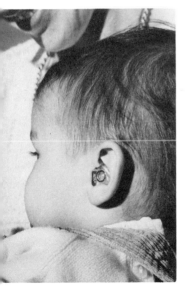 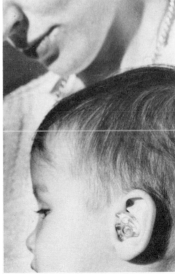

Using a long tip as a means of 'improving' the acoustic fit of the mould does not work and is not recommended.

The helix is the other important landmark in the external ear because it acts as an anchor point for the earmould. It is important for professionals to train parents on how to insert (and remove) the child' earmould − particularly attention should be paid to the helix anchor point which must be correctly located (Figure 5.2).

Positive Interaction

A confident workmanlike clinical approach is crucial in obtaining an accurate ear impression. The professional-parent-child interaction must be one of confidence and trust. It is vital with young children to turn the impression process into a pleasurable game and not something the child grows to dislike and fear. A child's confidence must be gained before proceeding with the process. Some children may be encourage to participate by first allowing them to look through the auroscope at the tips of their own fingers. With others an otoscopic examination of their teddy bear relaxes the situation, while others enjoy treating the light pen as a candle which is 'blown out' by a big puff of air. After the impression procedure is completed excess material may be dispersed on to the child's hand as a 'wiggly worm' − a very popular event with nearly all children. The aim should be to build up parent-child confidence so that future impression making becomes something t enjoy, not dread, on the part of both parent and child.

Ear Impression Technique

There are two approaches to 'taking' an ear impression. The *manual* method was used in the early days of audiology but has in most centres been replaced by the *syringing* technique. There are a number of basic steps to take prior to taking an ear impression:

(1) Organise the clinic so that the equipment is laid out neatly on the work bench.
(2) There is a common 'core' of useful equipment required regardless of which technique is employed. A good auroscope is vital so that the ear canal can be thoroughly examined. An earlight or light-pen is desirable for inserting the tamp into the ear canal. A selection of ready prepared tamps in either expanded foam or cotton wool with a few inches of thread attached should be on hand. The commercially available expanded foam tamps come in various sizes, however, and these often need trimming to fit a child's ear

igure 5.3: Examples of syringes (a) audiological and (b) dental based
hich may be used for ear impression work.

)

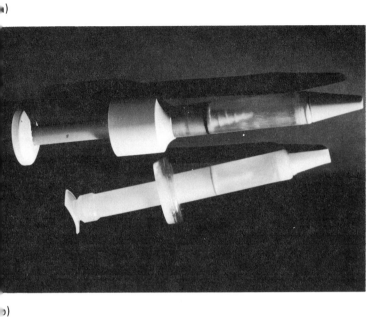

)

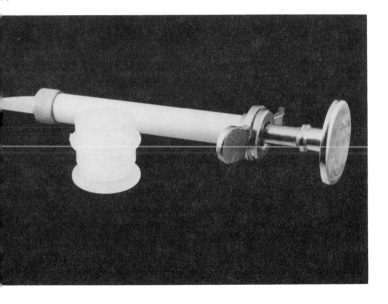

Figure 5.4: The ear impression process. (a) Ear examination; (b) positioning tamp; (c) injecting impression material; (d) excess injected on baby's hand; (e) awaiting curing-impression in ear.

(a)   (b)

(c)   (d)

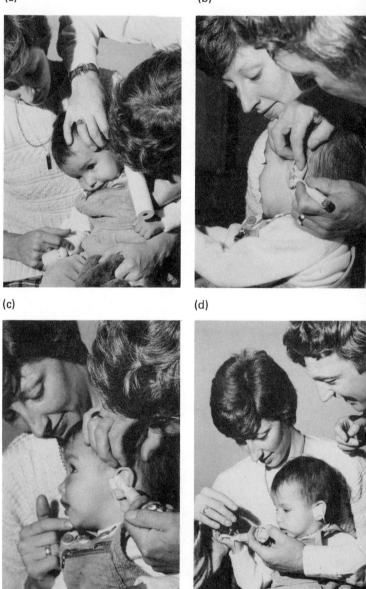

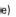

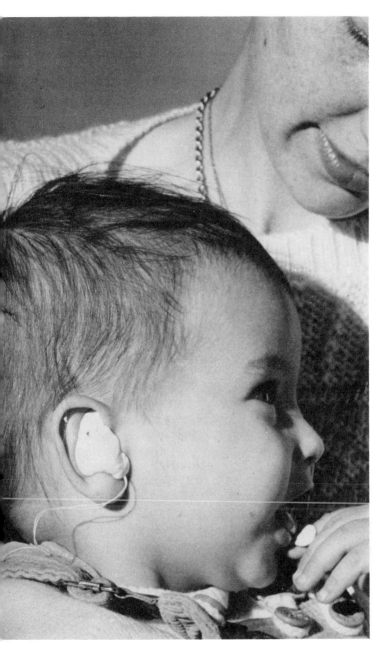

canal. A pair of scissors should therefore be on hand also.

Suitable mixing vessels and pads, a plastic and a metal bladed spatula and dedicated ear impression syringes with loading applicators will also be required. Syringes are available (Figure 5.3) in various configurations – the most appropriate for young children are the 'dental type' such as the 'IMPREGUM' syringe which has a disposable curved plastic tip which may be cut to a suitable size to suit the ear canal.

Once the child and parent have settled in the clinic the first step of the impression taking process is an examination of the external ear and ear canal by means of the auroscope (Figure 5.4). The canal should be clean and unobstructed. Small deposits of wax should cause no difficulty. However, if any heavy deposits of wax or a foreign body are observed, the child must be referred to the GP or ENT specialist for its removal. The auroscope, and subsequently, light-pen should be used by bracing one's hand against the side of the child's head so that any sudden movements of the head do not result in either instrument penetrating deep into the ear canal. The child (particularly youngsters) should be seated side-saddle on mother's knee with the head braced by mother on to her chest.

Figure 5.5: Comparison between a syringed tamp impression and a manually invested impression.

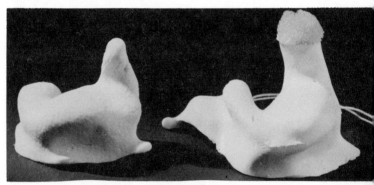

It is vital regardless of subsequent technique to tamp or block the ear canal. This prevents material travelling deep into the ear. The tamp should be placed on the cartilaginous bony canal junction so that when in position it sits at right angles to the canal walls and 'just fills' the cross-sectional area of the canal. Foam tamps make the most practical tamps and should be used wherever possible. The tamp should be pricked' with the fingers into a cone shape to aid correct insertion into he ear. The tamp is placed in position by means of the light-pen. The use of the tamp helps to ensure that the impression material fills the whole section of the external ear. It may be seen by reference to Figure 5.5 that one of the pitfalls of not tamping is lack of definition of the ear canal due to the 'cone-effect' which occurs whenever a material is pushed down a tube.

Once the tamp is in position, the ear impression material should be prepared. It is vital to measure out the correct proportions of impression paste and hardener. If this is not done, curing time may be much too short or alternatively curing may never occur. Equally important is the need to use sufficient material for one impression and not to mix far too much material which is simply wasted. It is not good practice to try to do impressions on both ears from the same mix. One should concentrate on one ear at a time.

Once the impression material has been prepared, it should be invested into the ear.

If the manual method (not recommended) is followed the material is formed into a sausage shape and 'fed' into the ear and pressed up. Distortion of the aural tissues may result from this approach which may mean some difficulty in fitting the final mould. By far the best approach is the syringing method. The syringe should be loaded and the head of the syringe then placed against the tamp in the ear canal. The material is gently invested into the ear – the head of the syringe being gradually withdrawn using a spiral action keeping it below the level of the material until the whole of the requisite parts of the ear have been filled. Particular attention should be paid to the helix and a 'full' concha bowl. The back of the material in the concha may be pressed up by application of thumb or palm pressure, so as to form a flat backplate. When post-aural aids are to be used it is advisable prior to investing material to place the aid on the ear so that the ear is in the 'wearing' position. Once the material has hardened, the impression should be carefully removed by a rocking motion. It should be inspected for flaws and scrapped if unsatisfactory.

The recommended procedure of ear examination, tamping and syringing of the ear impression material into the ear will in itself improve the quality of earmoulds by providing a superior cast on which the earmould laboratory can work. If the clinician wishes to obtain great accuracy and definition it is vital to have a knowledge of the properties of ear impression materials.

The Ear Impression Material

There are three main types of impression material in use. Acrylic, condensation silicone and addition silicone. The primary requisites of the ear impression material may be summarised as:

(i)   accurate and stable over long periods of time;
(ii) flexible;
(iii) easy to work with;
(iv) sets in a reasonable time with no undesirable side effects (no exotherm);
(v)   adequate flow properties;
(vi) sufficient mechanical strength not to tear or permanently deform upon removal.

The acrylic impression materials formerly used in audiology were shown to be unsuitable because of their dimensional instability (Nolan *et al.*, 1978). Nowadays the majority of ear impressions are taken in silicone rubber. The most popular currently used silicones set by a condensation polymerisation reaction. As a consequence these materials although accurate and far superior to the acrylic are not dimensionally stable, since shrinkage is associated with the polymerisation reaction. A new range of silicone materials is available based on an addition polymerisation reaction (Craig *et al.*, 1979). Their dimensional stability is excellent. The addition silicones although more expensive are now finding more widespread use and are to be recommended. These materials are available in a range of consistencies or 'body'. The regular and heavy body are appropriate for ear impression work.

Where a wash technique is applied (Fifield *et al.*, 1980) the wash material will be of light body consistency. Care must be exercised when using this approach as distortion of the aural tissues may occur.

If an ear impression is to be packaged for posting to the earmould laboratory it must be placed in a suitable rigid box. It is advisable to glue the mould to the bottom of the box and ensure that it is in no way being distorted by the box lid or accompanying order form.

Earmould Configuration – Ordering the Mould

It is possible to obtain earmoulds in a wide range of configurations. The most commonly used moulds for children are the '*solid*' (regular or standard) for pocket aids and radio hearing aids and the '*shell*'

Figure 5.6: Examples of commonly used earmoulds. (a) Solid (pocket aids); (b) shell (post-aural); (c) skeleton (post-aural).

(a)

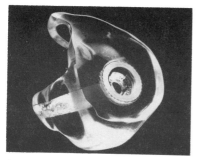

(b)

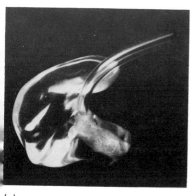

(c)

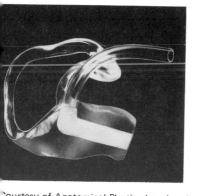

Courtesy of Anatomical Plastics London, Ltd, Washington, Tyne and Wear.

for post-aural aids (Figure 5.6). It is not advisable to use *'skeleton'* moulds with youngsters because these moulds tear or crack under the strain of the child user. The use of an insert (Figure 5.7) rather than a bonded tube with the shell mould permits regular changing of the plastic tubing between ear hook and insert. This tubing tends to 'dry out', discolour and split and can have a significant influence both on aid performance (because of feedback) and wearer attitude to the aid (cosmetic appearance).

Figure 5.7: The ear insert and the vented mould.

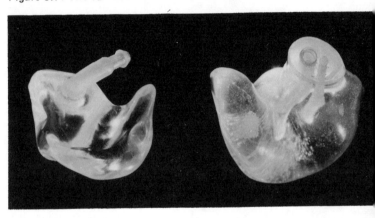

Earmould Management

The parents initially, and subsequently the child himself, must take the responsibility of ensuring that the earmould is kept clean. A nightly procedure of teeth cleaned-earmould cleaned should be adopted from the outset, so that this becomes routine for the child. The problem of wax blocking the sound tube with a resultant ineffective amplification system is not uncommon and often goes unnoticed, especially with young children who may not indicate a 'fault' on their hearing aid.

Parents must in the case of 'shell' moulds be given spare tubing so that hardened, discoloured or cracked tubing can be quickly replaced.

The professional adviser must appreciate that insertion and removal of earmoulds may present some difficulty 'early on' in the habilitative programme. It was suggested earlier that parents should be carefully advised and trained in this procedure. Equally, however, parents should encourage the child to do this himself so that he soon develops a fitting independence.

There are no absolute guidelines on replacement times for ear-moulds. Earmoulds should be replaced whenever they prove unsatis-factory either because of the growth and associated problem of acoustic feedback or perhaps because of damage (chewed tips) or loss. Parents and professionals must be ever vigilant in respect of earmoulds and never be prepared to 'accept' an inadequate product. The philosophy must be one of efficient and effective amplification at all times (Figure 5.8).

Some children chew their earmoulds or bite off the meatal tips. This is often associated with an uncomfortable mould due to an over-long tip. If the problem is purely habit it must be prevented perhaps by use of an 'anti-finger nail nibbler' application such as bitter aloes.

Clinicians must pay attention to the question of child allergy to certain earmould materials. Dry, flaking skin or itching of the concha and ear canal are clear signs of this problem. Use of an alternative material is essential in such cases as is referral to the GP. The improved performance of the modern generation of post-aural aids has resulted in an increasing number of children using such aids. The need for a good acoustic fit of the earmould is fundamental because of the proxi-mity of the transducers to the ear. One consequence of the fit is the problem of condensation in the tubing. This can cause intermittency of sound, and parents, teachers and children should be advised of this. It may be easily overcome by removal of the aid, the condensation being blown out of the tube after the mould has been disconnected. Routine checks by parents and teachers during the day are advisable.

Earmould Acoustics

The point was made at the beginning of this chapter that the earmould is an integral part of the wearable hearing aid. It is vital to realise that the earmould can and does influence the frequency range and fre-quency response delivered to the child's ear. The major factors of note in this respect are the length and diameter of the sound tube and in addition for 'solid' moulds the 'well depth' below the lock spring. It is reasonable to follow a rule of thumb that long sound tubes and narrow bores attenuate the higher speech frequencies. Obviously the longer the sound tube the higher (relatively) the sound pressure at the tympanic membrane. In general, the audiologist should aim to fit a child with an earmould having a meatal tip which lies at the junction of the cartilaginous and bony canal and a sound tube bore that is as wide as possible.

One of the dangers of using soft rubber materials such as silicone

Figure 5.8: The boom ear mould testing system (Siemens Instrument):
(a) close-up, (b) in operation.

(a)

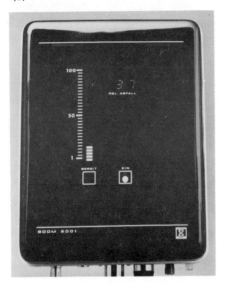

(b)

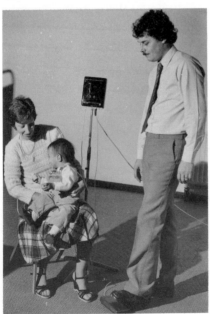

and vinyl is that the plastic tubing lining the sound bore can become 'strangled' or squashed by the material, that is, the sound tube collapses. This results in an occluded or much reduced sound bore — severely attenuating information from the higher speech frequencies (above 1000Hz). Parents and professionals must be alert to this danger and check for it. If this does occur, steps must be immediately taken to rectify it.

The problem can in fact be avoided in manufacture by means of 'wiring' the plaster cast so that the final mould is cured with a sound tube 'built in' — no drilling or core boring being necessary. Professionals should take this matter up with suppliers if it proves to be a recurrent problem.

The well depth below the lock spring should be as shallow as possible because unnecessarily deep wells attenuate the higher speech frequencies (Lybarger, 1967).

Adjusting the Frequency Response

It is now possible, especially with adults and teenage children whose ears are relatively large, to make adjustments to the frequency response of a hearing aid by attention to the earmould and associated plumbing. It may be seen by reference to Figure 5.9 that individual adjustments to low, mid and high frequencies may be achieved by the use of *venting*, *damping* and *horn effects* respectively. However, it must be emphasised that this should be interpreted with caution as the effects are not as clear cut as standard texts often imply. Furthermore, the earmould material may make it impossible to achieve the modification. Silicone rubber and vinyl are not easy materials to work. Acrylic moulds should present no problem.

Figure 5.9: Earmould modifications and frequencies of influence.

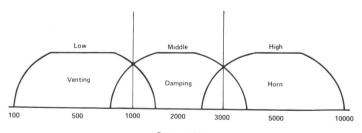

EARMOULD MODIFICATION – FREQUENCY REGION AFFECTED

Source: After P.C. Werth Ltd, London.

Venting

The term venting is used to describe the situation where a second hole is bored through the earmould. There are three main reasons why venting may be of benefit to a hearing aid user. It can increase the user's comfort by releasing sound pressure in the external auditory meatus. It can eliminate the 'blocked ear' effect about which some subjects complain when using a closed earmould. It can alter the frequency response of the hearing aid – primarily by low frequency reduction. It is difficult to quantify specifically the absolute effect of venting on frequency response. This will be a function of the length and diameter of the vent, whether the vent runs parallel or breaks into the sound tube (diagonal) and the characteristics of the hearing aid. However, very narrow vents (<1 mm) have little effect on frequency response but do help to overcome sound pressure and 'full ear' effects.

Figure 5.10: Venting and the effect on hearing aid frequency response.

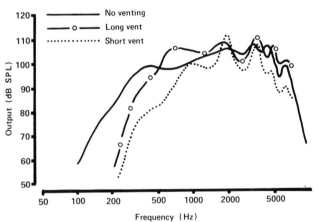

Source: After P.C. Werth Ltd, London.

For many hearing-impaired children conventional venting is undesirable. This is because of the risk of acoustic feedback and the children's amplification requirements. It is interesting to note that French St George and Barr-Hamilton (1978) recommend the use of a vent incorporating a sintered filter, which, it is reported, overcomes the 'full ear' effect and is less prone to acoustic feedback in comparison to the conventional vent. Practical problems of ear size, however, will militate against the implementation of this recommendation with young children.

Figure 5.11: Examples of damping elements (a) and (b); and (c) the resultant influence on the hearing aid frequency response.

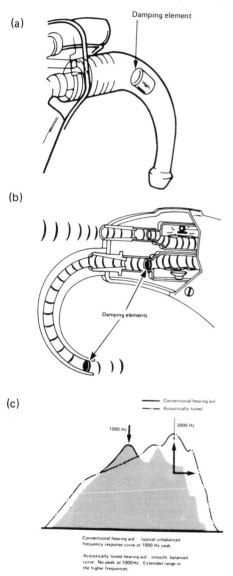

(a)

Damping element

(b)

Damping elements

(c)

Conventional hearing aid
Acoustically tuned

1000 Hz

3000 Hz

Conventional hearing aid : typical unbalanced frequency response curve at 1000 Hz peak

Acoustically tuned hearing aid : smooth, balanced curve. No peak at 1000 Hz. Extended range in the higher frequencies.

Source: after Phonak Ltd, Switzerland and Philips, Eindhoven.

Damping

The major problem associated with vented earmoulds is that of producing acoustic feedback. In the case of children who require significant gain, this approach to modifying the frequency response of the aid will be out of the question.

It is possible, however, to effect changes to the normal response of a post-aural aid by means of *damping* which is simply a mechanical procedure of introducing a resistive device (cotton, lamb's wool, sintered metal pellets) at one or more specific points in the earmould — ear hook plumbing (Figure 5.11). Nowadays, such devices (damping elements) are sometimes incorporated into commercial hearing aid designs — in the earphone acoustic chamber or connecting plastic ear hook, to provide a smooth frequency response — important in relation to acoustic feedback as discussed shortly. Alternatively, it is possible for the professional to achieve this by insertion of resistive damping elements in the aid plumbing. Some degree of trial and error may be necessary to obtain the desired effect. One particular use of damping elements could be in smoothing out the resonant peaks often seen in modern day post-aural aids.

Horn Effects

It has been found possible (Killion, 1980) to enhance and extend the high frequency performance of a hearing aid by use of a preformed tube having a horn configuration rather than a uniform regular diameter — the Libby horn (Figure 5.12). Unfortunately, such a device will generally be impractical for use with young children because of the physical size of the ear and associated earmould. However, it may prove advantageous for certain older children, particularly those with more severe high frequency hearing loss. Various experimental studies have highlighted the importance of a good extended high frequency response in relation to hearing-impaired children's speech discrimination abilities (Watson, 1960; Olsen, 1971; Pascoe *et al.*, 1973; Triantos and McCandles, 1974). Acoustic horns therefore have a valuable role to play in the ongoing management of the hearing-impaired.

Acoustic Feedback

Acoustic feedback is by definition the return of some of the energy of the output signal from a hearing aid receiver to the input transducer

Figure 5.12: The Libby horn.

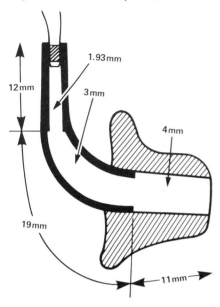

(the microphone). The result of this is howl or a characteristic high pitched whistle when the aid reaches oscillation point and a continuous saturation output is produced. An amplification system in this condition is totally unacceptable because of gross distortion of any processed signals, high output and distracting and sometimes embarrassing effects on the user. The cure for howl is reduction in the gain of the hearing aid, because howl occurs when the gain of the aid exceeds the attenuation present in the feedback path (see Table 5.2). The unfortunate consequence of this action for a child could be totally ineffective amplification because of inadequate usable gain.

The major factors that contribute to acoustic feedback may be summarised as:

(i) sound leakage from an acoustically poor fitting earmould. This is by far the most significant factor;
(ii) sound leakage as a result of the fact that the earmould has not been inserted properly into the ear. This usually occurs because of failure to locate the helix of the earmould and results in the mould standing proud in the ear;
(iii) sound leakage from the coupling point between earphone receiver

and lock spring for body worn aids;
(iv) sound radiating from the back of the receiver in the body worn aids;
(v) sound radiating from the sound tube in post aural aids;
(vi) sound radiating from the tube connections, earhook-receiver nozzle coupling point and other plumbing in post-aural aids;
(vii) sound radiating from the ear as a result of an increase in sound pressure level in the ear canal, because of a temporary conductive disorder or hard impacted wax.

Table 5.2: Electrical analogy of acoustic feedback assuming positive feedback modality.

OUTPUT = INPUT $\times$ GAIN (VOLTS)

  let   INPUT = 1 VOLT
        GAIN   = A
$\therefore$ OUTPUT = A VOLTS

Assume a fraction B of the output returns to input and adds to input (+ ve feedback)

  $\therefore$ Feedback = AB

To maintain output at a constant level one would have to reduce input

  Input = 1 $-$ AB
  $\therefore$ GAIN $A^1 = \dfrac{A}{1-AB}$ $\dfrac{OUTPUT}{INPUT}$ (VOLTS)

  as AB $\rightarrow$ 1
     1 $-$ AB $\rightarrow$ 0
  $\therefore A^1 \rightarrow \infty$

i.e. no input is required for a continuous saturation output — oscillation feedback howl results.

The increase in sound level results (in conductive disorders) from a reduction in ear drum compliance and in certain cases an increase in user gain.

Audiologists clearly have a very important role to play in the management of this problem, which if left unchecked can lead to total rejection of a hearing aid by a user. The following procedures are recommended in the management programme:

1. Acoustically good fitting earmoulds are made available.
2. Patients (parents in the case of young children) are given guidance on insertion, removal and day-to-day care of earmoulds. Particular

attention should be paid to the need for good aftercare of earmould plumbing in post-aural aids – spare lengths of tubing being provided.

3. Thick walled type tubing should be employed with high gain post-aural aids (wall thickness 0.8-1 mm).

4. In the case of body worn aids – earmoulds should be carefully examined to ensure that the lock ring is seated correctly and the backplate is flat, prior to fitting. Subminiature earphone receivers should be employed. The plastic washer on the back of the receiver should be replaced by a layer of 'blue tac'. Attention must be paid to the condition of the receiver nub which can be worn down over a period of time by a metal lock spring. Use of nylon lock springs as standard will overcome this problem.

5. Contralateral routing of signals (Figure 5.13) with twin body worn hearing aids is not a method to employ in trying to overcome the feedback problem (Markides, 1981).

6. Arrangements to be made for an examination of the ear canals and impedance bridge measurements in cases where feedback presents as a persistent problem or suddenly for no apparent reason.

Figure 5.13: Possible arrangement of twin pocket hearing aids.

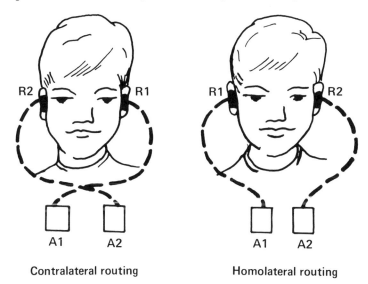

Contralateral routing   Homolateral routing

Other Areas of Attention in Relation to Feedback

The problem areas described thus far are of a practical nature and there is therefore no reason why they cannot be improved upon. It is of interest to note, however, that there are additional considerations, approaches, modifications which in theory may be employed to improve the prevailing feedback situation.

The idea of implanting the receiver of a post-auricular or body aid in the earmould has been suggested by a number of authors. One study by Ross and Crimo (1980) using a post-auricular hearing aid with the receiver implanted in the earmould reported an improvement in usable gain before feedback of 7-13 dB in the mid-frequencies in comparison to a conventional aid. The authors reasoned that this improvement was a result of overcoming the 'plumbing' factors discussed earlier, and in addition, the mechanical and electrical contributions to feedback which can arise. Although these results appear encouraging the practical application of this approach is very questionable. The integrity of the electrical connections to the receiver during everyday use, the job of keeping the mould clean while not damaging the receiver, the influence of condensation and any migration of body juices on the receiver and the physical problem of siting the receiver in the mould (particularly for young children) are all relevant in this respect.

The use of frequency shifting as a means of controlling acoustic feedback was originally developed by Schroeder (1959) for public address systems. Hartley Jones (1973) working on this approach reported an improvement in stability of a sound reinforcing system of 8 dB by incorporation of a frequency shift circuit which shifted frequency by 5 Hz.

Bennet *et al.* (1980) extended this approach for use in a hearing aid. Using a bench test rig they reported that a reduction in feedback was achieved by a progressive shift system. However, this was not quantified. Although interesting, this approach obviously warrants further investigation particularly into the effects on speech intelligibility for the user. One must not lose sight of the fact that the root problem still remains that when feedback is occurring the system is acoustically poor in fit and this can have very detrimental effects on the frequency response of the hearing aid.

Reference to Figure 5.14 may illustrate this problem more clearly. The acoustically poor system (which in Figure 5.14 is in the feedback mode) is effectively a vented system (Lybarger, 1967) and as a result low frequency performance is inferior to the situation where a good acoustically fitting system is employed with the same hearing aid. For children with profound hearing loss who rely heavily on such frequencies (who are generally 'at risk' with regards feedback) the loss of such frequencies could be very significant. It is imperative therefore to continue to seek to improve the quality of acoustic fit for these children and hence ensure that they are not deprived of important frequencies of speech.

Figure 5.14: The influence of acoustic feedback on the frequency response of a hearing aid.

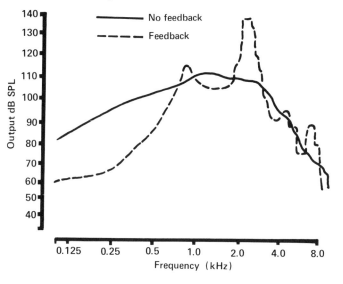

In any hearing system there will be one frequency at which loop gain (as described in Table 5.2) is a maximum and this will depend on the frequency characteristics of the complete feedback chain. Certain hearing aids lend themselves to feedback because of their very 'peaky' frequency response. In choosing a hearing aid system one should therefore give consideration to trying to provide a *smooth* rather than 'multi peak' response pattern for the child.

Recent Developments

Two-stage Earmoulds

The majority of children's earmoulds are fabricated in acrylic. While this material is easy to process its major weaknesses are quality of acoustic fit and texture. Even in the 'soft' form it is still relatively hard. There are alternatives to acrylic. PVC (vinyl) is one material that has found use in audiology. It is fabricated into earmoulds by injection-moulding techniques which require very specialised equipment. The cost of tooling up for this process is such that only a small number of manufacturers produce these moulds.

The present authors reasoned that two areas, dentistry and medical science, could provide other materials for earmould application not requiring specialised manufacturing equipment. Research was undertaken and the outcome was the development of two mould making procedures involving the use of silicone rubber (Nolan, 1982).

The research highlighted the fact that, whatever the earmould material, there was a definite need to follow certain well defined steps if the final product was to be satisfactory. These were:

(i) Use addition cure silicone impression material via a syringe.
(ii) 'De-air mix' the plaster prior to investing the impression.
(iii) Use a minimal amount of 'interaction' with the mould once it is removed from the plaster cast, that is, no polishing.

The two materials at the centre of the development work were a pourable, high strength, clean grade silicone rubber elastomer and a denture soft-lining material. The pourable silicone elastomer had been used as a flexible mould to facilitate the encapsulation of electronic components of biomedical devices. The silicone based denture soft-lining material had a novel property of bonding to acrylic which was considered to be very important particularly with respect to pocket aids.

The benefits of the silicone rubber moulds were found to be:

(a) No polishing required therefore no loss of accuracy.
(b) Soft and comfortable to wear.
(c) Consistently able to provide gain in excess of 60 dB if required.
(d) Resilient to earmould nibblers.
(e) Reliable over time.
(f) Easy to keep clean.
(g) Good cosmetic appearance.

It may be added that there are certain disadvantages in the use of these materials in relation to acrylic:

1. They require more skill in manufacture.
2. They are more expensive.

3. They are difficult to fabricate into alternatives to solid and shell format.
4. The shear strength (resistance to tearing) is reduced.

Despite this, these earmould materials have an important role to play, especially where a good acoustically fitting earmould is required. As with any earmould material, however, quality will only be as good as that of the ear impression.

Processing

A brief summary of the procedures involved in processing the two materials is presented. It should be noted that the procedures as outlined follow a process of 'zero interaction' with the mould once it is removed from the plaster cast. The process may be simplified by omission of the steps facilitating 'built in' sound tube and lock spring. This work can be carried out after the cured mould has been removed from the plaster. However, one danger of such an approach is that the sound tube may over a period of time close up and eventually become occluded. This is a result of the fact that both materials are difficult to drill. Similarly this sometimes occurs with vinyl moulds.

Processing of Pourable Silicone Elastomer

Dow Corning MDX 4-4210.
  (i) Prepare plaster — de-air
 (ii) Make plaster model
(iii) Wire sound tube through model using stainless steel or copper. Silicone tubing for sound tube covers wire. Seal plaster
 (iv) Mix elastomer plus curing agent
  (v) Add medical fluid for better consistency
 (vi) De-air silicone mix
(vii) Pour silicone into plaster model
(viii) Cure at 100°C for 15 minutes in warm air oven
 (ix) Remove and check
  (x) Fit.
Note:
    (a) For post-aural aids only.
    (b) No specialised equipment required.

Processing of Composite Mould

Molloplast — B silicone denture soft-lining material with acrylic backplate.

  (i) Prepare plaster — de-air
 (ii) Make plaster model
(iii) Wire sound tube
 (iv) Wax up for lock spring (pocket aid only)
  (v) Place in dental flask
 (vi) Separate flask — boil off wax
(vii) Pack in silicone. Press up
(viii) Paint on bonding agent (Primo)
 (ix) Put on acrylic backplate
  (x) Press up
 (xi) Cure for 2 hours at 100°C in water bath
(xii) Remove and check.

Conclusions

It may be concluded from the comments made in this chapter that professionals must see the earmould as a very important component of the wearable hearing aid. It is not to be lightly dismissed or ignored, because this will result in a marked reduction in the effectiveness of the habilitative programme. At its limits, the child can be totally deprived of linguistic input at levels which are within his capabilities of perception.

References

ADI Plastics Ltd (1967) *Cold Cure Ear Inserts*, Guidance Note, Blackpool, England

Bennet, M.J., Srikandan, S. and Brown, L.M.H. (1980) 'Controlled feedback hearing aid', *Hearing Aid Journal*, *42443*, 12

Corell, I.C. (1978) *The Earmould in Theory and Practice*, Oticon Library, Oticon, Denmark

Craig, R.C., O'Brien, W.J. and Powers, J.M. (1979) *Dental Materials, Properties and Manipulation*, 2nd edn, C.V. Mosby Company, St Louis

Curran, J. (1978) 'Earmould modification effects', *Hearing Instruments*, *29(12)*

Dawson, F. (1977) 'Earmould production in Vinyl — the end of feedback', *Journal British Association Teachers of the Deaf*, *1(6)*, 209

Ewertsen, H.W., Ipsen, J.B. and Nielsen, S.C. (1957) 'On acoustical characteristics of the earmould', *Acta Otolaryngologica*, *47*, 312

Fifield, D.B., Earnshaw, R. and Smither, M. (1980) 'A new ear impression technique to prevent acoustic feedback with high power hearing aids', *Volta Review*, *82(1)*, 33

French St George, M. and Barr-Hamilton, R.M. (1978) 'Relief of the occluded ear sensation to improve earmould comfort', *Journal American Audiology Society*, May

Hartley Jones, M. (1973) 'Frequency shifter for "howl suppression"', *Wireless World*, July, 317

Insta Mold Prosthetics Inc. (1979) *Insta-mold Silicone for Earmoulds*, Philadelphia, USA

Killion, M. (1980) 'Problems in the application of broadband hearing aid earphones' in G. Studebaker and I. Hochberg (eds.), *Acoustical Factors Affecting Hearing Aid Performance*, Ch. 11, University Park Press, Baltimore

Lybarger, S.F. (1967) 'Earmould acoustics', *Audecibel*, Winter, 1967

Markides, A. (1981) 'Effect of homolateral and contralateral routing of signals through body worn hearing aids on the localisation ability of hearing-impaired people', *Journal of the British Association of Teachers of the Deaf, 5(3)*, 68

Nolan, M., Elzemety, S., Tucker, I.G. and McDonough, D.F. (1978) 'An investigation into the problems involved in producing efficient earmoulds for children', *Scandinavian Audiology*, 7, 231

Nolan, M., Tucker, I.G. and Colclough, R.O. (1979) *Instruction Manual on the Production of the Composite Earmould*, Department of Audiology, University of Manchester, Manchester

Nolan, M. (1982) 'Modern developments in earmould technology – implications for the profoundly deaf'. Paper presented at XVI International Congress of Audiology, Helsinki, Finland

Nueva Espania, H. (1980) 'The influence of earmould characteristics on the frequency response of a hearing aid'. Unpublished MEd dissertation, Department of Audiology, University of Manchester, Manchester

Olsen, W.O. (1971) 'The influence of harmonic and intermodulation distortion on speech intelligibility', *Scandinavian Audiology*, Supplement, *1*, 109

Pascoe, D.P., Miemoeller, A.F. and Miller, J.D. (1973) 'Hearing aid design and evaluation for a presbycusic patient', Eighty-sixth meeting of Acoustic Society of America

Ross, M. and Crimo, R. (1980) 'Reducing feedback in a post-auricular hearing aid by implanting the receiver in the ear mould', *Volta Review, 82(1)*, 40

Schroeder, M.R. (1959) 'Improvement of acoustic feedback stability in public address systems', *Proceedings of Third International Congress in Acoustics*, Elsevier, Amsterdam, *11*, 771

Sneyd, A. (1979) 'Earmould technology', *Talk*, *93*, 20

Triantos, T.J. and McCandles, G.A. (1974) 'High frequency distortion', *Hearing Aid Journal, 27(9)*, 38

Tucker, I.G., Nolan, M. and Colclough, R.O. (1978) 'A new high-efficiency earmould', *Scandinavian Audiology*, 7, 225

Watson, T.J. (1960) 'Some factors affecting the successful use of hearing aids by deaf children' in A.W.G. Ewing (ed.), *The Modern Educational Treatment of Deafness*, Manchester University Press, Manchester

6 TECHNICAL ASPECTS RELATING TO THE EFFICIENT USE OF HEARING AIDS

Guidelines on the Effective Day-to-Day Use of Hearing Aids

A set of routine procedures should be followed in order to ensur
that the aid is always working at peak efficiency.

The first step is subjective and requires routine daily listenin
tests via the child's hearing aids. The message 'listen yourself befor
fitting a hearing aid to a child' should be ingrained into the minds o
all parents and teachers of hearing-impaired children. The listenin
tests are quick and easy to apply. A minimal amount of equipmen
is required. The necessary 'tools' comprise:

  (i) a stetoclip;
 (ii) a supply of spares − leads, batteries, receivers, tubing, hearin
      aid. It is our policy to provide a child with a spare aid of th
      same type as is being used, so that he is exposed to a consisten
      listening pattern which is not interrupted when a fault develop
      on the aid which warrants technical support. Most childre
      therefore receive three hearing aids;
(iii) toothbrush and pipe cleaners.

Parents and teachers require knowledge, confidence, a measure o
patience, a fair degree of determination to ensure effective use o
aids.

1. The first step in the listening tests is not one of listening but look
ing. The child's aid should be examined for any signs of damage (fo
example, cracked case, broken switches). Sound should be able to pas
freely into the microphone, no foreign bodies such as 'dinner' or dir
should be obstructing this pathway. The controls should be checke
and reset if they have been inadvertently disturbed (for example
M-MT-T switch). The receiver on the pocket aid should be checke
so as to ensure it is the correct one for the child.
2. The earmould should then be examined. Recall that moulds shoul
be cleaned each evening with a little warm soapy water and a tooth
brush (spare one!) or pipe cleaner. This should prevent build up of wa

in the sound tube. Blow through the tubing so as to ensure that it is completely clear of debris.

3. The battery should be replaced if the changing guideline demands it. The pocket aid should then be switched on and the receiver held the lead length from the microphone. The volume control should be turned up whereupon the characteristic squeal should be apparent. With post-aural aids the plastic elbow should be held at the ear, the volume control turned up whereupon squeal should again be in evidence. This crudely assesses the battery condition.

4. The aid should then be connected to the stetoclip (using the small adaptor and a short length of plastic tubing with post-aural aids). Parents and teachers should develop a familiarity with the hearing aid. They should adjust the volume control so that the aid is at their most comfortable listening level. By speaking into the microphone it should be possible to check for sound quality and loudness. If either quality or volume appears to be less than that usually experienced a query could be put against the aid's performance. With pocket aids it is advisable to check the integrity of the lead by wiggling at the weak spots.

It is desirable to evaluate subjectively what is known as 'aid noise' on all aids, that is, the background 'shush' from the aid when no input signal is present. Here again parents and teachers will quickly tune into an aid's performance and can often spot deviant levels of electronic noise.

The sound quality should be assessed, primarily because receiver abuse can be significant with child users. This can result in distortion of the processed signal.

If as a result of the simple listening tests all appears well, then the aids should be fitted to the child. With pocket aids a clean, well-fitting harness is desirable with leads tucked out of 'harms way'. The aids should be set to the desired level and switched on. They must deliver the necessary gain without acoustic feedback. If the feedback does occur and is a result of inadequate earmoulds then new ones must be obtained immediately. In the interim period the aids must be set to a level which prevents the occurrence of feedback. It is important for the professional adviser to impress upon parents and teachers the need for correct fitting of earmoulds. Their attention should also be drawn to the steps that can sometimes be taken so as to prevent the occurrence of feedback (see Chapter 5). Post-aural aids, for example, must be seated correctly on the ear with the correct length of tubing. If they persistently fall from the ear then they must be taped on using surgical tape.

If when checking an aid a fault is noted, there is a certain logical procedure to follow which often solves the problem and saves a visit to the hearing aid technician. This is why the supply of spares is so valuable. Various faults do arise but a basic routine fault-finding approach is advisable in each case. Obviously certain steps may be missed out depending upon the symptom:

(i) Re-examine the aid and check that it is switched on and that the M position is selected.

(ii) Ensure that the earmoulds are not blocked.

(iii) Shake the aid so as to determine whether any components have become loose internally. If so, the likelihood is that technical assistance will be necessary. However, proceed through to the end of the exercise as the loose component may not in fact be responsible for the fault.

(iv) Ensure that the battery is in correctly (not upside down as does occur on occasions).

(v) Ensure that the plastic elbow on the post-aural aid is patent. If the problem still persists proceed to:

(vi) Replace the battery – recheck the aid.

(vii) Replace the lead on the pocket aids – recheck the aid.

(viii) Replace the receiver on pocket aids – recheck the aid.

It is advisable to leave a replacement part in the aid when moving through the exercise. This results from the fact that dual faults occur and would otherwise be missed.

If the check proves fruitless then the advice of a hearing aid technician must be sought. The faulty aid should obviously be immediately replaced by the spare aid.

It is worthwhile noting that the above-mentioned procedure does help to speed up repairs of children's aids because it prevents the system becoming 'clogged' with aids having minor faults which could and should be rectified without recourse to the technical service.

Hand-held Hearing Aid Tester

A very useful and easy to operate device has been developed with the aim of enabling the class teacher or visiting support teacher to check in the free field situation certain aspects of hearing aid performance (Jessops Acoustics). The unit is a hand-held instrument weighing approximately 300gm. It will therefore easily store in a drawer or andbag. It is relatively inexpensive, a primary consideration nowadays. is powered by a replaceable PP3 battery. There is a battery indicator corporated into the unit which permits a quick and easy check of attery condition. The unit is designed to check all types of hearing ds that are in use with children (but not headphones). Its main pplication is in measuring the output of hearing aids and the field rength of the electromagnetic loop induction systems (for example, assroom loops). The aid check is made in the 'real world' situation a that with a pocket aid, for example, the child would wear the aid, he earphone receiver being taken from his ear and connected to the cc coupler which is built into the unit. The unit provides a read-out f the sound pressure developed in the coupler. It covers the complete nge of sound pressure delivered by hearing aids. The input to the d could, for example, be speech so that a rough idea of the amplified eech level being directed to the child could be obtained. The class acher should be guided as to the required volume setting for a young hild. By routine testing of the aid at the user setting it soon becomes bvious if deterioration in output has occurred for a speech input gnal.

Two examples of the application of the device in the day-to-day anagement of aids will be given.

esting a Child's Aid at the Normal Setting. The hearing aid should be onnected to the instrument while in the normal wearing position on he child. The teacher should then position herself at distance which is ypical for the lesson. She should speak at her usual voice level and ote the sound pressure reading developed in the coupler. This reading hould be compared with that suggested as desirable by the advisory acher. Should marked deviations from the 'target' occur, immediate teps must be taken to discover the reason (for example, phone advis- ry teacher or initiate fault finding programme).

esting the Field Strength of Loop Systems. The instrument has a oop' setting which should be selected. This setting energises the tele- oil that is a built-in feature of the device. For checking classroom ops the box should be held so that the meter is horizontal. Someone hould speak at a normal level into the loop microphone – a reading of ield strength will then be given on the meter. This check should be pplied routinely each day, the result being compared with that which ; desirable.

Where neck loops or inductive pads (as in all radio loop systems) are to be tested, the instrument should be situated within the loop field and held horizontally. The read-out will again indicate the value of the field strength.

Overall, this instrument is seen as a very useful tool in helping to maintain continuity of amplification. It has proven to be of value in identifying problems that could have otherwise gone unnoticed. It is not a substitute for a hearing aid test box, but nevertheless is something that the ordinary teacher or parent could quickly learn to use and apply. Unit teachers who are often isolated technically speaking would find it very valuable indeed.

The second step in ensuring efficiency of amplification is regular standardised electroacoustic assessment of the hearing aid by means of a hearing aid test box. It is a fact of life that 'normally hearing ears' are often insensitive to the gradually deteriorating hearing aid performance as a result of wear and tear and ageing of the various components. While our ears can identify more gross problems, they may 'miss' ones that can nevertheless significantly influence the effectiveness of the hearing aid for the child. This is why it is imperative that hearing aids are regularly checked on a test box (2-3 weekly intervals) so that they are maintained, electroacoustically speaking, in their optimal condition.

The Hearing Aid Test Box

A hearing aid is built to stringent specifications. In relation to the amplification of sound, these specifications, for example, apply to the maximum amount of gain the aid can deliver, the aids maximum power output capacity and the distortion introduced into the processed signal. All of the electroacoustic specifications of a hearing aid together with the procedures of measurement are laid down in British, International and American Standards (BSI, 1968; IEC, 1959; ANSI, 1976). Hearing aid manufacturers produce a comprehensive data sheet on each hearing aid. This provides details on all of the parameters demanded by the relevant Standards.

It is the responsibility of all audiologists working with hearing impaired children to ensure that a hearing aid does maintain its design criteria performance. The only way that this can be achieved is to test the aid using the procedures laid down. A comparison of the reference (manufacturer) data with a particular aid's measured data will highlight an aid whose performance is unacceptable. It is worthwhile noting that all manufacturer data is average data based on tests of a large number of aids. Small fluctuations in measured performance will inevitably occur, but the tolerances are narrow and should be no wider than 5 dB.

The basis for all electroacoustic data is measurement of hearing aid performance in a low noise cabinet. The reason for this is quite simply because it is necessary to place the hearing aid microphone in an environment which is as free from extraneous noise as possible. The basic aim of the electroacoustic procedures is to place the hearing aid in a precisely known sound field and, by manipulation of this field and the hearing aid controls, accurately measure the specifications of the aid as stipulated by the agreed Standards.

The test facility which is used to achieve this aim is a hearing aid test box (Figure 6.1). It is best understood by seeing it as comprising two distinct parts. One part is responsible for the input signal *to* the aid, the other is responsible for quantifying the output signal *from* the aid.

The test chamber is a sound-insulated enclosure which is designed (within the tolerances laid down) to be as free and insulated from extraneous noise as possible. In effect the chamber may be considered as a mini sound-treated room into which the hearing aid will be placed at a precise location. The loudspeaker directs sound into the chamber. The signals that are used for assessing hearing aids are pure tones covering a range of frequencies from approximately 200 Hz to 6000 Hz (this varies according to the particular system employed). The intensity of the signal is adjustable usually in 5 or 10 dB steps over a range from 50 to 90 dB SPL. Again this varies according to the particular system employed. The signals are produced by an oscillator and amplifier. The test frequencies are either selected by a switch or automatically. The signal level is adjusted by means of a volume control. All test chambers have a target area over which the sound field is defined. The microphone of the aid should always be placed at a precise spot in this target area. This is usually indicated in the chamber.

The output from the hearing aid is measured by means of a coupler and a sound level meter. The receiver of a hearing aid is connected to the coupler and feeds sound into it (Figure 6.2).

Confusion sometimes arises with respect to the term 'coupler' and it is pertinent to discuss it at this juncture. A coupler is simply a cavity of a predetermined form. It is connected to a microphone which permits the measurement of the sound pressure developed in the cavity.

There are two possible functions for a coupler in hearing aid measurements. The first is to portray as nearly as possible the true behaviour of the hearing aid worn by a subject; the second is to provide a simple and ready basis for the exchange of hearing aid specifications. The

Figure 6.1: Examples of hearing aid test boxes. (a) Bruel and Kjaer Audiotest Station 2116 with 4222 anechoic test chamber; (i) pocket aid set-up, (ii) post-aural aid set-up. (b) Phonic Ear HC 1000. (c) Fonix FP 20 portable system.

(a) i

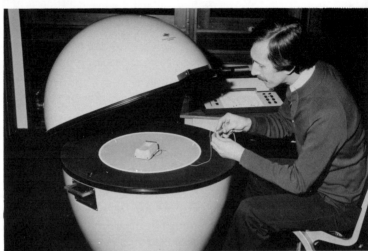

(a) ii

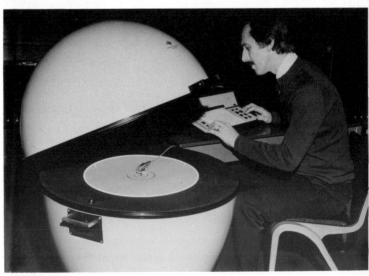

(b)

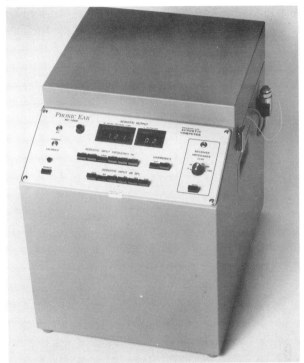

(c)

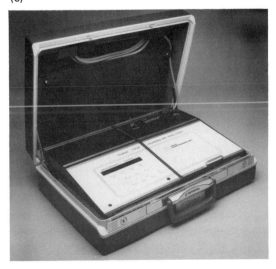

Figure 6.2: The 2cm³ coupler. (a) Pocket aid coupled; (b) post-aur

aid coupled; (c) 'in the ear' aid or 'through the mould' coupled.

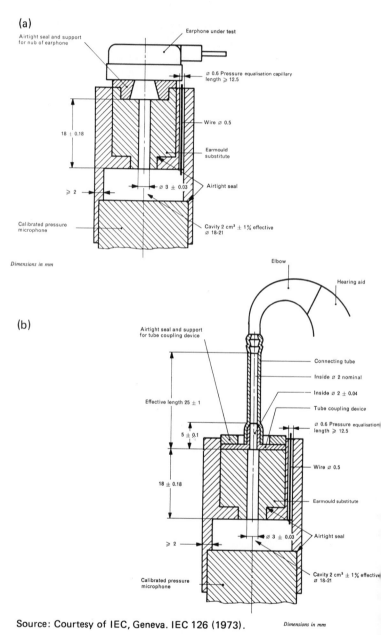

Source: Courtesy of IEC, Geneva. IEC 126 (1973).   *Dimensions in mm*

(c)

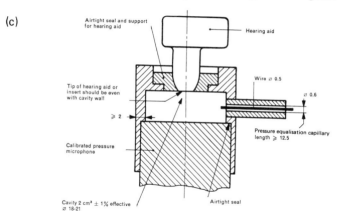

Airtight seal and support
for hearing aid

Hearing aid

Tip of hearing aid or
insert should be even
with cavity wall

Wire ⌀ 0.5

⌀ 0.6

≥ 2

Pressure equalisation capillary
length ≥ 12.5

Calibrated pressure
microphone

Cavity 2 cm³ ± 1% effective
⌀ 18-21

Airtight seal

Dimensions in mm

function that is relevant to hearing aid management is the second one, that is, the one that permits a comparison between the manufacturer's specifications and actual measured specifications. A particular coupler, the 2 cm³ coupler (IEC, 1981) has been accepted as standard for such measures. It has a sufficiently simple reproducible construction to permit a ready exchange of information between audiologist and hearing aid manufacturer. It is important to note, however, that 2 cm³ coupler specifications must not be interpreted as indicative of the performance of the hearing aid when worn by a child.

The 2 cm³ coupler as shown in Figure 6.2 comprises a number of components which permit measurements to be made using pocket and post-aural instruments. The output from the microphone of the 2 cm³ coupler is analysed by a sound level meter and associated filters. This system provides graphically or by digital read-out a measure of the sound pressure level developed in the coupler.

The modern generation of hearing aid test boxes are microprocessor controlled. They are available in both clinic-based and portable format (Figure 6.1). The development of portable test boxes is seen as a very important one in relation to efficient day-to-day use of hearing aids by children. Such a facility should constitute an integral part of any peripatetic audiological service. It provides the home and school visiting specialist with the opportunity of electroacoustically assessing hearing aids on a regular routine basis 'at source'. This is far more effective than the occasional check that very often occurs when test boxes are based centrally in an audiology unit when aids have to be brought in for checking.

Ear Simulator

The other category of coupler that has found application in audi
logy as a means of providing the audiologist with some idea of th
actual performance of a hearing aid when worn by a patient is usual
described as an ear simulator.

A true ear simulator would have to comprise not only the avera
external human ear but also the pinna, head and torso because a
these factors have been shown to influence the resultant sound pre
sure at the eardrum when an aid is being worn (Dalsgaard and Jense
1976). The fact that the head and body reflect and diffract soun
results in differences in the relative intensity of the signals arrivin
at the hearing aid microphone in relation to that which would occ
if the aid was suspended in free space. These differences are frequenc
dependent. There is as yet no international agreement on a true art
ficial ear which could be used as a means of quantifying the sour
pressure at a person's eardrum when using a hearing aid. Even if th
agreement ever came about such information would only be usef
as a rough guideline as to what the hearing aid was doing, quite simp
because of the very large number of variables that occur betwee
individual subjects.

At the present time there is agreement internationally on the spec
fication for an occluded ear simulator (IEC, 1981). The occluded ea
simulator is a device for measuring the output sound pressure of a hea
ing aid receiver under well-defined testing conditions in a specific
frequency range. It consists essentially of a principal cavity, acoust
loading networks and a calibrated microphone. It simulates the inn
part of the ear canal from the tip of the earmould to the eardrun
having the relevant acoustical characteristics similar to the average c
normal adults human ears. The location of the microphone is chose
so that the measured sound pressure corresponds approximately t
that existing at the normal adult human eardrum for a known inp
into the hearing aid microphone. This device therefore provides a mo
real ear-oriented guide to hearing aid performance in comparison t
that provided by the $2cm^3$ coupler, when the input into the micr
phone is known. However, this information should be treated as provic
ing only a very rough guideline because of the effects of individu
variability between ears (noting particularly that children may diffe
considerably from adults) and the interaction of ears with hearing aic
(for example, earmould fit). The occluded ear simulator can be use
instead of the $2cm^3$ coupler in conjunction with a test box facility
Both are couplers — one having properties like the occluded human ea

The Zwislocki coupler and the Bruel and Kjaer Ear Simulator type 4157 are commercially available occluded ear simulators. Hearing aid manufacturers are now beginning to supply information on hearing aid specifications based on both 2cm^3 coupler and occluded ear simulator. At the present time, however, 2cm^3 coupler data are perfectly satisfactory for the management programme. The main point of note with regards occluded ear simulators is that audiologists must not fall into the trap of believing that tests with an occluded ear simulator provide absolute information on how a hearing aid performs in a child's ear. The real ear performance may be significantly different (Berland, 1982). Occluded ear simulators do not take account of the influence of the wearer on the behaviour of sound arriving at the microphone inlet. These simulators simply give a more real ear idea of sound pressure developed at the eardrum for a known input into the microphone.

It may be of interest to note that certain hearing aid manufacturers sometimes provide specifications on a hearing aid in a form that may be interpreted as being the real ear performance of the aid as determined from measures on a 'true' artificial ear. Such information includes the effects of the wearer on the performance of the hearing aid. This information is in fact obtained by use of a manikin and an occluded ear simulator in an anechoic chamber. A manikin is simply a replica of the human head and torso which behaves in similar way in relation to interaction with sound (reflection and diffraction) as that of the average human adult. The Knowles Electronics Manikin for Acoustic Research (Kemar) has been shown to replicate this behaviour quite well and is normally used in such measures. An occluded ear simulator, the Zwislocki coupler, attaches to Kemar and together they are used to replicate the average adult human's hearing system. The hearing aid is mounted on Kemar and coupled to the simulator. While information from such an approach is 'real ear' oriented, it is nothing more than a guideline as to the performance of an aid when worn by a subject (Berland, 1982). As with any artificial object the design is based on an average and individuals can and will deviate from this average. This will be particularly so when considering child hearing aid users because 'the average' relates to the adult form.

Every effort should be made in the ongoing management of hearing-impaired children to quantify the real ear performance of the hearing aid. This is achieved by taking measures on the child with and without hearing aids as will be described shortly.

Let us now return to the hearing aid test box and summarise the situation. It is conventional to use a $2\,cm^3$ coupler for determination of hearing aid specifications. Both manufacturers and audiologists use this coupler and can therefore compare their findings so as to assess the performance of a particular hearing aid.

Real Ear and Coupler Measures – A Summary of Differences

The frequency response of a hearing aid when actually worn by a child is considerably different from that indicated by a 2cc coupler (Dalsgaard and Jensen, 1976). This results from the fact that the volume of the ear of a young child is likely to be significantly less than 2cc. Further the affects of the baffle and sound diffraction and the interaction of the ear with the earmould all add to the differences between real ears and couplers. There are a number of possible ways of measuring the performance of a hearing aid. These may be considered as:

(1) via a 2cc coupler;
(2) via a modified 2cc coupler where the earmould simulator is replaced by the child's earmould;
(3) via an occluded ear simulator;
(4) via an occluded ear simulator plus mannequin (for example Kemar);
(5) via the probe tube or miniature microphone mounted on the child in the ear canal;
(6) by warble tone sound field aided verses unaided subjective measures.

The procedures under categories 1-3 measure what is known as transmission gain of the aid, that is, for a known input to the hearing aid microphone an output figure is produced leading to the determination of gain. The effect of the child on the actual sound field at the microphone of the aid (for example, body baffle, diffraction) is not considered nor is the fact that couplers are not necessarily accurate representations of the child's ear – particularly the 2cc coupler. The effect of the child's earmould is not considered in 1 and may not be in 3 either. Measures 4 to 6 define the insertion gain of the hearing aid, that is, the actual change in sound pressure that occurs in the ear canal as a result of fitting the hearing aid. Measure 4 is the least accurate because it is based on an 'artificial person' who may differ significantly from the actual child. Measures 5 and 6 provide the most meaningful information n just what gain and frequency response is being made available to he hearing aid user.

If one therefore wishes to know the actual amplification change hat occurs at the tympanic membrane when a child is fitted with a earing aid then one must make direct measures on the child to obtain his real ear information.

The most meaningful way of doing this is to compare a child's ubjective thresholds to warble tones in a free field listening situation oth with and without a hearing aid. The sound pressure level is meaured at the point where the child is to be situated but without the hild there. This difference in sound pressure is known as the real ear ain of the aid. Recall that it is also referred to as the insertion gain f the aid — which is defined as the difference in the sound pressure t a specified point in the ear canal (measured by a probe microphone) or unaided and aided listening. While the actual values of sound presure were not measured in the ear canal the assumption was made that hey had been, and their differences would have been equal to the subective threshold differences — which are after all directly related to ar canal sound pressure level.

This leads us on to the second method of determining real ear nsertion gain of a hearing aid, that is, by means of a probe microhone. While this method is totally impractical at present, certainly vith children below the age of eleven years it is nevertheless worth xplaining. The real ear insertion gain is determined by placing a tiny nicrophone in the ear canal at a specific point (Harford, 1980). The ubject is situated in a known sound field and the sound level at the pecified point is recorded. The aid is then fitted, with the probe nicrophone still in position and the new sound pressure level is noted. he difference is the real ear insertion gain. This measure takes account f the effect that the subject and the hearing aid have in interacting vith the sound field.

The other technique for measuring the performance of a hearing id which is facilitated by use of an artificial ear and mannequin follows he procedure described above, the measuring microphone being ituated in the occluded ear simulator.

erminology

he parameters which are used in the specifications of a hearing aid vill now be defined.

ir to Air Gain or Acoustic Gain. The amount by which the sound pressure level developed by the hearing aid receiver in the coupler exceeds the sound pressure level in the free field into which the hearing aid microphone is introduced.

Gain (dB) = Output from aid (dB) minus Input to aid (dB).

Maximum Air to Air Gain or Maximum Acoustic Gain. The maximum value of the air to air gain obtainable from hearing aid allowing all possible settings of the hearing aid controls. This is often specified for a particular test frequency.

Frequency Response. The air to air gain of the hearing aid expressed as a function of the frequency under specified test conditions. This is usually presented graphically.

Comprehensive Frequency Response. A family of frequency response curves arranged in such a way as to exhibit the input characteristic of the hearing aid over a full range of operation.

Basic Frequency Response. One of the family of frequency responses of the comprehensive frequency response which is chosen as a reference condition for purposes of description.

Saturation Sound Pressure Level. The maximum r.m.s. sound pressure level obtainable in the coupler from the receiver of the hearing aid allowing all possible values of input sound pressure level. This is usually quoted for a specified frequency under specified operating conditions.

Rated Maximum Sound Pressure Level. The lowest value of sound pressure level in the coupler at which the total harmonic distortion reaches 10 per cent.

Using the Hearing Aid Test Box

Calibration. It is vitally important to calibrate a hearing aid test box before it is used. When calibrating the operator has two jobs to do. Firstly, it is necessary to check the accuracy of the coupler pressure microphone and associated sound level meter network, that is, the accuracy of the output measuring system. This is achieved by use of a sound level calibrator – a device that produces a very precise sound output at a specified frequency. The sound calibrator should be coupled to the cavity pressure microphone (without 2cm^3 cavity attached) in a particular manner. This will depend upon the test box in use. The

Bruel and Kjaer 4220 Pistonphone which produces a 250 Hz tone at 124 dB SPL (STP) or the Bruel and Kjaer 4230 Sound Level Calibrator which produces a 1000 Hz tone at 94 dB SPL are two examples of commercially available calibrators that are used with hearing aid test boxes. The reading on the sound output display should be checked and adjustments made should the system be out of calibration. One point of note with reference to the ordering of a hearing aid test box relates to the fact that the sound level calibrator is provided as an 'optional extra'. It is important that this is obtained at the same time as the test box. Otherwise calibration will not be possible.

The second stage of calibration involves that of the test chamber itself. In this case the precision of the input to the hearing aid is being assessed and adjusted to the necessary requirements. This is achieved by placement of the previously calibrated pressure microphone in the chamber at a precise location where the hearing aid microphone will be subsequently positioned (subsequently referred to as the target spot). The sound pressure should then be monitored across the range of test frequencies. Adjustments should be made either manually or automatically so that the sound pressure level across frequency is consistent and at the level indicated by the signal level control of the test box facility.

Calibration of the hearing aid test box ensures that both the input signal and the output signal from a hearing aid are known precisely.

The procedure of measurement that is commonly employed in hearing aid specification work is known as the substitution method. The hearing aid microphone replaces or is substituted for the pressure microphone used in the chamber calibration procedure.

An alternative approach is the comparison method where the hearing aid microphone and a microphone to measure and monitor the free field sound pressure are placed simultaneously at two different points in the test chamber. This approach and its method of calibration are described in IEC (1959). The substitution method will be followed in the subsequent discussion.

Testing the Pocket Aid. The set up for determining the specifications of a pocket aid are shown in Figure 6.1a(i). The rule of thumb to follow when testing any hearing aid is to place the microphone of the aid at the target spot in the test chamber. As little hardware as possible should be placed in the chamber. This is why in the case of pocket aids the aid is in the chamber, but the coupler and receiver are outside being linked to the aid by the lead.

Post-aural Aid. The set-up for the post-aural aid is shown in Figure 6.1a(ii). It should be noted that the aid is linked to the coupler by means of a special adaptor and plastic tubing (Figure 6.1b). The dimensions of both of these elements are laid down in the relevant standards for example, IEC (1973). The adaptor is normally supplied with the coupler. The aid microphone must again be sited at the target spot In this set-up both aid and coupler are placed in the chamber because there is no external lead. It is suggested that the orientation of the aid and coupler when placed in the chamber is such that the couple interacts as little as possible with the aid. This is why the aid has been rotated on the plastic elbow in the test set-up of Figure 6.2. Once the aid has been correctly located in the test chamber the measurement procedure may begin. The measurement procedures and definition of parameters are presented in the relevant standards. These should be carefully studied so that the specifications are correctly determined This then permits a meaningful comparison between manufacturer and measured specifications.

It is suggested that certain characteristics of a hearing aid are measured routinely during clinical practice so as to ensure that the aid' performance is maintained at an optimal level. These characteristic will differ depending upon whether British and International (identical) or American Standards for testing the performance of a hearing aid are followed. Manufacturers are now beginning to provide information on one data sheet covering both standards.

When checking the performance of a hearing aid for comparison with standard data from the manufacturer it is recommended that a new battery be employed. The usual method of measurement is that a certain constant intensity signal is presented over a range of frequencies and the output signal is either recorded by hand or automatically on graph paper.

Specifications Related to the International Electrotechnical Commission (IEC) and British Standards Institute (BSI)

The specifications of interest in routine clinical practice should relate to:

(a) maximum gain
(b) maximum gain at 1000 Hz
(c) maximum output

(d) maximum output at 1000 Hz
(e) basic frequency response
(f) harmonic distortion
(g) random noise.

Determination of Specifications

Specifications Related to Maximum Gain. Whenever maximum gain values are to be determined it is necessary to ensure that the input signal is not so strong as to drive the aid into saturation, otherwise an underestimation of gain will occur. The input should therefore be set to 50 dB SPL. The aid should be situated in the test chamber with its volume control on maximum and all other controls in the most usual positions (for example, N tone control, minimum peak clipping). The output of the aid across the test frequency range should then be determined. Gain is defined as Output minus Input (dB). The frequency where the output is greatest should be noted together with the value of this output. The output at 1000 Hz should be noted. Subtraction of 50 dB from these values of output give values of maximum gain and maximum gain at 1000 Hz.

Specifications Related to Maximum Output. The maximum output values are determined by use of the same test set-up as above, with the exception of the level of input signal. The input signal to the aid should be increased to 90 dB and the output across frequency recorded. The value of maximum output at 1000 Hz may be obtained from this information.

Specifications Related to the Basic Frequency Response. The procedure for determining this parameter is presented under HAIC specifications.

Specifications Related to Harmonic Distortion. It is important to monitor this parameter so that a child is never presented with unnecessarily distorted sound resulting from hearing aid dysfunction. Distortion is perhaps the most difficult parameter to quantify by the subjective listening tests. This electroacoustic test is therefore important. The subject of harmonic distortion is covered under a separate section and reference should be made to this. The procedure of measurement should be to set the aid to the child user's level. The input to the aid should be set to 60 dB SPL. Second and then third harmonic distortion should be determined (alternatively total harmonic distortion may be measured) at frequencies of 400, 1000 and 1500 Hz (function of test box). A criterion that this distortion never exceeds 10 per cent (that is, is at least 20dB weaker) in relation to the user frequency response should be applied. Aids with distortion values above 10 per cent should be replaced. It has been suggested that there is no point in applying this measure to a hearing aid where the frequency response curve rises 12dB or more between a distortion test frequency and its second harmonic because the greater relative amplification of the higher frequencies will cause any harmonic distortion to be exaggerated. This seems odd as the distortion product will be audible.

Specifications Related to Random Noise. The hearing aid electronics generate random noise and it is important to ensure that this does not present as a potential source of masking for a child.

(i)   The hearing aid should be placed in the test box and with an input of 60dB SPL at 1000Hz the gain should be adjusted so that the coupler output is 100dB SPL (that is, gain equals 40dB – aid is set to basic frequency response). The frequency response should be recorded.

(ii)   The sound source should be then switched off and the noise sound pressure level in the test chamber should be negligible.

(iii) The total sound pressure level in the coupler should then be measured and must be at least 30dB below the basic frequency response curve.

Specifications Related to the American National Standards Institute (ANSI)

In 1976 ANSI published new standards for testing hearing aids. This section explains the terminology and methods of determination of the parameters of that standard. It is worthy of note that where in the past test frequencies 500, 1000 and 2000Hz have been of particular interest in hearing aid specifications (for example, HAIC) this new American Standard specifies use of 1000, 1600 and 2500Hz in many of the tests. The parameters of interest are again covered by the sections (a) to (g) of the previous section. The differences between ANSI and IEC specifications arise in the definitions and methods of determination of certain of these parameters.

It is necessary to set the aid with all controls other than the volume control in the usual position (for example, N tone control, etc.).

Specifications Related to Maximum Gain. The term 'full-on' gain is used to define the maximum gain of the aid. This is determined in exactly the same manner as in the IEC and BSI Standards.

The term 'HF-Average Full-on Gain' is determined by averaging the 1000, 1600 and 2500 Hz full-on gain values.

Specifications Related to Maximum Output. The term 'SSPL 90' is used to define the maximum output of the hearing aid. It is equivalent to maximum output as described for the other standards.

The 'HF-Average SSPL 90' parameter is determined by taking an average of the outputs determined from the above at test frequencies 1000, 1600 and 2500 Hz.

Specifications Related to Frequency Response. It is necessary to set the volume control of the hearing aid to a 'reference test gain-control position' before certain measurements such as frequency response and harmonic distortion are taken. This position is determined in the following way:

(i) The HF-Average SSPL 90 value should be determined.
(ii) 17 dB should be subtracted from this value. This value is Reference Test Position.
(iii) The input to the hearing aid should be set to 60 dB SPL.
(iv) The volume control of the hearing aid should be adjusted so that the average output (of 1000, 1600 and 2500 Hz test frequencies) corresponds to the value determined in step (ii). If the aid does not have enough gain to permit this it should be left on full volume. Aids with a compression facility should be left on full volume.

The frequency response of the hearing aid should then be determined across the test frequency range (that is, graph of output verses frequency). The part of the graph which is above a baseline determined by subtracting 20 dB from the HF-Average SSPL 90 is considered to be the frequency response curve.

The frequency range is determined by noting the two points which are the intersection of the curve and the baseline mentioned above.

Specifications Related to Harmonic Distortion. The volume control of the aid should be set to the Reference Test Gain Control position. The input to the aid should be set at 70 dB SPL. The total harmonic distortion should be recorded in the coupler for 500, 800 and 1600 Hz test frequencies. The comments relating to the criteria of acceptability of an aid for a child and the fact that steeply rising frequency response curves may militate against measurement of this parameter at certain frequencies are discussed under the previous Standard.

Specifications Relating to Random Noise of the Aid. The term 'Equivalent input noise level' is used as an expression of the internal noise of the hearing aid. This is measured by setting the aid to the reference test gain control position. The average pressure level of 1000, 1600 and 2500 Hz should be determined for a 60 dB SPL input. The input signal to the aid should be switched off and the Sound Pressure Level in the coupler caused by inherent noise of the aid recorded.

If *Ln* is used to denote the equivalent input noise level, *Lavg* is used to denote the coupler sound pressure level for a 60 dB SPL input as defined above and *Lni* is used to denote the coupler sound pressure level with no input to the hearing aid then:

$$Ln = Lni - (Lavg - 60)\, dB$$

For example, if:

> *Lavg = 100 dB SPL*
> *Lni = 50 dB SPL*
> Then, *Ln = 50 − (100 − 60) dB*
> *= 10 dB SPL*

that is, the noise level from the aid is equivalent to an input signal to the aid of 10 dB SPL. This measure is only specified for linear gain hearing aids (that is, not for aids where compression is in use).

HAIC Specifications

Hearing aid manufacturers usually provide information under the heading HAIC specifications. These specifications were proposed by the Hearing Aid Industry Conference. Three parameters are defined under the HAIC heading.

The *HAIC gain* is the mean value of maximum gain for 500 Hz, 1000 Hz and 2000 Hz test frequencies. The *HAIC output* is the mean value of maximum output for 500 Hz, 1000 Hz and 2000 Hz test frequencies. *The HAIC frequency range* is determined from the basic frequency response characteristic of the hearing aid. The values of output as 500 Hz, 1000 Hz and 2000 Hz are averaged and this value is marked on the characteristic at 1000 Hz. A line is then drawn along the horizontal 15 dB below this point. The frequency values at the points where this line crosses the characteristic are the limits of this frequency range.

Determining the HAIC Specifications

Maximum Gain. The test box should be set to give an input of 50 dB SPL. The aid should be placed in the box, microphone at target spot with the volume control set to maximum. Determine the output of the aid at 500, 1000 and 2000 Hz. Subtract 50 dB from these values to give maximum gain values. The average of these gain values is the HAIC gain.

Maximum Output. The volume control of the aid should be set to maximum. The input to the aid should be increased until the maximum output is reached for 500, 1000 and 2000 Hz. The average of these values is the HAIC maximum output.

Frequency Range. The basic frequency response of an aid is determined for an input of 60 dB. The volume control of the aid should be adjusted so that for a 1000 Hz input frequency the output sound pressure level is 100 dB SPL. The frequency response of the aid (that is, output across the range of test frequencies) should then be determined at this setting. This is defined as the basic frequency response. This graph is then used to determine the HAIC frequency range as described above.

Testing the Aid at the User Volume Setting

It is recommended that the child's aid be tested via a test box at the 'user level' because this does provide information over time on the continuity of the amplification package.

The parameters of interest relate to gain, output, harmonic distortion and random noise of the hearing aid.

Procedures

The aid should be placed in the test chamber and set to the user level (including any tone control, compression, peak clipping, etc.). The input to the aid should be set to 60 dB SPL. The frequency response of the aid (output across frequency) should then be determined. Gain may be calculated by subtraction of 60 dB from these output values. It is recommended that whenever a child is provided with new earmoulds a measure of frequency response is made using the above test procedure, but with the earmould included. Many modern test boxes have available a range of adaptors which attach to the 2cc coupler and permit measures on 'in the ear' aids, for example. This 'in the ear' adaptor should be used instead of the conventional set-up.

The earmould should be mounted on the adaptor and secured in position with 'blu tac' so that no acoustic leakage between adaptor and mould exists. The test then proceeds in the usual manner with hearing aid coupled to earmould and the resultant frequency response is recorded. This information is useful because it does highlight the influence of the earmould plumbing (particularly sound tube diameter) on a hearing aid's frequency response. It does, for example, highlight the dangers of very narrow sound bores and strangled sound bores (see Chapter 5). If at any time there is a suspicion that the sound tube of an earmould (for example, vinyl, silicone) is being strangled, then it could be checked by this frequency response measure. The aim in all hearing aid fitting is to provide a child with as wide an experience of speech sounds as possible. The 'through the mould' test and free field aided threshold tests (described later) when put together do help to pin-point the detrimental influences of an earmould.

The maximum output of the aid 90dB input at user level should be checked so as to ensure that it does not exceed the child's upper tolerance limit.

It may prove more practical to check harmonic distortion and random noise of the hearing aid at the user level (in relation to ANSI). By keeping a detailed record of these parameters from issue of the aid (the aid having satisfied manufacturers' specifications) any deterioration in performance will be obvious. The harmonic distortion for second and third harmonic (or total value) may therefore be measured using the set-up that has just been described (that is, aid set to user gain level and 60dB SPL into aid). A criterion of 10 per cent harmonic distortion being the maximum acceptable should be applied. The random noise from the hearing aid may also be monitored by the set-up described. Once the user frequency response has been determined, the signal should be switched off and the resultant sound pressure output in the coupler measured across the test frequency range. This must be at least 30dB down (quieter) on the user frequency response. It is important that there is no significant 'noise' in the test chamber due to the facility being used in a relatively noisy environment (a noisy clinic, for example). If noise does 'leak' into the chamber it will be picked up by the hearing aid microphone with the result that the random noise from the aid will be overestimated.

Regardless of which Standards are adhered to, a regular comparison between hearing aid specifications as laid down by the manufacturer and the actual measured values on a hearing aid do help to prevent a child from being exposed to a degraded signal. A child should therefore have every chance of enjoying efficient amplification, when daily listening tests are coupled to routine electroacoustic measures.

The Influence of the Wearer on the Frequency Response of a Hearing Aid

When the specifications of a hearing aid are being considered by the audiologist it is important to recall how they were obtained. The standardised method involves use of a hearing aid test box and coupler. The hearing aid is placed in the test box, attached to the coupler and certain standardised measures are then made. The performance of a hearing aid when actually worn by a person will be significantly different to the results from a test box measure. This is partly due to the differences between coupler and real ears in their reaction to sound-waves, and partly to the sound source location because of the influence of the head and body on the behaviour of sound in the vicinity of the hearing aid microphone.

When a sound-wave encounters a person, absorption, reflection and diffraction of sound occur.

Reflection of Sound. A sound-wave reflects from an object that is large in comparison to the sound's wavelength (wavelength = velocity of sound ÷ frequency of sound). Reflection of sound is similar in its behaviour properties to reflection of light in that the angle of incidence is equal to the angle of reflection. Head baffle and body baffle result from sound reflection (Nichols, 1947; Christen, 1979).

Diffraction of Sound. Diffraction of sound may be thought of as a 'bending' of the sound-wave around an obstacle. When a sound-wave encounters an obstacle a number of possibilities related to sound diffraction may result. If the obstacle is small in relation to the sound's wavelength then the sound effectively washes over the obstacle and proceeds as if the object didn't exist, (that is, the sound diffracts around the obstacle). However, if the object is large relative to the wavelength of the sound, a distinct shadow region occurs behind the obstacle. The extent of the shadow zone depends on the dimensions of the object relative to the wavelength of the sound. The human head will — as will all other objects — produce a shadow effect disturbing the transmission of the sound of frequencies with adequately small wave-length. The parameter of head shadow results from diffraction effects (Christen, 1979).

Sound Reflection and the Hearing Aid

Body Baffle. When a sound-wave encounters the human body some of the incident energy is absorbed and some reflected. The reflected sound interacts with the incident sound, this interaction varying as a function of frequency. The sound pressure at the microphone of a pocket aid will be influenced by body baffle effects. This means that changes will occur in the relative levels of the input sound pressure as a function of frequency. It has been reported (Erber, 1973) that when a pocket aid is worn on the chest three distinct frequency regions are influenced by body baffle.

(i) The sound pressure at the hearing aid microphone is increased 2-6 dB in the range 200-800 Hz.
(ii) The sound pressure at the microphone is decreased 5-15 dB in the range 1000-2500 Hz.
(iii) The sound pressure is not significantly affected above 3000 Hz unless the aid is covered by clothing when a decrease in sound pressure of 2-3 dB occurs.

Interestingly, body baffle effects are 1-5 dB greater for adults than for children in the frequency ranges 200-400 Hz and 1000-1500 Hz. Body baffle effects are not included in test box specifications on hearing aids. It is important for audiologists to try and quantify this effect and as a result include the information in hearing aid fitting deliberations. The best way to approach this is by free field aided versus unaided threshold work as will be discussed later. The point to bear in mind with reference to the pocket aid is that body baffle effects will act to alter the shape of the frequency response of the aid as measured in a test box, when the aid is worn by the child. Some increase in amplification occurs in the low frequencies, and some decrease occurs in the mid to higher frequencies (Dalsgaard and Jensen, 1976).

Head Baffle. The head like the body will act to reflect sound and this can lead to variations in the output sound pressure level at the hearing aid microphone, which will be a function of frequency, microphone location and also source orientation. Head baffle effects differ from body baffle. Head baffle acts to enhance the sound pressure at the microphone by up to 5 dB in the 1-3 kHz region particularly for top-mounted microphones when the source is on the aided side of the head (Shaw, 1966; Tonisson, 1975).

Sound Diffraction and the Hearing Aid

The fact that diffraction of sound leads to a shadow effect has significant implications for hearing aid use. The first consequence of head shadow is that there will be significant differences between the sound pressure level at the two ears, this being a function of source location and frequency. This therefore means that the sound pressure level at the microphone of a post-aural aid will be affected by diffraction effects. It has been found that sound diffraction can lead to differences of 15 dB or more in the sound pressure level at the two ears — this being most pronounced when the head is directly between one ear and the source (Sivian and White, 1933). The effect is most pronounced for the frequencies 2000-3500 Hz. The most obvious situation where sound diffraction effects could cause a deterioration in the effectiveness of a hearing aid is when the child uses one aid and the speaker is situated on the unaided side of the head. It has been found that speech is attenuated by approximately 6 dB (Tillman *et al.*, 1963) in such circumstances which may lead to a decrease in the child's discrimination ability.

The point was made earlier that it has been proposed that the optimum position for the microphone of a post-aural aid is top front. This results from the research findings which suggest that diffraction effects are smallest and head baffle effects largest for this microphone location (Olsen and Carhart, 1975).

Distortion in Hearing Aids

When a speech signal is amplified by a hearing aid it inevitably becomes distorted. This distortion occurs in the form of changes in the relative frequency and intensity relationships and bandwidth (range of frequencies in signal) of the input signal. The reason this distortion arises is a result of the fact that the hearing aid comprises of a series of building blocks with their own built-in characteristics. These characteristics act to introduce changes in the make-up of the processed signal so that the output is not a simple amplified version of the input. The amount of distortion that is introduced into the amplified signal is a function of the fidelity of the amplification system — fidelity being an expression of how accurately a signal is reproduced. High-fidelity equates with very accurate reproduction while low-fidelity equates with poor reproduction. Hearing aids in general would be considered as 'middle to low' fidelity instruments. When one recalls the previous discussion on the components of a hearing aid it should become obvious why such a comment applies: the bandwidth of the speech signal may be 'narrowed' considerably by receiver and earmould; the receiver may act to introduce peaks and troughs in the frequency range covered by the aid; the amplifier may produce non-linear amplification which results in the generation of harmonics (harmonic distortion) and intermodulation products (Pollack, 1980) (intermodulation distortion), that is, sounds in the output signal that were not present at the input. Hearing aids may also have difficulty in mirroring the rapid changes (sharp attack or sudden decay) of sound energy that occurs in running speech, such that formant transitions, for example, are sluggishly reproduced. Finally, the introduction of noise (for example, clothes' rub, wind noise, electrical noise) into the processed signal acts to degrade the signal and is therefore also considered as a distortion factor.

The basic aim of any hearing aid programme is obviously to provide a child with as distortion-free a signal as possible. It is important for audiologists to take note of and appreciate the importance of the comments relating to distortion discussed in the above paragraphs. The main point of note is that various forms of distortion can arise in a hearing aid and each can have a significant influence on the effectiveness of the aid for a hearing-impaired child. Any steps that can be taken to reduce distortion will be of benefit to the child. Interestingly, with the exception of 'electronic noise', only one specific type of distortion, harmonic distortion, is usually considered and quantified in relation to the performance of a hearing aid. It is in fact the only type of true distortion for which standards of measure have been agreed and laid down. The likely reason for this is that harmonic distortion is the easiest type of distortion to measure.

Harmonic Distortion

When a signal of frequency f_1 is processed by a hearing aid, integer multiple frequencies may be produced at the output, that is, $2f_1$, $3f_1$, $4f_1$, etc. in addition to the amplified f_1 component. This means that signals appear in the output which were not present at the input and distortion has therefore occurred. A harmonic is simply a tone whose frequency is an integer multiple of the fundamental frequency

(f_1). The second harmonic has a frequency of $2f_1$, the third harmonic a frequency of $3f_1$. Harmonic distortion in a hearing aid may originate in the transducers (microphone, receiver) or the amplifier. In addition, it should be recalled that the deliberate act of limiting a signal by peak clipping inevitably introduces harmonic (and intermodulation) distortion. This is because the sinusoidal input pattern of the sine wave or pure tone is not reproduced at the output of the hearing aid. It is in fact possible to generate a waveform similar to the one shown in Figure 4.9 by means of a synthesiser. This machine combines large numbers of pure tones and produces a resultant waveform. If this is done, it will be found that the waveform comprises a fundamental pure tone of frequency equal to the input frequency plus a large number of integer multiples (harmonics), of different amplitude (weaker for higher order). Thus harmonic distortion would result.

When considering the behaviour of the harmonics as produced by a hearing aid, the even harmonics usually show similar behaviour as do the odd harmonics. A basic difference, however, usually exists between the behaviour of even and odd harmonics. The harmonics do get weaker with increasing order and as a rule it is sufficient to determine second and third harmonic distortion when measuring the distortion level of the hearing aid. Alternatively, the total harmonic distortion, which is the sum of the second and third harmonic components may be determined. While there is no absolute maximum level of acceptable total harmonic distortion, a level of 10 per cent is usually set as the ceiling value. It has been reported that subjects can tolerate quite high levels of harmonic distortion without any significant influence on their speech discrimination ability (Staab, 1972). However, the fact that such studies were applied to adults means that the findings do not necessarily apply to pre-lingually deaf children who, one must remember, are learning the language. The goal must be 'a minimal amount of distortion' so that within the constraints of present-day hearing aids the hearing-impaired child is furnished with as natural an experience of language as possible. One factor which can significantly influence this goal, is that of selection and setting of the hearing aid for the child. Studies have highlighted the fact that many hearing aids display a behaviour of: the greater the gain setting of the aid the greater the harmonic distortion in the processed signal (Lotteman and Kasten, 1967). It is therefore inadvisable to select and fit a hearing aid to a child where gain has to be set at or near the maximum in order to reach the child's desired listening level. As a rule of thumb a gain reserve of 5 dB should be available on all hearing aids.

Determining Harmonic Distortion

Most of the modern generation of hearing aid test boxes have a facility which enables the user to measure the degree of harmonic distortion generated by a hearing aid. The method of measurement has already been described but it is important to stress the fact that a standardised method of measure must be followed if sensible results are to be obtained. For example, there is little point in applying such measures with the aid saturated because this will inevitably lead to a high degree of distortion, regardless as to the 'well-being' of the components of the hearing aid. If results at this setting are taken as an indication of the distortion level of the aid in use and compared with manufacturers' specifications, then this will inevitably lead to the rejection of the aid, probably unnecessarily. Normally, second and third order harmonic distortion can be measured separately on a hearing aid test box. Alternatively the total harmonic distortion (sum of second and third order) may be recorded.

It is possible to express harmonic distortion in two ways. Either the sound pressure level of the distortion product is expressed as a certain number of decibels below the sound pressure level of the total output signal from the hearing aid or the distortion product sound pressure level is expressed as a percentage of the sound pressure level of the total signal. For example, the Bruel and Kjaer 2116 system quantifies in decibels, while the Phonic Ear HC1000 and Fonix FP20 quantify in per cent. When the result is quantified in decibels we call it a distortion ratio and when it is quantified in per cent we call it a distortion factor. These two parameters are related and it is a simple matter to convert from one to the other (see Table 6.1). For example, if the harmonic distortion ratio is 20 decibels this means that in percentage terms the distortion factor is 10 per cent.

Consider the following example:

Let f_1 be a fundamental tone which is to be fed into the hearing aid (that is, the test tone). Let f_2, f_3 be the frequencies of the second and third harmonics which will appear in the output signal together with f_1 (assuming harmonic distortion occurs and that higher order harmonics are negligible). Let P_1 be the r.m.s. sound pressure level of the f_1 signal developed in the 2 cc coupler. Let P_2, P_3 be the r.m.s. sound pressures of the second (f_2) and third (f_3) harmonics developed in the 2 cc coupler.

Let P_c represent the total sound pressure of the output signal (comprising f_1, f_2 and f_3) developed in the 2 cc coupler. By definition:

$$P_c = \sqrt{P_1^2 + P_2^2 + P_3^2}$$

The Harmonic distortion factor for second order: $= d_2 = \dfrac{P_2}{P_c} \times 100\%$.

The Harmonic distortion factor for third order: $= d_3 = \dfrac{P_3}{P_c} \times 100\%$.

Table 6.1: Conversion from distortion ratio (dB) to distortion factor (%)

Distortion ratio (dB)	Distortion factor (%)
0	100
5	56
10	32
15	18
20	10
30	3·2
40	1

The harmonic distortion ratios are determined by first expressing the coupler sound pressures in decibels:

Thus, $H_1 = 20 \log \dfrac{P_1}{Pref}$ dB

$H_2 = 20 \log \dfrac{P_2}{Pref}$ dB

$H_3 = 20 \log \dfrac{P_3}{Pref}$ dB

$H_c = 20 \log \dfrac{P_c}{Pref}$ dB

$(Pref = 20 \, \mu Pa)$

The sound pressures are therefore expressed in dB SPL.

The harmonic distortion ratio for second order $= H_c - H_2$.

The harmonic distortion ratio for third harmonic $= H_c - H_3$.

Example (Figures chosen simply for ease of manipulation)

Let $P_1 = 100 \, \mu Pa$ $f_1 = 500 \, Hz$

$P_2 = 20 \, \mu Pa$ $f_2 = 1000 \, Hz$

$P_3 = 10 \, \mu Pa$ $f_3 = 1500 \, Hz$

Now $P_c = \sqrt{P_1^2 + P_2^2 + P_3^2}$

$P_c = 102 \cdot 5 \, \mu Pa$

(i) DISTORTION FACTORS

Second harmonic distortion:

$$d_2 = \frac{P_2}{P_c} \times 100 \qquad \%$$

$$d_2 = \frac{20}{102 \cdot 5} \times 100 \qquad = 19 \cdot 5\%$$

Third harmonic distortion:

$$d_3 = \frac{P_3}{P_c} \times 100 \qquad \%$$

$$d_3 = \frac{10}{102.5} \times 100 \qquad = 9 \cdot 75\%$$

Total harmonic distortion:

$$d_T = \sqrt{d_2{}^2 + d_3{}^2} \qquad = 21.8\%$$

Quite often the harmonics are very different in magnitude and a good rule of thumb to follow is to take the total harmonic distortion factor as equal to the larger of the individual harmonics when they differ by more than a factor of 2. If they are equal in magnitude the total will be greater by a factor of $1 \cdot 4$ (that is, $\sqrt{2}$) because

$$d_T = \sqrt{d_2{}^2 + d_3{}^2}$$

$$d_T = \sqrt{d_2{}^2 + d_2{}^2}$$

$$= \sqrt{2d_2{}^2}$$

$$= \sqrt{2}\, d_2$$

$$= 1 \cdot 4 \quad d_2$$

(ii) HARMONIC DISTORTION RATIOS

$$H_1 = 20 \log \frac{100}{20} \qquad dB\ SPL$$

$$H_2 = 20 \log \frac{20}{20} \qquad dB\ SPL$$

$$H_3 = 20 \log \frac{10}{20} \qquad dB\ SPL$$

$$H_c = 20 \log \frac{102 \cdot 5}{20} \qquad dB\ SPL$$

The harmonic distortion ratio of second order:

$$H_c - H_2 = 20 \left(\log \frac{102 \cdot 5}{20} - \log \frac{20}{20}\right)$$
$$= 20 \log \frac{102 \cdot 5}{20}$$
$$= 14 \; dB$$

Note that: $20 \log \dfrac{102 \cdot 5}{20} = 20 \log \dfrac{P_c}{P_2}$

$$= 20 \log \frac{100}{d_2}$$

so $H_c - H_2$ can be calculated from a knowledge of d_2.

The harmonic distortion ratio of third order:

$$H_c - H_3 = 20 \left(\log \frac{102 \cdot 5}{20} - \log \frac{10}{20}\right)$$
$$= 20 \log \frac{102 \cdot 5}{10}$$
$$= 20 \; dB$$

Note again that:

$$20 \log \frac{102 \cdot 5}{10} = 20 \log \frac{100}{d_3}$$

So $H_c - H_3$ can be determined from a knowledge of P_3. Note too that $H_c - H_{2+3} = 20 \log \dfrac{100}{d_T}$ = total harmonic distortion ratio.

In the above example the second harmonic has a distortion factor of approximately 20 per cent which means it is 14 dB weaker than the total signal. The third harmonic has a distortion factor of approximately 10 per cent which means it is 20 dB weaker than the total signal. The total harmonic distortion factor in this example is approximately 22 per cent which means that the sound pressure of the combined distortion products is 13 dB below the total signal.

A final point of information with respect to this section is to draw the readers attention to the fact that the majority of hearing aid test boxes use values of P_1 and H_1 rather than P_c and H_c for expressing distortion. In other words, instead of relating the distortion product to the overall sound pressure of the total signal developed in the coupler, reference is made to the sound level of the fundamental. If, for example, the second order distortion factor was 10 per cent, it would mean that the second harmonic was 10 per cent of the fundamental or 20 dB weaker than the fundamental. This approach changes nothing in the aforementioned examples other than replacing P_c and H_c by P_1 and H_1.

The rule of thumb to apply when dealing with harmonic distortion is not to accept an aid for a child where total harmonic distortion is at or in excess of 10 per cent level.

References

American National Standards Institute (1976) *Specifications for Hearing Aid Characteristics*, ANSI S 3.22, American National Standards Institute

Berland, O. (1982) *On Simulated In-situ Performance Data*, Oticon Information Series, Oticon, Denmark

British Standards Institute (1968) *Methods of Test of Air Conduction Hearing Aids*, BS 3171, British Standards Institute, London

Christen, R. (1979) 'Selecting amplification characteristics for auditory training equipment' in *Proceedings of the Third Conference for the Audiological Society of Australia*, Sydney

Dalsgaard, S.C. and Jensen, O. (1976) 'Measurement of insertion gain of hearing aids', *Journal of Audiological Technique, 15*, 171

Erber, N.P. (1973) 'Body-baffle and real-ear effects in the selection of hearing aids for deaf children', *Journal of Speech and Hearing Disorders, 38*, 224

Gengal, R.W., Pascoe, D. and Shore, I. (1971) 'A frequency response procedure for evaluating and selecting hearing aids for severely hearing-impaired children', *Journal of Speech and Hearing Disorders, 36*, 341

Harford, E.R. (1980) 'A microphone in the ear canal to measure hearing aid performance', *Hearing Instruments, 31(11)*, 14

International Electrotechnical Commission (1959) *Recommended Methods for Measurements of the Electroacoustical Characteristics of Hearing Aid*. Publication 118, Geneva

International Electrotechnical Commission (1973) *IEC Reference Coupler for the Measurement of Hearing Aids Using Earphones Coupled to the Ear by Means of Ear Inserts*, IEC 126, International Electrotechnical Commission, Geneva

International Electrochemical Commission (1981) *Occluded Ear Simulator for the Measurement of Earphones Coupled to the Ear by Ear Inserts*, IEC 711, International Electrotechnical Commission, Geneva

Jessops Acoustics Surveyor 1, *Hand-held Hearing Aid Tester*, Jessops Ltd, London

Lotteman, S.H. and Kasten, R.N. (1967) 'The influence of gain control rotation on non-linear distortion in hearing aids', *Journal of Speech and Hearing Research, 10*, 593

Nichols, R.H. (Jr) (1947) 'The influence of body baffle effects on the performance of hearing aid's', *Journal of the Acoustical Society of America, 19*, 943

Olsen, W. and Carhart, R. (1975) 'Head diffraction effects on ear level hearing aids', *Audiology, 14*, 244

Pollack, M.C. (1980) *Amplification for the hearing-impaired*, Grune and Stratton, New York

Shaw, E.A.G. (1966) 'Earcanal pressure generated by a free sound field', *Journal Acoustical Society of America, 39*, 465

Sivian, L. and White, S. (1933) 'On minimum audible sound fields', *Journal Acoustical Society of America, 4*, 288

Staab, W.J. (1972) 'Hearing aid compression amplification: Fittings', *National Hearing Aid Journal, 25(12)*, 34 illman, T., Kasten, R. and Horner, J. (1963) 'Effect of head shadow on reception of speech'. Paper presented at the American Speech and Hearing Association Convention, Chicago

onisson, W. (1975) 'Measuring in the ear gain of hearing aids by the acoustic reflex method', *Journal of Speech and Hearing Research, 18,* 17

7 HEARING AIDS NOT ENTIRELY WORN ON THE LISTENER

Hearing-impaired children inevitably find themselves in situations where listening conditions are far from ideal. As a result the effectiveness of their hearing aids can be significantly reduced. Two factors, background noise and reverberation, have been shown by numerous studies to have a very deleterious influence on the speech discrimination abilities of hearing-impaired children (John, 1957; Gengel, 1971 Gengel and Faust, 1975). The reasons for this are a direct result of the properties of sound-waves.

The background noise in the vicinity of a hearing-impaired child originates from two main sources — noise from within the room where the child is situated and noise from other rooms and from the outside Noise may be considered as any sound that is of no interest to the listener and is in effect in competition with the message, that is, the sound of interest.

Reverberation is simply a means of expressing the persistence of a sound in a room once the source is switched off. It is defined as the time taken in seconds from the instant a source ceases until the sound pressure has fallen by 60dB. The reverberation time of a room is a function of frequency.

The reason sound persists in a room is a result of the fact that the boundary walls do not absorb all of the sound energy hitting them. Some sound energy is reflected back into the room, the amount being a function of the constituent materials of the boundary walls and the frequency of the sound (B & K, 1979, 1982). The harder and denser the material the greater the proportion of incident sound energy reflected. The reflected sound arrives at the ear later in time than the direct sound (because it has travelled further). If the absorption of sound energy is relatively small upon reflection, it will require a number of reflections before the sound becomes so weak as to be inaudible. The more the reflections the later in time the sound will arrive at the ear and therefore the longer the sound will persist.

Effects of Background Noise

The energy generated by a sound source such as the vocal organs

ecomes weaker as it travels through the air. The further away we are
rom the source the quieter the sound is perceived. A hearing aid
microphone does not choose which sounds to convert into electric
ignals. It converts background noise as well as speech. It is as a result
f the fact that the difference between the background noise and the
peech signals becomes smaller (signal-to-noise ratio (S/N) will decrease)
s the speaker moves away from the hearing aid, that hearing-aid users
o find great difficulty in understanding speech at a distance.

Reverberation

he fact that sound can persist in a room has significant implications
or the hearing-impaired. The first consequence of this is that the
tronger vowel-like components of the speech message can act to mask
ut following weaker consonant information and thus reduce speech
ntelligibility (John, 1957). The second consequence is that the rever-
erant room is more 'noisy' than the sound-treated room because it is
ive' and reflective and acts to emphasise all unwanted sounds rather
han dampen them out.

Controlling Noise and Reverberation

t is possible to control background noise and reverberation. This is
ar more easily achieved by definition of the required acoustic environ-
nent prior to the construction of a building rather than after comple-
ion. Guidelines and building regulations on the design of educational
acilities for the hearing-impaired are available for this very reason
RNID, 1980). Three factors are of primary importance:

   (i) sound insulation;
  (ii) sound treatment;
 (iii) noise source control.

ound insulation acts to reduce the amount of noise permeating into
he room. Sound treatment shortens the reverberation time and also
cts to reduce the internal noise level. Attention to the internal and
xternal sources of noise, for example by carpeting floors, using rubber-
op tables, not siting rooms adjacent to major roads or factories, will
bviously have a significant effect on the prevailing noise level in a
oom.

   It is of interest to note that reverberation times of no more than 0·5 seconds from frequencies 125-4000 Hz and noise levels of the order of 30 dBA across the same frequency range are recommended for classrooms where hearing-impaired children are being educated (Borrild 1978).

The basic aim of controlling noise level and reverberation is to furnish a hearing-impaired child with a favourable signal to noise ratio. However, it is often difficult or impossible to achieve this goal in the manner outlined. Audiologists must therefore realise that the noise levels and reverberation times (perhaps simply because of financial constraints) will often be higher than is desirable, particularly in mainstream education. Children in such placement will therefore be at risk in relation to the effective use of their residual hearing regardless as to the degree of hearing loss. Work by Gengel (1971) and Gengel and Faust (1975) has indicated that a signal to noise ratio of +24 dB is essential for optimal auditory reception by hearing-impaired children in education.

Alternative Approaches to a Favourable S/N Ratio

Alternative approaches to achieving favourable signal-to-noise ratio have therefore been devised. The solution to the problem is to present stronger speech signals to the hearing aid microphone. This is achieved by speaking close to the microphone (within 20 cm). Research has shown that the use of a short microphone distance does help to avert or minimise the deleterious effects of background noise and reverberation (Ross and Giolas, 1971; Ross *et al.*, 1973; Markides *et al.*, 1980). The systems that have been developed attempt to render constant the level of the signal delivered to the hearing-impaired child — regardless of the relative position of the teacher (or parent) and child, and in certain systems, 'child to child' in the classroom. One characteristic of such a system is that a part of it is not worn by the child (that is, the user). This is why the term 'Hearing aids not entirely worn on the listener' has been adopted (IEC, 1979) as a means of categorising such equipment. While such systems can and do find application outside school they will be considered as 'amplification systems for education' in the subsequent discussion.

Amplification Systems for Education

The reason why amplification systems for education are not entirely worn by the child results from the practicalities of ensuring that the child is furnished with a favourable signal regardless of the distance between the teacher and child. Teachers of hearing-impaired children would find it very difficult indeed to provide speech close to the microphone of a conventional hearing aid. The teacher must therefore be fitted with a separate microphone which is linked to the child's hearing aid (Figure 7.1). This linkage and the actual aid worn by the child differs according to the system in use. The group hearing aid which is a classroom based amplification system uses wires as the linkage (that is, a visible link). Other systems employ electromagnetic induction (the loop system), radio transmission or infra-red light as the 'carrier' of the speech information between teacher and child (that is, an invisible link). The auditory link between child and child in the classroom will be at risk if it is achieved in the conventional manner of sound travelling through the air from speaker to hearing aid user (air-borne linkage). Certain educational amplification systems do facilitate effective child-child linkage by use of the same format as is used to link teacher-child (for example, group aid). Others, however, such as the radio aid employ the conventional air-borne linkage. Teaching style in such situations will be critical in ensuring that effective child to child communication occurs.

Figure 7.1: The theoretical idea behind short microphone distance — teacher microphone linked to child's aid.

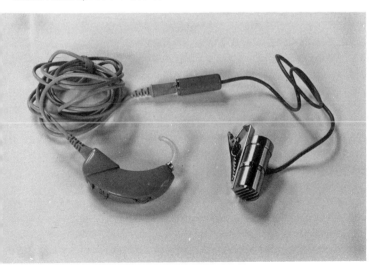

Before going on to describe the currently used 'amplification system for education' it will be useful to draw up a design specification for the 'ideal' system. This will help in highlighting the drawbacks and limitations of the various systems.

1. Effective teacher-child communication.
2. Effective child-child communication.
3. The teacher must be able to move freely around the classroom.
4. The children must be able to move freely around the classroom.
5. There must be no limitation on the number of systems in use in a school and no interference between systems in the different classrooms.
6. It must be possible for a number of activities to be carried out at the same time in the classroom.

The Group Hearing Aid

The group hearing aid is a classroom based amplification system. It is either 'desk fixed', the pupil 'stations' being linked together and to the teacher 'station' by wire leads, or is housed in a trolley cabinet (that is, mobile). This cabinet has space for storage of pupil microphones and headsets. Each child station comprises: an amplifier allowing individual adjustment of frequency response, output level and microphone level; a microphone which is usually linked to the headset to facilitate close talk (this microphone provides the child with a good ear-voice link and a means of communicating with other children); headsets which provide a much broader frequency response than is available via conventional hearing aids and help in particular in extending the higher frequencies possibly out to 10 kHz and in preventing acoustic feedback; a four position programme switch which permits the selection of the appropriate transmission from the teacher. The teacher station has up to 4 programmes of transmission incorporating two microphone amplifiers and two auxiliary input jacks. These jacks may be used for things such as tape recordings or records. Each pupil can be switched to any of these input programmes so that a number of activities can be carried out at the same time. The teacher is fitted with a close talking microphone which can if required be free of a trailing lead by use of a radio-microphone. The group hearing aid does achieve the desired goal of facilitating effective teacher-pupil and pupil-pupil communication. It can be used in adjacent classrooms without problems of interference and does facilitate a number of activities in the classroom at any one time. Its major drawbacks are lack of mobility particularly for the children and the fact that it is only useful for groups of hearing-impaired children. Its main application nowadays is in special schools for hearing-impaired children and on occasions in unit placements.

Overall, the system is far superior in fidelity terms to a conventional hearing aid. The basic frequency response from 70 Hz to 10,000 Hz has the potential of providing children with a greatly extended frequency response. Acoustic feedback is avoided by the use of headsets, which nowadays have supra-aural cushions and a lightweight plastic construction and are very acceptable to hearing-impaired children. There is no doubt that the principle of the group hearing aid is well established in the education of hearing-impaired children. Such systems should continue to play an important role, particularly with those children who are functioning on a very restricted auditory signal (Markides *et al.*, 1980). This last comment is important because in certain quarters there does now appear to be less emphasis placed on fidelity and more on mobility than perhaps is absolutely necessary for education of groups of hearing-impaired children. We believe that while modern developments in amplification systems are to be applauded this does not mean that established systems, which have proven to be very effective tools in the habilitative programme, should be simply discarded. Modern hearing aids including the FM radio systems described shortly still lack the fidelity of the group aid and auditory training unit (Nolan, 1982a) and are more vulnerable to the effects of background noise.

The Infra-red System

Portable Wire-less Mono Infra-red Pulse System

The major drawback of the hard-wire group hearing aid is lack of mobility for teacher and children. This is an important consideration in the education of the hearing-impaired. In order to overcome this problem while retaining short microphone distance it is necessary to couple the teacher-child by an invisible lead or wire-less link. Ideally, the same should apply to child-child linkage but at the present moment no satisfactory solution to this demand has been found. Children still have to rely on air-borne linkage for inter-child communication.

The link between teacher and child can be facilitated by the use of light waves. It is necessary to use a specific part of the light spectrum which will not suffer significant interference from daylight or classroom illumination systems. The solution is to use infra-red light (that is, light in the invisible spectrum) which acts to 'carry' the speech signal from the teacher to the child (Siemens Hearing Instruments). The major advantage of using light as a carrier relates to the fact that the signal is contained within the classroom and there is therefore no spillover. Any number of classrooms in a school can be fitted on the same carrier frequency without interference (Figure 7.2).

Figure 7.2: Siemens mono infra-red wire-less system and operational possibilities.

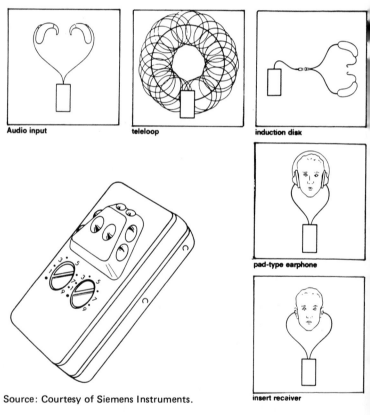

Audio input   teleloop   induction disk

pad-type earphone

Source: Courtesy of Siemens Instruments.   insert receiver

The disadvantage of the system is that it cannot be used outdoors. Further, direct sunlight can introduce noise into the system. Windows in classrooms where the system is to be used should be fitted with unfilters, curtains or blinds to prevent this problem.

The basic principle of the infra-red system is that the teacher's speech is sensed by a microphone worn close to the mouth which then delivers the signal to a pocket aid sized infra-red transmitter also worn on the chest. This transmitter radiates the invisible light upon which the speech signal is carried (the light is FM modulated). The room is flooded with the light which reflects from walls and ceilings and should therefore ensure uniform distribution of signal throughout the room. If problems do arise, it is possible to employ wall or stand mounted 'slave' transponders which increase the coverage of the room. The children are fitted with a pocket type unit which acts as a conventional hearing aid and an infra-red receiver. This is worn on the chest outside the clothing. A hemispherical transparent plastic receiving lens situated on the casing acts to focus the light on to silicon photo diodes. The speech information is then recovered in an electrical format, directed to the amplifier and subsequently passed through the hearing aid in the normal manner. The child's unit has an environmental microphone which provides a good ear-voice link and also acts to pick up the speech of other children. This makes it possible for the child to use the unit as a conventional aid both in and out of doors when the infra-red system is off. Children and teachers are able to move freely around the classroom without degradation of the speech signal. Children can in fact turn their backs on the transmitter since the infra-red light that is reflected from the walls and ceiling will be adequate to ensure proper reception. Both transmitter and receiver are powered by rechargeable Ni-Cd batteries. The average daily battery life is approximately 5½ hours for the transmitter and 15 hours for the receiver (Siemens Hearing Instruments). An auxiliary input for tapes and cassettes is available on the transmitter.

The child's unit can be used in various ways. It may be used in conjunction with a headset or insert receivers and therefore constitute the child's hearing aid. Alternatively, it can link up with the child's conventional hearing aids by means of direct input (that is, galvanic coupling) or electromagnetic induction via a neck loop or inductive pad. This area will be discussed in more detail under FM radio systems. The use of headphones does furnish the child with a broader frequency response (out to 7 kHz) than would be possible using conventional aids with earmoulds. This may be an important factor particularly where acoustic feedback or the degree of hearing loss means that a child is operating on an extremely limited auditory signal via his hearing aids. The advantage of using the galvanic or electromagnetic coupling configuration is that the child simply disconnects the infra-red system when it is not required and continues on his own hearing aids. He is not therefore changing from one system to another during the day.

The infra-red system has found application in the schools for hearing-impaired children but at the present time it is seldom used outside this environment. It is worthy of note that a second type of infra-red device which is specific to the education of groups of hearing-impaired children and is a fixed classroom based system is available (Siemens Hearing Instruments). The principle of operation is the same as the mono system, the major differences being in the layout of the components (the transmitter is mains operated), the improved fidelity and the fact that the system is stereo rather than mono. This system does not use the close microphone format but two free standing microphones separated in space by the approximate distance between the ears (that is, 20 cm). These microphones are situated between teacher and children and attempt to link child-teacher, child-child by infra-red light. The microphones feed the infra-red 'stereo' transmitters, which are wall-mounted around the classroom. The body-worn infra-red receivers have two environmental microphones (one for each ear) and therefore act as the child's hearing aids. They drive headphones and provide an excellent fidelity signal. The major drawback of this system relates to the free standing nature of the microphones which are very susceptible to background noise (Markides *et al.*, 1980). Teaching style and the particular classroom activity are fundamental considerations to the successful use of such a system in a school for the hearing impaired.

Electromagnetic Induction

Audio-loop Systems

The principle of electromagnetic induction was discussed earlier under telecoil. This is another means of facilitating an invisible link between teacher-child, thus providing for mobility for the child while retaining a short microphone distance for the teacher. The loop induction system comprises a microphone which is connected to a loop drive amplifier. This microphone is usually desk-mounted (resulting in lack of mobility for the teacher) or may be of a radio microphone type (providing mobility for the teacher). The radio microphone mode would necessitate that a radio receiver be connected to the input of the loop amplifier. The amplifier drives current (from the microphone) through a wire which is placed around the entire classroom (Figure 7.3) (that is, the loop). While it is acceptable to site the wire at any convenient height, ideally it should be sited slightly out of plane with the hearing aid when the aid is worn by the seated child. This helps to facilitate a more uniform magnetic field in the teaching situation where children will often be mobile.

Figure 7.3: Format of a classroom based loop induction system.

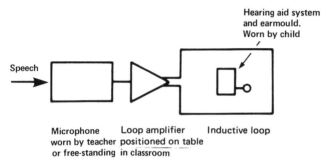

When a teacher talks into the desk microphone, current flows through the loop in synchrony with the speech. This current sets up a synchronous magnetic field in the classroom. The telecoil in the child's aid is able to sense the fluctuating magnetic field and transforms it into an equivalent electrical signal which is directed to the amplifier. This signal runs in parallel with signals coming from the child's environmental microphone. As far as the child is concerned, his hearing aid has been stimulated by a teacher talking close to the microphone (that is, the desk or radio microphone invisibly linked to the hearing aid).

The use of electromagnetic induction does permit a good teacher-child link, but not child-child link. This is why it is normally desirable to use an aid on the MT setting in a classroom situation, so that the child receives both teacher via T and his own voice and those of the other children (perhaps not very satisfactorily) via M. Classroom based loop induction systems have fallen into disrepute, the reasons being outlined as follows:

1. The major drawback of the classroom loop relates to the fact that the electromagnetic waves are unaffected by brick walls. This results in the problem of spillover into adjacent classrooms. No satisfactory

method of overcoming this problem has been found.

2. The frequency response of a hearing aid on the T mode can be different to that on the M mode. This may cause significant problems for certain children.

3. The actual mode of operation and use of the system in schools for the hearing-impaired has presented problems. Many systems were installed prior to the publication of recommended standards for the magnetic field strength of loop systems (IEC, 1978). This has resulted in considerable variation in performance of loops even within a school (Huntington, 1976). The consequence of this has been wide inter-classroom variations in hearing aid performance on the T mode.

4. Weak or dead spots can and do arise in a classroom loop system. This can result in children receiving no effective signal via the loop modality.

5. The loop induction system may generate a high level of random internal noise in an aid (Hawkins and Van Tasell, 1982). This can act to mask out certain speech information.

Despite the above comments the principle of the loop system still plays a very major role in the education of hearing-impaired children. However, modern day systems are child based rather than classroom based — each child having his own personal loop. This has been achieved primarily as a result of the rapid growth in the use of FM radio transmission systems which employ neck loops or inductive pads. The same format may also be employed with the infra-red mono wire-less system. The personal loop systems overcome the problem of spillover because the magnetic field is very localised around the child. Equally the problem of weak or dead spots is also overcome. The most significant factors that remain are the differences in hearing aid performance on M and T modes and the possible problem of a higher random noise level from the aid when operating on T than on M mode (Hawkins and Van Tasell 1982). It is important for audiologists to apply a very thorough evaluation of a radio loop system prior to issue to a child. Every possible attempt must be made to furnish the child with as 'noise free' a signal as possible.

FM Radio Transmission System

Over the last few years there has been a sharp increase in the number of wire-less FM radio amplification systems. This solution to the wire-less link between teacher and child has been widely taken up by educational audiologists and has found application across the whole cross section of educational provision. This type of system is rapidly becoming seen as an essential part of a child's amplification requirements. In certain services for the hearing-impaired it is now provided routinely as part of a child's personal hearing aid package.

The basic format of the FM radio system is two units. The teacher's transmitter unit (worn by the teacher) is a small box about the size of a pocket aid. It comprises a microphone (for short microphone distance) coupled to a radio transmitter antenna. The electrical signals from the microphone frequency modulate a radio frequency carrier wave which is broadcast through the air. The child's unit, a radio receiver, which 'decodes' the radio transmission, recovers the speech signal in an electrical format and amplifies it ready for delivery to the ear. There is a wide range of FM systems on the market. They can be divided into two main groups which will be denoted as type 1 and type 2. They differ in the facilities offered by the child's receiver unit.

All of the FM systems in use are one-way radio transmission devices. Herein lies one potential weakness of these systems in relation, say, to hard-wire group hearing aids of the multiple microphone type. The teacher in an educational setting will be the one with the radio transmitter. Clearly in any teaching situation other children will contribute and it is therefore vital that the teacher reinforces student contributions either verbally or by effective use of the radio transmitter. Children in integrated educational programmes require particular attention in this respect. This is clearly a matter for advisory teachers to discuss with the class teacher.

The Radio Microphone Hearing Aid – Type 1

Type 1 systems comprise the conventional radio hearing aid which is both a personal hearing aid *and* a conventional radio receiver (for example, see Figure 4.2). The child wears one box containing both of these facilities. It is interesting to note that these systems are usually considered as the personal hearing aid of the child and are not specific to classroom use. Examples of the type 1 systems currently in use in the UK are:

a) Phonic Ear: HC 431 Stereo
b) Jessops: FM Radio Hearing Aid
c) Cubex: Radio Link.

The basic function of a radio hearing aid is outlined in Figure 7.4. The child's unit containing both conventional hearing aid and radio receiver is normally worn on the chest.

Figure 7.4: Format of the radio microphone hearing aid system.

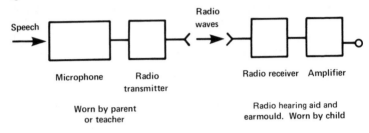

The teacher is fitted with a radio microphone transmitter which is 'tuned' to the frequency of the child's receiver. The child's unit may be used in one of three ways:

(a) as a normal hearing aid with no radio facility functioning;
(b) as both a normal hearing aid and a radio receiver, that is, the conventional type 1 radio microphone hearing aid;
(c) as a radio receiver without the environmental microphone of the system operating.

Use of facility (a) helps to extend battery life. It is not desirable to use the system in mode (b) all the time. There will be times during the day when the radio facility will not be required, for example, close up work with the child when the aid's environmental microphone is employed; play time or lunch breaks at school where the system would be simply used as a normal hearing aid; periods during the day when in pre-school years the child's mother is actively engaged in noisy domestic duties or is well away from the child conversing with a neighbour or on the telephone, that is, not directing communication to the child. In the latter situations it would be better for her simply to switch her own transmitter OFF but leave the child's radio receiver ON, so that she can easily switch ON again when she *wants to communicate with the child*. This will avoid her having to find the child in order to switch the radio receiver on but will obviously not help to conserve the battery. It is also important to note that children need time and opportunity to develop a familiarity and knowledge of their auditory environment. Radio received information simply appears 'in the head' without dimension or direction. Hence, periods when the environmental microphones of the system are used will help to nuture this need, particularly so when stereophonic amplification is applied.

The use of the system in mode (c) is sometimes adopted when problems of acoustic feedback arise. This mode of operation should be used with care, because one must remember that the child will be unable to hear his own voice or sounds in his vicinity unless he is close to the radio transmitter. It is a mode of operation to use perhaps as one would a speech training unit. Students in school, further and higher education also use this mode in some lecture situations.

The performance of a radio microphone hearing aid system in terms of frequency response and output capacity should be equivalent on both audio (that is, via the aid's environmental microphone) and radio (that is, via the radio transmitter) channels. This means that the signal output to the child is satisfactory for both input channels. It is important to be aware of the need to 'balance' both input channels so that the child is listening at a comfortable level to radio and audio received information. In general everyday situations the audio received information will be weaker than that received via radio (~10dB) because of the proximity of the radio transmitter to the teacher or parent (6 ins). Voice level going into the transmitter will be of the order of 75 dB SPL (Ross, 1977) while speech picked up by the microphone of the child's unit will be approximately 60-65 dB SPL (Nolan, 1977).

Some systems, which have one control for the level of the signal delivered to the child, take account of this effect in that the output from the child's unit is 'balanced' for radio and direct audio received information when the signal level on the radio channel is 10dB greater than that on the audio channel (that is, 75 dB SPL signal via radio is equivalent to a 65 dB SPL signal via audio (microphone)). This means that in everyday situations the teacher's voice level via radio will be 'just above' the child's own voice level picked up by the aid's environmental microphone.

On other systems the levels of the two channels of input to the child's ear (that is, direct audio via the aid's environmental microphone and radio) may be adjusted separately by independent volume controls. It is necessary to remember the difference in input for the two modes when setting a system up for a young child. Use of aided thresholds is advisable in such cases. For older children it is possible for them to optimise listening conditions by fine adjustments of microphone and FM volume controls.

Figure 7.5: Battery slide-packs on transmitter and receiver units (Cubex Radio Link MK III).

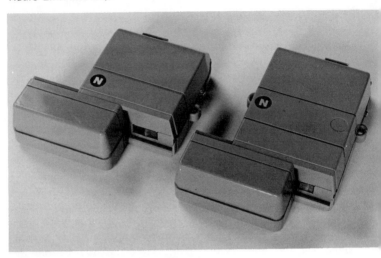

Figure 7.6: Lapel microphone (Jessops Acoustics).

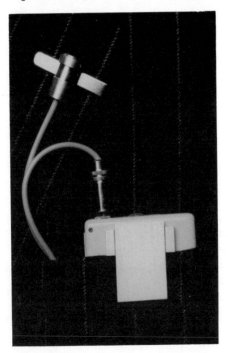

Features of the Systems

Batteries

1. All systems employ rechargeable nickel-cadmium (Ni-Cd) batteries.
2. The batteries are NOT removable on certain systems.
3. Other systems employ a 'slide-pack' battery which can be replaced as required. This is a very desirable facility in aids of this type because of battery life (Figure 7.5).
4. Most systems will require battery recharge or replacement after 8-10 hours of general use (Table 7.1). Battery life will vary depending on how the aid is used. The discharge characteristic of nickel-cadmium batteries is such (Ever Ready, 1980) that it is *not* good practice to develop a policy of 'topping up' followed by another wearing session in the late afternoon. Once the output performance of the aid begins to fall off and reaches an unsatisfactory level as a result of exhausted batteries then those batteries should be put on recharge for 8-12 hours (Table 7.2).

Table 7.1: Hours in use using rechargeable batteries (manufacturers' information).

System	Hours
Cubex Radio Link Mk III	10
Jessops FM Radio	8/10
Phonic Ear HC 44 system	7/8
Phonic Ear 421, 432 stereo	8/10
Phonic Ear 455 mono	8/10
Connevans system	8
Jessops Syncom	8

The following points should be noted:

a) Certain battery chargers take the battery to its end-point *before* beginning its recharge cycle. Hence, 'topping up' is impossible. It is of interest to note that complete discharge of these cells prior to recharge is not recommended (Philips, 1982) as it reduces the number of possible recharges. Rechargeable nickel-cadmium batteries may be recharged hundreds and even thousands of times (Ever Ready, 1980).
b) In slide-pack systems, an exhausted battery can be replaced with a fully charged slide-pack. It is therefore advisable to have a set of four slide-packs so that two are always fully charged.

Table 7.2: Battery charger charging time for full capacity from end-point (manufacturers' information).

System	Charging time (hours)
Cubex Radio Link Mk III	14
Jessops FM Radio	8
Phonic Ear HC 44 system	14
Phonic Ear 421, 431 stereo	10
Phonic Ear 455 mono	10
Connevans system	15
Jessops Syncom	12

(c) On systems with non-replaceable batteries, the problem of exhausted cells and low output will necessitate removal of the aid from the child so that the cells can be fully recharged for the following day. The child must have stand-by aids in such circumstances. Although this is not a policy to be encouraged it is the only way of ensuring that a child does not miss out on auditory input in the latter part of the day. The major weakness of such a policy is the change in amplification pattern enjoyed by the child. Ideally, therefore, two systems should be available to the child. Battery life can be extended by thoughtful use of the system. Switching OFF the radio side of the child's system when not required can extend battery life to 12 hours.

Leads

The leads on type 1 systems (the radio microphone hearing aid) do differ. It is important that the correct type of lead is used with each system.

Phonic Ear – 2 pin leads. The output socket of the hearing aid connects to a right angle non-polarised connector on the lead (that is, pins same size). The receiver transducer connects via a polarised straight connector on the lead (that is, one wide diameter, one narrow pin).

Cubex Radio Link Mk III – 2 pin leads. The output socket of the hearing aid connects to a straight polarised connector on the lead. The receiver transducer connects via a straight polarised connector to the lead.

Jessops FM Radio System – 2 pin leads. The output socket of the hearing aid connects to a straight polarised connector on the lead. The receiver transducer connects via a straight polarised connector to the lead.

All leads should be of child and not adult length.

Earphone-receiver

It is important to note that the earphone-receiver transducer will significantly influence the frequency response of the systems. It is vital that a record is kept of the receiver in use and that steps are taken to ensure it is not swopped or replaced with an inappropriate receiver. Spare leads and receivers should be kept on hand at all times. Subminiature receivers should be used with children. There is no real advantage in fitting children with power push-pull (PP) standard sized receivers because of the interaction of the receiver with the child's soft small ear (Nolan, 1979). As a general rule National Health Service receivers are compatible with these radio aids. One simply needs to match an NHS receiver to that supplied with the aid.

General Features of Note

Lapel Microphone

Certain systems have a facility for lapel microphone use with the transmitter. Use of a lapel microphone mutes the microphone that is built into the transmitter. It is important to check whether the gain of the system alters when the lapel microphone is used instead of the built-in microphone. This may occur and should warrant advice to parents on the required settings of the child's aid (particularly with young children who rely on their parents to set up their aid), so as to ensure continuity of amplification. A simple check on a hearing aid test box will answer this question. Lapel microphone facility is a very desirable feature of a radio hearing aid system because it enables parents or teachers to wear the transmitter on a belt at waist level rather than around the neck (Figure 7.6).

These same systems usually have a lapel microphone facility for use with the child's unit. This is a very attractive feature because it means that the body worn unit can be worn on a belt or beneath the clothes (concealed) without interfering with the reception of the child's own sound making activities or environmental sounds around the microphone. Removal of the aid from the chest to a belt or concealed position obviously helps to child-proof a system from everyday enemies such as food and drink (Powell, 1975). Clearly the lapel microphone lead must be carefully positioned under the clothes. The microphone itself must be secured by a suitable clip. The question of using the lapel microphone facility more generally with children is one which requires investigation and field study trials. Binaural amplification by means of stereo hearing aids — which is far more desirable — will necessitate two lapel microphones, but the siting of these is another area of study. The currently available systems, with lapel facility, are mono; that is, one microphone is employed with the systems.

Crystal Oscillator Module

The crystal module which 'tunes' the child's unit to a particular radio frequency on which the parent or teacher is transmitting is replaceable on all units. Certain systems can be issued with either a single channel or dual channel oscillator. The dual channel oscillator enables the child to switch over to a second radio frequency which, for example, could be 'common' throughout the school and used for school gatherings such as assembly. The other frequency would be specific to a particular class. Dual oscillators eliminate the need for children to remove their class module and replace with a 'common' one for assembly, etc. The other systems employ single channel detachable modules.

Various radio frequencies are reserved for use with the deaf (Table 7.3). This stops children unnecessarily listening in on taxi or police conversations. The supplier should be advised on the frequencies in use in a school and on which frequency is required when a new system is ordered. Further information is available from the DHSS Radio Regulatory Division on the radio frequencies that are reserved for the deaf and the categorisation of such frequencies. This is perhaps the major weakness of the FM radio system in that as with electro magnetic induction, radio waves are hardly affected by brick walls. The range of radio transmitters from 30 m up to 100 m means that different classes in a school must use separate carrier frequencies.

Low Battery Indicator

The problem of low battery with resultant low gain performance was highlighted earlier. There is an obvious need in view of the relatively short battery life for a 'low voltage' indicator, particularly on the child's unit, which will draw attention to this problem (Nolan, 1980). This type of indicator is available on certain systems (Figure 4.2). How ever, in the light of comments by Fulbeck *et al.* (1979), further improve ments are still desirable. An audiovisual alarm is necessary for all systems and should be extended into all types of hearing aids used by

Table 7.3: Radio aid frequencies (United Kingdom).

| Classification | Frequencies MHz | Manufacturer code | | |
		Cubex + Connevans	Phonic Ear	Jessops
W	171.100			
P	173.350	N	red/brown	mauve
P	173.400	A	red/red	red
P	173.465	B	blue/red	green
P	173.545	C	blue/orange	yellow
P	173.640	D	blue/yellow	blue
S	173.695	P	white/grey	mauve/white
S	173.755	Q	white/brown	red/white
W	173.800			
S	173.825	R	white/red	
S	173.950	S	orange/blue	yellow/white
S	174.070	T	black/grey	blue/white
S	174.120	U	black/brown	mauve/blue
S	174.185	V	black/red	red/blue
S	174.270	W	black/green	gold
S	174.360	X	black/orange	green/blue
S	174.415	Z	black/yellow	yellow/blue
W	174.500	M		
P	174.600	E	green/blue	mauve/gold
P	174.675	F	pink/orange	red/gold
P	174.770	G	pink/yellow	green/gold
W	174.800	O		
P	174.885	H	pink/green	yellow/gold
W	175.000			
P	175.020	J	pink/blue	blue/gold

Note: P = primary allocation, S = secondary allocation, W = wideband.

children. Such a device has been developed for use initially with Phonic Ear systems (Nolan, 1980).

One other point of interest in relation to batteries for type 1 and 2 systems is that of recharge time. As indicated in Table 7.2, this is a function of the system. Many chargers provided by manufacturers have no time function in them.

A digital electronic plug-in timer is very useful and will switch devices on and off at precisely set times on a 24-hour clock. It simply plugs into a 13 amp socket providing a similar socket itself and can handle an electrical loading of up to 3 kW. It will therefore prove very valuable in schools and the home — for example, switching chargers on and off each evening-morning — and also at weekends in schools.

Radio Transmitter

There are a number of pitfalls related to inappropriate use of the radio transmitter. It is not good policy for a teacher to wear and use more than one transmitter on the same frequency at the same time. Considerable distortion may ensue with consequent unacceptable performance of the children's hearing aids because of the lack of 'birdie' filters on the radio receivers. Such a situation may arise if a teacher is faced with a small group of children using different makes a radio system all on the same frequency. The answer to this situation is to use one manufacturer's transmitter to which all the children are tuned. It is advisable to check the performance of each child's system as transmitters may differ in power, but as a rule no problem should occur. Alternatively, the problem can be foreseen and avoided by standardisation, using only one particular manufacturer's product.

If more than one system is in use on different frequencies in the same room, the teacher will again have to wear a number of transmitters. Problems may arise here when one transmitter is switched off and the child tuned to that frequency comes within two feet of the teacher with his radio facility still ON. A considerable amount of 'noise' may be generated in the child's system. Hence, in 'close up' group work such a problem may arise and must be avoided. The simple answer to this is to switch OFF the child's radio facility when the radio transmitter is OFF.

Type 2 Radio Hearing Aid Systems

'The Personal System'

Type 2 systems comprise a radio transmitter-receiver system which is used in conjunction with the child's own personal hearing aids of either body worn or post-aural type (Figure 4.2). The radio facility can be dispensed with when not required. The child, therefore, need not carry it around in such situations as is necessary with type 1 FM systems. *It is important to note* that a type 1 system as described may be used as a type 2 system, although size and weight may well be a problem. Examples of the type 2 systems that are currently available in the UK are:

(1) Phonic Ear 441T   442 R
              441T   445 R
(2) Connevans CRM-R-100   T-100

CRM-R-100/M T-100
(3) Jessops Syncom – S
Syncom + Sel
Syncom + Mic
Syncom + Sel + Mic

Mode of operation – Type 2 system

The 'radio received' information is passed on from the radio receiver to the child's own hearing aids for amplification in one of two ways:

(i) By direct connection (audio input) to the child's hearing aid via a lead (Figure 7.7). The child's hearing aid must have an audio input facility – many hearing aids do not possess such a facility. Various manufacturers now produce aids with direct audio input facility and many children are successfully using them. A limited range of pocket aids is available with this facility. These aids are to be seen as high power body instruments (Figure 7.8).

Figure 7.7: Format of the personal radio hearing aid system using direct input.

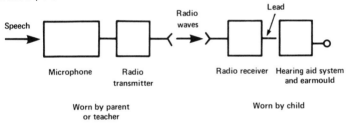

Speech

Microphone

Radio transmitter

Radio waves

Radio receiver

Lead

Hearing aid system and earmould

Worn by parent or teacher

Worn by child

A wider range of post-aural aids with this facility is available. It would appear from reference to Figure 7.9 that children and teachers will have difficulty mating the cable with the audio input connector on some systems. The need for standardisation on one audio input connector to the post-aural aid is obvious.

It is important to note that the correct audio input lead must be obtained. The various Personal radio systems may be used with the range of aids having an audio input facility provided that the correct audio input lead is used. The audio input lead is therefore an integral part of the amplification system. This comment applies equally when the infra-red mono system is used. Audio input leads are specific to a particular hearing aid and must not be employed with the aids

Figure 7.8: Examples of pocket aids with direct input facility. (a) Dana-vox 787PP and Viennatone 2000 AX-PP using a 2.5mm jack plug; (b) Widex S21 and Maico Windsor EL. MK II using standard hearing aid leads.

(a)

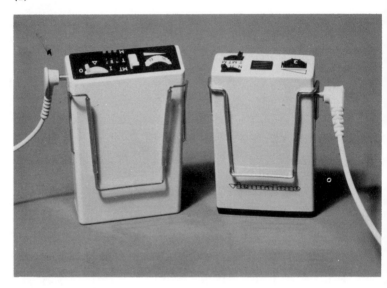

(b)

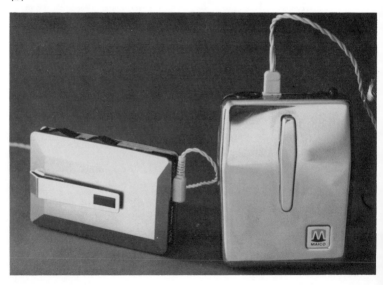

Figure 7.9: Examples of post-aural aids with direct input facility. (a) Phonak PPCL; (b) Danavox 775; (c) Oticon E22P; (d) Oticon E28P; (e) Viennatone AO/PP/AU; (f) Unitron E1P.

(a)

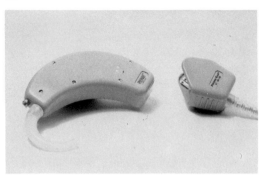

(b)

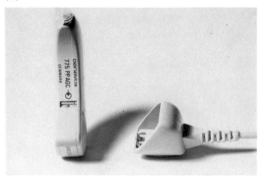

(c)

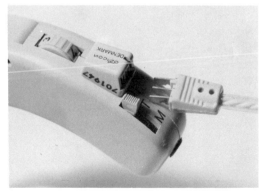

(d) Figure 7.9 (cont'd)

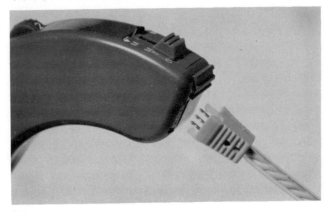

(e)

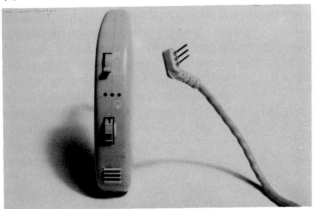

(f)

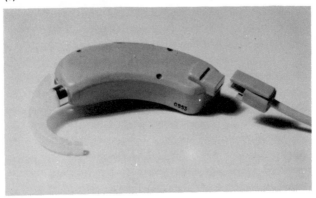

of other companies even when the connector plugs are the same.

(ii) Aids without audio input facility are used with the type 2 radio system by means of loop induction (Figure 7.10). The child's radio receiver drives a loop which may be a neck loop or inductive radiator – for use with post-aural aids (Nolan and Tucker, 1981), or a body coupler (Figure 7.11). The child's aids must be set to be sensitive to loop induction signals (T or MT mode).

It has been shown by recent research that direct input does ensure a more equivalent performance on both microphone and radio received 'channels' of the child's hearing aid (Hawkins and Van Tasell, 1982). This is to be expected in the light of the earlier comments related to telecoil and loop systems.

There are a number of possible problems to be faced by children using loop systems:

(a) The performance of a hearing aid on loop mode can be significantly inferior, particularly in the low frequency region, in comparison to the microphone performance. This is of particular importance to profoundly deaf children who rely heavily on this frequency region (Nolan, 1982b; Huntington, 1976; Ling, 1964). This may be assessed by use of aided thresholds for M and T modes of listening.

(b) Many post-aural hearing aids do not have an MT mode, that is, the child's microphone and loop sensitivity cannot both be on at the same time. This means that the child must switch to loop (T) to receive radio information via neck loop. As a result he no longer receives information from his own voice or those of his classmates. So in order to overcome this problem his radio receiver *must* have an environmental microphone facility which will do the job of the aid's microphone. The information from this environmental microphone will come 'down the line' via the neck loop as with radio information. This receiver should be worn on the chest to ensure a good ear-voice link, not under clothes or at waist level unless a lapel microphone is provided. Such provision is desirable for children because it does then enable concealment of the receiver unit. The use in binaural fitting of one ear on M, the other on T, is not recommended.

(c) The orientation of the telecoil of a post-aural hearing aid will vary with head movement within the localised loop field set up by a neck loop. This variation in telecoil orientation has been investigated. The results for a range of post-aural aids revealed gain variation for the extreme of telecoil orientation of ~15 dB. In normal everyday situations

Figure 7.10: Format of the radio loop system.

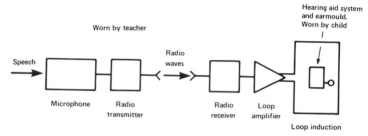

(a)

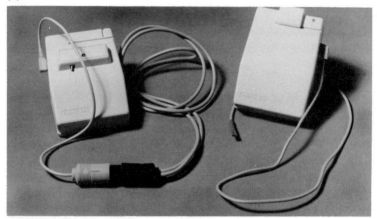

(b)

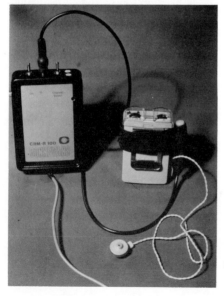

Figure 7.11: (a) Radio neck loop system (Phonic Ear 44 system). (b) Radio pocket loop system (Connevans Ltd).

his variation should not exceed 10 dB in response to head posture changes. It is important to advise mature children of this characteristic of neck loop systems.

Certain radio receivers have a control facility which enables the user (or the person responsible for the use of the system) to set the level of the signal coming from the radio receiver. This means that the level of the signal driving the neck loop or going directly into the hearing aid via the audio input lead can be adjusted and set to a predetermined level. This facility is extremely useful because it enables the radio received information to be adjusted to a satisfactory level independently of the hearing aid setting used normally by the child. This system therefore enables teachers and parents, for example, to set up relatively quickly a system for a young child without disturbing the settings of the child's personal aids. When setting up such systems the initial procedure to follow is similar to that adopted with type 1 systems allowing a 75 dB SPL signal on the radio channel to equate with a 65 dB SPL signal on the audio channel. Aided threshold measures should then be applied. This will ensure that the teacher's signal will be received at a comfortable level. Older children should be encouraged to set the hearing aid microphone and FM radio signal ratio to meet their particular listening needs.

Other radio receiver units do not have a signal control facility. These systems provide a fixed output for a given input to the radio transmitter. The signal strength of the output from the radio receiver is too strong to be simply directed into the hearing aid. It is therefore necessary to reduce the strength of the signal from the radio receiver prior to it being fed into the aid. In *fixed* output systems this *must* therefore be done *in* the audio input lead. Hence, it is necessary to obtain a specific audio input lead for a particular hearing aid to match the output of the radio receiver to the direct input requirements of the hearing aid. This point is of particular importance because manufacturers of audio input leads having built in attenuators do not as yet appear to be agreed upon what constitutes an acceptable level of signal into the child's hearing aid. Some manufacturers are designing audio input leads so that a 65 dB SPL signal into the transmitter (teacher signal) balances with a 65 dB SPL signal into the aids microphone (child's voice), while others are using the convention of a 75 dB SPL signal into the microphone. From the observations of Ross (1977) and Powell (1982) this latter procedure would seem more appropriate. However, what is really desirable is the flexibility of the adjustable output radio receiver, which permits children to 'fine tune' the FM signal to best meet their needs. Similar comments relate to the use of radio loop systems (Nolan, 1983).

Problems in Use

Muting Problems. One problem associated with type 2 systems which has been noted is that related to the squelch or muting circuit. This problem arises when the teacher's transmitter is switched off while the child's receiver unit is left on. In normally functioning systems a muting or squelch circuit in the receiver unit ensures that the receiver is quiet and does not generate noise when the transmitter is switched off. However, if this circuit is inappropriately set by the manufacturer the result is one of white noise (similar to that produced by a transistor radio when 'off channel' at high volume setting), which is generated by the receiver and hence amplified by the child's aid. This noise will act to mask speech information. It is vitally important to check all systems and return those producing such problems for adjustment. The simplest way to check for this problem is:

(a) Switch on the child's transmitter — place in another room by a radio or with another person.
(b) Couple an appropriate lead to an earphone receiver and plug into the output socket of the radio receiver.
(c) Set the receiver to receive radio transmissions. Listen via the stetoclip and adjust to a comfortable level (if a volume control is provided on the receiver).
(d) Switch the transmitter off. If white noise is audible which then goes off when the transmitter is switched on again then the fault is present and the system requires adjustment.
(e) If, when the transmitter is OFF and the child's system is ON, no significant white noise is apparent then the system is satisfactory.

Battery Contact. The type 2 radio systems employ replaceable rechargeable batteries. It has been noted that the battery contacts on some systems gradually lose their 'elasticity' and fail to make contact with the battery when it is inserted. It is important for the audiologist to ensure that a regular check is made to ensure that this problem does not go unnoticed. The problem can be overcome by 'packing' the battery compartment with a piece of foam or polystyrene.

Work by Ross and Giolas (1971) and Ross *et al.* (1973) has demonstrated the superiority of FM amplification over the hearing

mpaired child's personal hearing aid when used in a normal school
lassroom, in terms of speech discrimination ability. However, Markides
t al. (1980) did not report such dramatic improvement. The dif-
erence in research findings is important because it does highlight
wo factors: (i) the importance of a child's personal hearing aid to
which he will become accustomed and 'tuned'; and (ii) the fact that
ecause radio hearing aids of type 1 configuration (Nolan and Tucker,
981) have a limited flexibility of frequency response, they will not
ecessarily suit all children. It is very short-sighted to view radio hearing
ids as only suitable for severe hearing loss, but it is equally short-
ighted to adopt a policy of providing type 1 radio systems 'blanket
ashion' for all children. Type 1 radio systems have a limited frequency
esponse which may be considerably different from that of the child's
wn personal hearing aid and amplification requirements.

Overall, it may be concluded at this juncture that while radio hearing
id systems do offer hearing-impaired children opportunities which
hould be seized upon, such systems must be chosen with great thought
nd care. There is clearly a need for greater consideration to be given
o the provision of radio systems for partially hearing children. Perhaps
he most significant development in this area that has opened up new
orizons is the growth in provision of type 2 radio systems (Nolan and
'ucker, 1981). This system which is used together with a child's
ersonal hearing aid certainly presents as the optimal FM system at
his time and does overcome the above-mentioned weakness of the type
  radio system. Type 2 systems are without doubt practical amplifica-
ion systems for education which may be used by a wide range of chil-
lren with varying degrees of hearing-impairment.

Day-to-day Management of the Systems

Whilst all of the systems described can undoubtedly offer potential
enefits in terms of enabling a child to maximise the educational use
f residual hearing, their correct utilisation is often 'a pain in the neck'
Ross, 1977). It is therefore vitally important for management staff
o be familiar with the range of systems available, and capable of
nsuring continuing effective use once a system is obtained for a child.
rovision of such a system for a child is no guarantee of success, parti-
ularly if steps are not taken to ensure efficient and effective ampli-
ication subsequent to provision. Another important point to note
elates to repairs. Teachers and others responsible for the systems must

ensure that a thorough check takes place when a system returns from being repaired. This must be done before reuse. Cases where aids were sent back for repair, the repair was carried out, but the system arrive back still not working, another fault having arisen in transit, do occur. This is obviously an important point of note.

The Group Aid

The major cause of dysfunction with this system is related to headset. Broken contacts are not uncommon. Teachers must ensure that the apply a regular check to the system. This is best done by subjective listening. Obviously one would hope that the more mature child use would indicate when faults arise — but this cannot be taken for grante as research has clearly demonstrated (Martin and Lodge, 1969).

Infra-red Systems

Listening tests are advisable with both the portable mono system an the classroom based group aid. It is also suggested that users of th mono equipment discuss with their suppliers techniques of determinin electroacoustic parameters which can be cross-checked by means of test box in a similar manner as is used to check conventional hearin aids. It would be useful to consult the document (IEC, 1979) whic outlines the standards for measurement of equipment 'not entirel worn on the person'. A hand-held hearing aid tester as described earlie can be used to check that the transmitter-receiver is operating and tha the signal level is appropriate for the child.

Electromagnetic Induction

The classroom based loop systems are most easily evaluated by use c a hearing aid on the T mode. The teacher should listen through 'he aid, as she moves around the room. This check can be made with eithe a colleague or an auxiliary source of input to the loop microphone.

   An alternative to the listening test is to use a hand-held tester whicl has a loop facility and which can therefore provide a direct readin related to the electromagnetic field strength in the classroom. Thi clearly indicates when a fault is present. The instrument is also usefu for teachers in that by walking around the classroom while holdin the tester (set to loop) they can find the areas where field strengt is weak and avoid sitting children in such positions.

   Routine checks on the performance of the children's aids on T mod must be made by the audiological advisor. The standard method of mea surement for telecoils is laid down in International Standards (IEC, 1975)

The Management of Radio Hearing Aid Systems

Radio Hearing Aid systems must be regularly tested so as to ensure that they are maintained in a state of maximum efficiency. It is desirable to apply two categories of test — daily subjective listening tests and regular (for example, monthly) electroacoustic measures on a hearing aid test box.

Radio systems are produced in different formats by a number of manufacturers. Audiologists must familiarise themselves with the control layout and mode of operation of each system in use in their service. This information is vitally important and must be passed on to the parents and teachers so that they can properly fit and effectively use these systems with hearing-impaired children.

The subjective listening tests are relatively easy for parents and teachers to apply, particularly when the audiologist has taken time carefully to explain the methods of application. A stetoclip is the only piece of equipment that is required during tests.

It is useful when describing these tests to divide radio systems into two types. The tests for use with the type 1 system — the conventional radio hearing aid will be described first, followed by the tests for the type 2 system — the personal radio aid which is used in conjunction with the child's conventional hearing aids.

Type 1 Systems

Listening Tests. The radio hearing aid comprises both a conventional hearing aid (or 2 aids for stereo model) and a radio receiver in the one box. Testing of the system therefore involves:

1. Checking the system as an ordinary hearing aid with the radio facility OFF.
2. Checking the system as a radio transmitter-receiver with the environmental microphone of the child's unit OFF.

Step by Step Listening Check

(1) The first step involves a visual check of the whole system. The child's unit should be examined for any signs of damage. The microphone inlets should be free of debris. The crystal oscillator should be removed (if externally situated) and wiped clean with a cloth. The oscillator socket area should also be wiped clean as this is a perfect trap for food and drink. The radio microphone transmitter should be inspected. The inlet grill of the microphone should be free of debris.

The integrity of the aerial should be checked.

(2) Attention should now concentrate on the child's unit which should be treated as a conventional pocket hearing aid. The radio microphone should be OFF as should the radio facility on the child's unit.

(3) The volume control should be adjusted to full. The characteristic acoustic howl should be present when the earphone receivers are held lead length from the microphone. This assesses battery condition.

(4) The volume control should be set to the listener's most comfortable level. The left and then right channel (earphone receiver) should be connected to the stetoclip. By talking or singing into the microphone (6 ins from mouth) the integrity of the leads can be checked by wiggling at the connector weak spots and listening for intermittency

(5) The quality of sound should be noted.

(6) The power of the sound should be compared with that normally experienced. Once each channel has been checked and found to be satisfactory it is then in order to proceed to check the radio facility. If a fault is noted in the initial tests it may prove necessary to resolve it before the radio system can be assessed. Fault finding will be discussed shortly.

Checking the Radio Facility

(1) The crystal oscillator should be in position in the child's unit. The unit should be set to receive radio transmission, the environmental microphones should be off.

(2) The radio transmitter should be placed in an adjacent room with another person or by a source of sound (for example, a transistor radio).

(3) The transmitter should be switched on and the quality of the radio transmission should be assessed by connecting first left then right earphone to the stetoclip.

(4) A check should be made so as to ensure that the problem of muting (described earlier) is not present.

Electroacoustic Measures. The electroacoustic measures using a hearing aid test box follow a similar test format to that used in the subjective listening tests. It is always advisable to listen subjectively to a system before proceeding to check it on a test box. These listening tests help to highlight faults and reduce time wasted in trying to assess a faulty system.

(1) The first step of the electroacoustic test involves the child's unit

which is treated as a conventional hearing aid. The radio facility should be OFF.

(2) The test format is the same as that described for the pocket aid. The child's unit is placed in the test box with the microphone at the target spot.

(3) The earphone receiver of left and then right channel should be connected to the 2 cc coupler. The other channel when not being tested should be left connected to the aid. It is suggested that the earmould be coupled to the earphone of this channel. The mould should be occluded by a blob of 'blu tac' so that problems of acoustic feedback don't arise. The standardised measures (which were described earlier) for the pocket aid should then be applied.

(4) Once the system has been assessed as an ordinary hearing aid it is then in order to proceed to assess the radio facility.

(5) The aim of the test is to assess the integrity of a system comprising a microphone worn close to the speaker's mouth which picks up speech and directs it to a radio transmitter. The signal is then broadcast to a radio receiver worn by the child. This decodes the signal and directs it to the amplifier of the hearing aid. The signal is then processed by amplifier and earphone receiver and directed into the child's ear.

The microphone that is sensitive to sound in the above is the microphone on the radio transmitter. It should therefore be placed at the target spot in the test box. The radio transmitter should be switched on. The child's unit should be set to receive radio transmissions and switched on. This unit should be placed on the table by the 2 cc coupler. It is advisable when checking the radio facility to switch the environmental microphones on the child's unit OFF, or if this is not possible to set them to minimum sensitivity. Otherwise, the results will be influenced by the ambient noise around the child's unit which will be 'picked up' by these microphones and delivered via the hearing aid to the 2 cc coupler. First left then right channel should be connected to the coupler. Measurements on the performance of the system should be applied as in the first set of tests when the system was considered as a conventional hearing aid. It is suggested that reference be made to the published hearing aid standards for measurement of the electroacoustical characteristics of hearing aids – see 'Hearing aid equipment not entirely worn on the person' (IEC, 1979) for a fuller discussion of this area.

One particular measure that is important to check is the relative sensitivity of the audio (that is, via the child's environmental microphones) and radio (that is, via radio transmission) channels of the child's system. It was mentioned earlier that there may be a 'built-in' sensitivity difference to account for the differences in teacher voice input and child voice input to the radio aid system. It is important to advise parents and teachers of young children as to the appropriate setting of the volume control particularly when radio and audio channels have separate volume controls. As a guideline a 65 dB SPL input into the audio channel should be compared with a 75 dB SPL input to the radio channel when measures are made on the 2 cc coupler.

Type 2 Systems

Listening Tests. When a child presents with a type 2 radio hearing aid system he will be using conventional hearing aids together with a radio transmitter-receiver system. The radio system will be coupled to the conventional aids in one of two ways. Either (i) by direct connection that is, audio input, or (ii) by loop induction.

The subjective tests will be described separately for the above two formats.

When a child presents with an 'audio input' system the listening tests follow a logical procedure.

(1) The conventional aid or aids should be checked in the manner described earlier via the stetoclip. Once these tests have been applied the radio system can be tested.

(2) The radio system comprising transmitter and receiver should be checked as an independent unit before being coupled to the child's aid in the audio input format. A lead plus earphone receiver should be connected to the output socket on the radio receiver. This socket normally takes the audio input lead or neck loop connector. The audiologist must provide the parent and teacher with an appropriate lead and receiver. A subminiature wide range earphone receiver of appropriate impedance should be used for the listening test. This plugs into the stetoclip.

(3) If the radio receiver has an environmental microphone facility then this should be switched on. (If not step 4 may be applied.) By talking or singing into this microphone (with stetoclip in ear) the integrity of the microphone and the battery in the radio receiver can be assessed. The microphone should then be switched off.

(4) The radio transmitter should be switched on and as with type 1 systems placed in an adjacent room with a person or other source of sound. The listening test via stetoclip should then assess the quality of

radio transmission to the radio receiver.

(5) If the radio system is functioning satisfactorily it may then be coupled to the child's aids — each in turn being assessed via audio input.

(6) The transmitter should be situated by a source of sound as in step 4. The radio receiver should be connected to the child's hearing aids via the audio input lead. The stetoclip should be connected in turn to the output transducer of each of the child's aids. The integrity of the audio input lead should be thoroughly checked out by wiggling at the connector weak spots and by listening for intermittency of sound.

This approach of listening to aid, radio system and then 'total' system does help to isolate faults and makes correction of certain ones a relatively easy task.

The listening tests to be applied when loop induction is employed as the link between hearing aids and radio system follow similar lines to those described for the direct input system.

(1) The child's hearing aids must be assessed.

(2) The radio system should then be treated as a separate independent system and checked.

(3) Once these tests, which are common to both 'connection formats', have been applied the integrity of the loop induction system can then be assessed.

(4) The radio transmitter should be positioned close to a source of sound and switched on.

(5) The neck loop should be connected to the radio receiver. The radio receiver should be set to receive radio signals. The loop should be placed around the neck with the radio receiver coupled to a belt or the clothes.

(6) Each aid in turn should be set to T. They should be coupled to the stetoclip and situated by the ear in the normal user orientation. The quality of sound reception should then be assessed by listening via the stetoclip. The neck loop is prone to faults, particularly intermittency or breakage in the wire of the loop or at the connector sockets. The loop lead at the connector socket should be wiggled and a check made for intermittency of sound. The loop itself should also be wiggled at various points and checked for sound cut-out. The hand-held hearing aid tester may also prove useful here — it being set to T mode, placed within the loop and a check made on the loop field strength.

Electroacoustic Measures. The electroacoustic measures comprise tests on the child's conventional hearing aids followed by tests on the radio system and finally tests on the complete system either via direct input or neck loop. The tests on the child's conventional aids are as described earlier for either pocket or post-aural model.

The second category of test involves two measures on the radio system, one of which is only carried out when the radio receiver incorporates an environmental microphone. The tests are intended as a means of assessing the performance of the radio receiver when it is 'driven' by an audio signal (via the environmental microphone) and by a radio signal (from the radio transmitter). The tests require provision of an appropriate lead and earphone receiver which plug into the output socket of the radio receiver. It is important to use the appropriate type of earphone receiver which will have been used by the manufacturer in the production of the radio aid specifications. The methods employed in obtaining these specifications are laid down in the relevant standards.

The measures relating to the built-in environmental microphone simply involve setting the radio receiver so that this microphone is operating. The radio transmitter should be off. The receiver unit should be placed in the test box with the microphone at the test spot. The earphone receiver should be connected to the 2 cc coupler as with a pocket aid. It is recommended that measures of the basic frequency response of the radio receiver for a 60 dB input together with a frequency response specification for a 90 dB SPL input to be made. Application of these measures is described earlier and also in the relevant standards. The results should be compared with manufacturers' specifications.

The second test involves measures on the radio microphone transmitter-receiver system. The radio microphone transmitter should be placed in the test box. The radio receiver (environmental microphone off) should be set to receive radio transmissions. The earphone should be connected via the lead to the 2 cc coupler. The standardisation measures may then be applied. The measures of basic frequency response for a 60 dB SPL input and a frequency response for a 90 dB SPL input are again recommended. These should also be compared with the manufacturers' specifications.

The final measures relate to tests on the whole system comprising hearing aids, radio system and audio input connectors or neck loop.

The format for direct input aids comprises:

- (i) Place radio transmitter in test box.
- (ii) Place child's conventional aids on a bench adjacent to test box.
- (iii) Connect these aids via appropriate lead to the radio receiver.
- (iv) Connect in turn the child's aids to the 2 cc coupler. (Occlude other aid to prevent feedback whistle.)
- (v) The radio microphone should be switched on.
- (vi) The radio receiver should be on but with the conventional microphone (if fitted) off.
- (vii) The aid under test should be set to receive signals via audio input.

Measures of performance of the aid when used with the radio system may then be applied. It is important to make measures on the relative sensitivity of the hearing aid when used as an ordinary aid and in the radio mode. A useful measure is to determine the required volume setting of the radio receiver (if a feature of the system) so that an equivalent output from the hearing aid is achieved for both audio and radio input channels. As a starting point a 65 dB SPL input into the hearing aid microphone should equate with a 75 dB SPL into the radio microphone transmitter. Parents and teachers of young children should be advised as to both the required hearing aid volume setting and the volume setting of the radio receiver. These settings should be subsequently determined by real-ear measures.

It is recommended that the random noise of the complete system be compared with that of the hearing aid alone. This is considered important particularly in the light of comments relating to muting on radio systems.

When a loop induction system is employed it is useful to obtain a tailor's dummy (ideally a mannequin such as Kemar could be used but costs may prohibit this). Obviously, Kemar together with an occluded ear simulator could provide useful information on 'real ear' performance. It is also suggested that an extra long lead from the measuring microphone of the test box be obtained. The test format may be summarised as:

1. The loop should be placed around the dummy's neck and connected to the radio receiver which should be clipped onto clothing or a belt.
2. The hearing aid should be connected to the 2 cc coupler and held in place on the dummy's head in the usual wearing format.
3. The aid should be set to T mode and switched on.
4. The radio microphone should be placed in the test box.

5. The performance of the system may then be assessed.

A useful measure is to compare the basic frequency response of the hearing aid when used normally with that when used with the radio loop system. The radio loop measure is achieved by use of a 60 dB SPL input to the radio microphone. The hearing aid should be at the same volume setting as was used for measurement of the microphones basic frequency response. The volume control on the radio receiver should be adjusted until the hearing aid output at 1000 Hz is 100 dB SPL. This measure helps to highlight the changes in hearing aid frequency response in going from microphone to loop setting (although these are not absolute real ear differences).

The random noise of the radio loop system should be measured and compared with that of the aid when in the microphone mode. The same criteria of acceptable noise level should be applied to this system as with the conventional aid.

Fault Finding

One of the consequences of applying daily listening tests is that faulty systems will be identified. While certain faults will require technical support, some can be rectified on the spot by correct application of a fault finding procedure. The necessary 'tools' that will be needed comprise:

1. Stetoclip.
2. Spare leads, receivers, battery packs (if batteries are replaceable).

The procedure for the type 1 hearing aid will be considered first.

Fault 1. No output from the child's unit on either audio or radio channel. This could be due to:

  (i) low battery in transmitter and/or receiver;
 (ii) broken leads;
(iii) broken receivers;
(iv) internal fault.

The likelihood is that it will be a battery fault. It is advisable to work through a logical testing procedure when trying to isolate the fault.

. Replace the battery in radio receiver unit and check again, treating
the unit as a pocket aid. If this step cures the problem on the audio
channel then proceed to use the radio transmitter and check the radio
channel. If the radio channel is still dead replace the battery in the
radio transmitter and check again. If this then cures the problem on
the radio channel the fault was battery condition in radio transmitter
and receiver. Some radio aid systems do not have replaceable battery
packs. For such systems it is suggested that battery condition is measured by an AVO meter. If this indicates low batteries then the aid
should be put on recharge and rechecked after a full charging cycle.
If the batteries are not coming up to full charge or if the aid becomes
dead again very quickly, that is, within one hour, the indications are
faulty batteries or a faulty charger. Both of these possibilities should be
investigated by the technical service.

. If the system fails to function with good batteries proceed to change
the leads on the child's unit and listen again.

. If this does not cure the problem change the earphone receivers and
listen again.

. If all these measures fail to resolve the problem seek technical advice.

It is useful, in cases where the fault cannot be isolated, to check
the condition of the radio transmitter independently of the radio
receiver because the fault on the system may be specific to the radio
receiver unit. This may be done by the use of the transmitter with
another radio receiver on the appropriate radio frequency. If the second
receiver performs satisfactorily then the fault must lie in the child's
radio receiver.

Fault 2. Normal performance on audio channel, no output on the radio
channel. The possible causes of this fault are:

  (i) battery in radio microphone;
 (ii) crystal oscillator in radio receiver;
(iii) aerial on radio microphone;
(iv) internal fault.

. If the radio system uses replaceable batteries then the first step
would be to change the battery in the radio microphone and recheck.

. If this fails to cure the problem then technical help must be sought.
If access can be gained to a second radio system operating on the same
radio frequency as the faulty one, it may be possible to isolate the fault

to transmitter or receiver unit and hence facilitate a speedy re pair.

One possible reason for the fault could be the crystal oscillato module which plugs into the child's unit. This can be checked b using it with a second system provided of course that both system are on the same frequency. If the second system works satisfactoril with this oscillator then the indications would be a faulty transmitte on the child's system. This too may be checked by using it with th second radio receiver. If the second system doesn't work on radi then the fault must be in the radio microphone transmitter. On common fault is the integrity of the aerial connection. This can b quickly resolved by a competent technician. If the transmitter doe work in the above test then this would indicate an internal fault in th radio receiver.

Systems which do not use replaceable batteries cannot be as easil checked. Nevertheless the integrity of the crystal oscillator and radi transmitter can be assessed if access can be gained to a second system This check will at least point to the site of the problem (that is, i transmitter or receiver).

Fault 3. Very low output on audio channel, normal performance o radio channel. Here, the first check to be made is a visual one. Examin the microphone inlet grill and check for debris. This should be cleane out if present and the system then rechecked. If this fails to rectify th fault, or if cleaning is not possible without dismantling the aid case then technical support must be sought.

Type 2 Systems

The faults that occur in these systems arise in the child's individua aids, the radio system or the connecting link between aid and radi system. The listening tests must be applied logically so that fault can be isolated and rectified.

The aids themselves must be checked first and if a fault is foun then it can be tackled in the manner outlined for conventional aids The radio system must then be checked in isolation and the approac to fault finding follows that just described for the radio system. Finally the whole system is checked. If a fault occurs here it is very likely t be in the link between aid and radio receiver (that is, audio input lea or neck loop) and this can therefore be checked by replacement o these components.

Auxiliary Aids for the Hearing-impaired

Hearing-impaired children face many difficulties when they attempt to augment their listening experience by use of 'add on' electronic equipment. Yet such equipment is essential if items like television, radio or telephones are to be used effectively. For the sake of convenience we propose to use the term auxiliary aid for all these additional pieces of equipment.

Television Aids

The television fulfils a central function in many people's lives and has an important role in schools, too. Sound quality from the average television is relatively poor, it being fair to say that the television does a good job of turning an excellent audio received signal into a very poor sound signal at the listener's ear. This is because of the poor amplifier/speaker combination in the set. Hearing aid users face great difficulty in that they may wish to turn up the sound volume to a level which, if left, would be intolerable for other listeners. There are various ways of overcoming this problem when there are hearing aid users in the family.

a) Loop Induction. With this system the signal is either collected directly from the television speaker terminals (in which case unless there is already an isolated output then an electrician must fit an isolating transformer) or via a microphone which is 'stuck' to the speaker grill. The signal is amplified and passed round a simple loop of wire, thus creating the magnetic field required by the loop induction setting of the hearing aid. Here, of course, the signal is converted back into sound to be relayed at an appropriate volume to the hearing aid user's ear (see Figure 7.12). The main drawbacks of this system are:

(1) If modification of the television set is undertaken this will need to be done each time a set is purchased.
(2) The loop field will vary in strength and it will be important to know the best positions in the room for listening.
(3) The frequency response of the hearing aid on the loop setting may differ considerably from that on the normal microphone as will the basic signal to noise ratio. Certain severely impaired users will find this system totally unsuitable for their needs.
(4) If the loop signal comes from a microphone stuck to the speaker grill an already poor signal will be further degraded for the hearing aid user.

Figure 7.12: Format of a TV loop system.

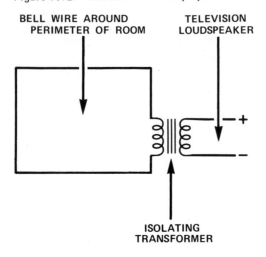

(5) Children who use ear-level aids may not be able to listen to both television and other people in the room because many such aids do not have an MT setting.

Whilst the loop system does have the drawbacks mentioned above it does at least have the major advantage over some systems in that the hearing aid user can be mobile in the room.

(b) A Microphone Amplifier System. This system comprises a microphone that stands by or is stuck to the speaker grill of the television set. This microphone connects via a long lead to a small amplifier with volume control, and then the ear. Figure 7.13 shows this system being used with a stetoclip to deliver the sound to the ear. The system is lightweight and portable, it replaces the hearing aid and therefore provides a different amplification pattern for the child. It is possible to organise the system so that the signal is fed into the transmitter unit of a radio hearing aid or auditory training unit. In the conventional format, sound quality from the television speaker, the problem of background noise and the fact that the child is 'wired' to the system will be major drawbacks for child use. (Mobility problems can be overcome via the radio system.)

(c) The Television Adaptor. Television adaptors are small control boxes directly connected to the sound source. In the case of a television

Figure 7.13: The TV adaptor.

(a)

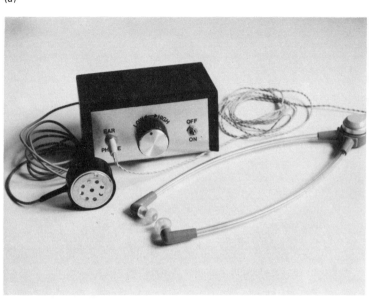

(b)

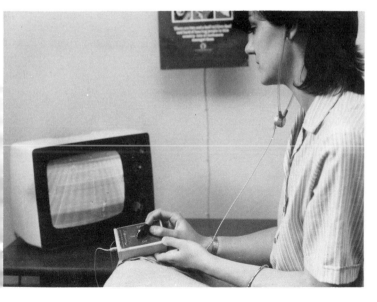

without an isolated socket the connection must be via an isolation transformer fitted to the set. This can either be inside the set or as a unit outside the set. The adaptor connects via a long lead to the isolated output and rests on the arm of a chair. The user is linked to the adaptor by a further lead and earpiece. It is possible to arrange for children with direct audio-input aids to have the signal from the unit fed directly into their aids. However, it is ESSENTIAL that teachers realise the potential dangers of audio-input and always ensure that the child is isolated from the electrical source with an appropriate isolator. If in doubt ALWAYS check with a competent engineer. The weakness of the system is, as with microphone-amplifier systems, that the user is anchored to the unit.

(d) Isolated Socket with Radio Microphone. The isolated socket may be used in conjunction with a conventional radio microphone transmitter. An appropriate matching lead will be required to link the socket to the auxiliary input on the radio microphone. The child would then use his radio receiver-hearing aid to pick up the sound track. Mobility with such a system is obviously guaranteed. Mode (d) is far more desirable if a radio system is available relative to (b) or (c).

(e) The Television Sound Tuner. The sound tuner is separate and independent of the television and is a more radical attempt to solve the problem of poor sound quality from televisions (see Figure 7.14). The device is mains operated and obtains its signal via the aerial. Installation is very simple and only involves splitting the incoming aerial signal using an aerial splitter (see Figure 7.14a). One output from this connector feeds into the television as usual, the other supplies the tuner with the audio sound track of the programmes. The tuner can therefore be used to feed television sound directly to a hearing-impaired child, or group of children, via a radio transmitter (see Figure 7.14b). This clearly achieves the goal of mobility for the children, but what is perhaps more important is that it retains the very high quality of the signal received via the aerial of the television set. If a simple amplifier is built into the tuner this can enable it to drive a loop system or to drive headphones directly. A great advantage of this system is that the child can be mobile. Also no mains isolator is required for the television set. Push button channel selectors are used to tune in the various television channels. The device may also be used via a hi-fi system, thus providing the whole family with a high-fidelity sound quality (albeit mono at present) and allowing the poor quality sound of the television

Figure 7.14: The TV adaptor: (a) in conjunction with a loop drive amplifier; (b) in conjunction with a radio microphone transmitter.

(a)

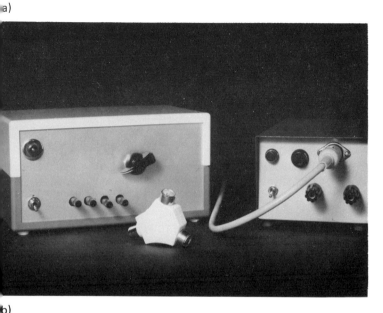

(b)

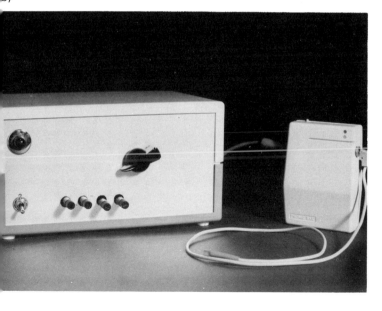

to be turned down altogether. It seems very likely that future genera
tions of television sets will incorporate an output from the tuner.

Presently available television tuners are marketed primarily for use
with hi-fi systems, but it is a relatively simple task to adapt them for
use with, say, a radio transmitter. All that is required is a connecting
cable between the tuner and the transmitter appropriately matched so
that the input signal to the transmitter is at the optimal level.

(f) Infra-red. The most recent development in television technology
which should be generally available at a realistic price in the not too
distant future is that of using an infra-red emitter from the built in
TV tuner. A set of relatively inexpensive receiver units which could
be used, for example, as 'straight' listening devices (low power) or as
a means of providing direct input to the child's aid would form part
of the kit comprising the TV unit.

Radio Set Aids

Radio sets in current use often have portability advantages over tele
visions in that they are frequently battery powered. They usually
have an isolated socket for earphone or extension speaker use. Even
the mains powered units are usually fitted with such sockets, but if
not any connections would need to be made via an isolating trans
former. Radios can be used via:

1. A button earphone as used in a pocket aid (better than the
supplied versions).
2. Headphones.
3. Adaptor as in the case of television (for mains operation).
4. As a source for feeding into aids such as auditory training units.
5. To feed a loop induction system. The power from the isolated
socket may not be sufficient for children with more than a moderate
hearing loss. Recent developments of miniature stereo radio cassette
machines using lightweight headphones offer some possibilities
particularly for less severely hearing-impaired children.

The Telephone

Many parents like their hearing-impaired children to be able to use
the telephone and there are now more facilities available to make this
possible. British Telecom provide details of specialised telephones and

equipment which can be used in conjunction with the telephone to aid the hearing-impaired.

Amplifying Handset. A handset which contains a transistorised amplifier replaces the normal telephone handset. The sound in the earpiece can be increased from normal by turning a volume control on the side of the earpiece. This may be of some use particularly to children with partial hearing loss who may choose to use the system with or without their hearing aid, although it is fair to say that users find it difficult to use in conjunction with their body aid since the handset needs to be held near the chest. Background noise around the telephone, however, will be a problem and non hearing-impaired users need to beware when they pick up the handset that the volume has not been left on full.

Inductive Coupler. Inductive couplers are devices that attach to the handset of the telephone. They produce a strong localised magnetic field around the handset in response to the incoming signals (much like the loop system described earlier). The hearing aid user sets the aid to the T position, hence overcoming the problem of background noise around the telephone. The inductive coupler can be either built into the handset or, where the user needs to use several different telephones in the course of the day, it can be attached on the outside of the handset – held on by an elastic strap (see Figure 7.15).

Handset with a Visual Call Indicator. A handset which incorporates a volume control in the side of the earpiece for increasing the level of the incoming signal and a neon lamp in the coupler can be fitted if required.

Extension Bells. A range of extension bells can be obtained which may aid the hearing-impaired to hear the call alarm.

Loudspeaking Telephones. These devices remove the need to hold the telephone handset. The call is reproduced via a loud speaker and may therefore be more easily received by certain hearing-impaired users.

Viewdata Services

Both the television companies (BBC and ITV) and British Telecom now provide television text in the form of pages of information, each page being selected by the user which is then displayed on the television screen. BBC's Ceefax and ITV's Oracle contain information on wide

Figure 7.15: A telephone induction coupler (Rastronics TA 80).

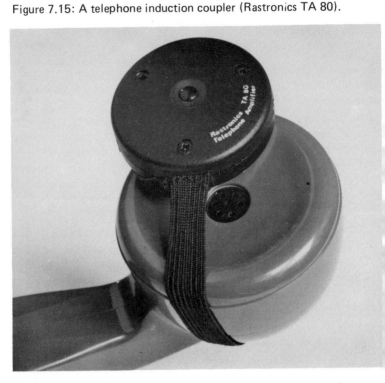

ranging topics — news and current affairs as well as matters relating to specific programmes. As the information is presented visually it is of particular interest to the hearing-impaired. The television text is generated or transmitted through the air with the television pictures. It cannot be displayed on the television set until the set is modified by fitting with a decoder. The page selector is a small keyboard or keypad which looks like a pocket calculator operated either by remote control or via a lead to the set.

The British Telecom viewdata service is called Prestel. It is effectively a giant in comparison to the television viewdata — being generated by a central computer containing many thousands of pages of information (Ceefax and Oracle are a few hundred pages in size). However, the Prestel system does not come through the air but down the telephone line and on to a 'Prestel television' set. One important point of note is that once a Ceefax-Oracle decoder has been bought and fitted the service is free other than the cost of the television licence. The Prestel system is not free, the user must pay — much like using the phone for a call — the user effectively calls up the computer. The present-day cost of a Prestel system is very high and in addition 'line time' must also be paid for. However, there are grounds for optimism in that as demand for new systems grows, costs (as with video) tend to come down. Further details on Prestel may be obtained from local British Telecom offices and by obtaining the booklet, *Teletext and Prestel*, from the RNID.

Perhaps the most useful form of special help via the television at present is the provision of subtitling for ordinary programmes. These are displayed rather like subtitles on foreign-language films. This is currently only carried out on a relatively limited scale. It takes approximately two days of a person's time to subtitle a half-hour programme though experiments are underway with synchronous subtitling as was used at the wedding of the Prince of Wales and Lady Diana Spencer.

The BBC and the RNID co-operated in a joint scheme to distribute summaries of BBC television programmes to hearing-impaired people. The service covers drama serials and one-off plays for adults and occasionally situation comedy. The summaries are written from programme scripts.

A useful directory of suppliers of auxiliary aids for the hearing-impaired is presented in the article by Tucker and Nolan (1983).

References

Borrild, K. (1978) 'Classroom acoustics' in M. Ross and T. Giolas (eds.), *Auditory Management of Hearing-Impaired Children*, University Park Press, Baltimore

Bruel and Kjaer (B&K) (1979) *Architectural Acoustics,* B&K Labs, Denmark

Bruel and Kjaer (B&K) (1982) *Noise control,* B&K Labs, Denmark

Ever Ready (1980) *Modern Portable Electricity*, the Ever Ready Company, London

Fulbeck, C.J.E., Nolan, M. and Powell, C.A. (1979) 'Battery use in hearing aids', *Journal of British Assoc. Teachers of the Deaf, 3(2)*, 30

Gengel, R. (1971) 'Acceptable speech to noise ratios for aided speech discrimination by the hearing impaired', *Journal of Auditory Research, 11*, 219

Gengel, R. and Faust, K. (1975) 'Some implications of listening level for speech recognition by sensori-neural hearing impaired children', *Language and Hearing Services in Schools, 6*, 14

Hawkins, D.B. and Van Tasell, D.J. (1982) 'Electroacoustic characteristics of personal FM systems', *Journal of Speech and Hearing Disorders, 47*, 335

Huntington, A. (1976) 'Tests on induction loops in current use in schools for the deaf', *Teacher of the Deaf, 74*, 7

International Electrotechnical Commission (1975) *Methods of Measurement of Characteristics of Hearing Aids with Induction Pick-up Coil Input*, IEC 118-1, Geneva

International Electrotechnical Commission (1978) *Magnetic Field Strength in Induction Loops*, IEC 118-4, Geneva

International Electrotechnical Commission (1979) *Methods of Measurement of Electroacoustical Characteristics of Hearing Aids – Hearing Aid Equipment not Entirely Worn on the Listener*, IEC, 118 Part 3, Geneva

John, J.E.J. (1957) 'Acoustics in the use of hearing aids' in A.W.G. Ewing (ed.), *Educational Guidance and the Deaf Child*, Manchester University Press, Manchester

Ling, D. (1964) 'Implications of hearing aid amplification below 300cps', *Volta Review, 66*, 723

Markides, A., Huntingdon, A. and Kettley, A. (1980) 'Comparative speech discrimination abilities of hearing-impaired children achieved through infrared radio and conventional aids', *Journal of British Assoc. Teachers of the Deaf, 4(1)*, 5

Martin, M.C. and Lodge, J.J. (1969) 'A survey of hearing aids in schools for the deaf and partially hearing units', *Sound, 3*, 2

Nolan, M. (1977) 'The performance of a wide range of hearing aids', *Journal of British Assoc. Teachers of the Deaf, 2(3)*, 98

Nolan, M. (1979) 'Subminiature receivers for use with DHSS call off contract body worn hearing aids', *Journal of British Assoc. Teachers of the Deaf, 2(3)*, 98

Nolan, M. (1980) 'Battery use in hearing aids'. Paper presented at British Society Audiology Meeting, Manchester

Nolan, M. (1982a) 'The method of evaluating hearing aids for infants'. Paper presented at the Conference of Heads of Schools and Services for the Hearing Impaired, Department of Audiology and Education of the Deaf, University of Manchester, Manchester

Nolan, M. (1982b) 'Hearing aids for children', *Journal of British Assoc. Teachers of the Deaf, 6(5)*, 118

Nolan, M. (1983) 'Radio hearing aid systems', *Journal British Assoc. Teachers of the Deaf, 7(4)*, 105

Nolan, M. and Tucker, I.G. (1981) *The Hearing Impaired Child and the Family*, Human Horizon Series, Souvenir Press, London

Philips (1982) *Batteries in Hearing Aids*, Product Information Services Hearing Aids, Philips, Eindhoven

Powell, C.A. (1975) 'The ergonomic design of hearing aids for children', International Congress on Education of the Deaf, Tokyo

Powell, C.A. (1982) Private communication

Royal National Institute for the Deaf (1980) 'Design of educational facilities for the deaf children', *British Journal of Audiology*, Supplement no. 3

Ross, M. (1977) 'Classroom amplification' in W. Hodgson and P. Skinner (eds.), *Hearing Aid Assessment and Use in Audiologic Habilitation*, Williams and Wilkins, Baltimore, pp. 221-43

Ross, M. and Giolas, T. (1971) 'Effect of three classroom listening conditions on speech intelligibility', *American Annals of the Deaf, 116*, 580

Ross, M., Giolas, T. and Carver, P. (1973) 'Effect of three classroom listening conditions on speech intelligibility: A replication in part', *Speech Hearing Service in Schools, 4*, 72

Schmaehl, O. (1958) 'The use and benefits of hearing aids in german schools for the deaf', *The Modern Educational Treatment of Deafness*, Manchester University Press, Manchester

Siemens Hearing Instruments 'Mono Infra-red System', Phonophore Acoustics, Aylesbury, Bucks

Siemens Hearing Instruments 'Stereo Infra-red Auditory Training System', Phono-

phore Acoustics, Aylesbury, Bucks
Tucker, I.G. and Nolan, M. (1983) 'Auxiliary aids for the hearing-impaired', *Journal British Assoc. Teachers of the Deaf*, *7(5)*, 155

8 AID FITTING PROCEDURES AND AMPLI- FICATION REQUIREMENTS OF CHILDREN

Introduction

The optimum starting point of a habilitative programme for hearing-impaired infants is one where diagnosis is early and appropriate amplification is then provided. This should be the goal.

The programme, however, must be a team approach (Grammatico, 1975) involving teachers, parents and clinicians. It must be seen as an ongoing picture of the overall child being built up over a long period of time — from observation, assessment and interpretation.

When consideration is given, for example, to decisions on amplification for a young hearing-impaired child, such decisions will be based on measurement, clinical interpretations and compromise — and these decisions are obviously open to modification as more information becomes available.

There are numerous issues with respect to wearable amplification for hearing-impaired children which are controversial (Rubin, 1975; Ross, 1975; Matkin, 1981) but there does seem to be universal agreement upon (i) the importance of maximum utilisation of residual hearing regardless of the prevailing educational philosophy, and (ii) its provision as early as possible.

Although no one would dispute the need for the optimum starting point for a habilitative programme this is no guarantee of success in the long term. If professionals are to have any chance of achieving success they must provide the family unit with appropriate and effective support, guidance and counselling. Professionals must never underestimate the importance of the parents' role in the successful application of the habilitative programme. As Madell (1975) stated 'Kids do better when their aids are working'. As parents are the ones who will have to fit and carry out day-to-day management of hearing aids, it is obvious that they need to be motivated, assisted and trained to do this — and convinced of its importance. The most frustrating aspect of hearing aid provision for young children is not being able to quantify the accuracy of the decisions taken.

It is worthwhile summarising a number of salient points in relation to hearing aid selection and provision for young children. These will be developed subsequently.

Jobs to be Done, Points to be Noted by the Audiologist

1. Identify hearing loss across frequency, that is, obtain an audiological data base — develop testing strategies as the child matures.

2. Instigate investigations into the child's upper tolerance limit (UTL) or loudness discomfort level (LDL).

3. Realise that the hearing aid performance data as reported for the 2 cc coupler (that is, gain, frequency response and range, maximum power output) is not representative of that received by a child wearing the aid (Dalsgaard and Jensen, 1976). The effects of the child's earmould, his head and body and his ear canal will result in significant differences between the real ear and coupler performance. The most meaningful way of measuring real ear hearing aid performance is on the child.

4. Begin investigations as to the performance of the hearing aid when worn by the child (that is, obtain a 'real ear' data base).

5. This 'real ear' data base may take time to build up. There may therefore be a need to provide a hearing aid on the basis of the available audiological data using a prescriptive procedure, which takes some account of real ear versus 2 cc coupler differences, although this will be very approximate (that is, from the available audiological information select an aid on the basis of its 2 cc coupler response).

6. Have a clear understanding of what one is trying to achieve with a hearing aid fitting. In our opinion, one is trying to furnish a hearing-impaired child with as wide and effective an experience of sound as possible. This should apply throughout the whole of the child's waking day. In having this aim there must be a realisation that the fitting of a hearing aid cannot be optimal for all communication distances, situations and environments. Initially we set out to furnish the child with a hearing aid that provides effective linguistic stimulation in favourable listening conditions. We must then seek to preserve the signal in relation to the noise in less favourable settings perhaps by use of educational amplification systems, so that we do maintain the quality of the speech input at a favourable level.

7. As speech is the input signal with which we are primarily concerned, it would seem sensible to consider any research evidence which is of relevance in relation to those components of the signal which influence speech intelligibility.

8. We must appreciate that the speech signal is a rapidly changing auditory input. It has time, frequency and intensity domains (that is,

it is in fact a speech spectrum). The normal human ear is tuned to receive the 'speech spectrum' at an optimal level. The time averaged sensation level (SL) of conversational speech (that is, level above threshold) varies across frequency. We should seek to preserve this relative frequency-intensity relationship when presenting amplified speech to the hearing-impaired ear. The overall presentation level should be at the most comfortable level for the user (MCL). It would obviously be hoped that this would also be as close as possible to the Optimum Listening Level (OLL).

9. We can estimate the sensation level (SL) of the speech signal by comparison of the unaided auditory thresholds in the free field with the 'real ear' sound level of the amplified speech signal. The SL may be manipulated by attention to the hearing aid and earmould characteristics.

10. Prescriptive approaches seek to achieve this goal without direct measurement (for example, with very young children, physical and mentally handicapped persons).

11. As children mature we seek to develop our knowledge on the effectiveness of the fitting by use of our ongoing parent-child interactive studies, speech discrimination testing with and without lip-reading (Markides, 1980a) both in quiet and in conditions of background noise. We employ 'speech babble' or 'cocktail party' noise (Nielsen, 1974) when doing these tests. We obviously develop our knowledge on residual hearing capacity.

12. The initial hearing aid provision should not be seen as necessarily being an absolute fitting. The aid must have built in flexibility so that, for example, manipulation of the frequency response and hence 'real ear' sensation level (SL) of the speech signal can be facilitated.

13. It is advisable to record all the information on hearing levels speech input, amplified speech level and loudness discomfort levels in dB SPL (re 20 μPa) rather than the audiometric dBHL format. This approach facilitates a more ready exchange of information on patient-hearing aid performance.

Audiological Information — Hearing Thresholds — Loudness Discomfort Levels

The information upon which early management is based is that related to the audiological picture of the child. It must be accurate because it will form the basis for hearing aid selection. It will also indicate whether any middle ear involvement is present. However, all children must be examined by an otologist prior to hearing aid fitting regardless of middle ear condition.

The aims of the diagnostic procedures should be: to quantify hearing across the speech frequencies; to assess middle ear function; and to instigate investigations into aetiology of the deafness. Once the diagnostic investigations have been applied and a hearing-impairment has been identified, then the procedures leading to the provision of amplification will begin. Herein lies the clinicians first problem – the wish to fit amplification as early as possible but at an early age being provided with limited information on auditory acuity across the speech frequency range. This information will undoubtedly be free field in nature, unless of course the diagnosis is very late or very early. Recall that children below the age of 30 months rarely carry out pure tone audiometry successfully.

The clinician responsible for hearing aid fitting will wish to develop a very thorough 'information base' on acuity across frequency. This will take time to achieve. More extensive tests than those employed in identification of the hearing-impairment may be necessary. For example, the free field measures could be extended to provide more frequency specific information by use of warble tone or narrow band noise stimuli. These measures would be applied using either distraction or performance format depending upon the age of the child. An intensity-amplitude function may be developed using BSER audiometry (Kiessling, 1982).

Investigations into the child's dynamic range of hearing must begin. This is often a very difficult area particularly with young children. The aim here is to find the child's usable range of hearing, that is, what is the range in decibels between the child's awareness of speech and his intolerance of speech (IDL). This information is required because children are not likely to adjust to amplification if the amplified sound proves to be an unpleasant experience. The maximum power output (MPO) of the aid must be limited so that it is below the child's upper tolerance limit. One approach at estimating upper tolerance levels is to look at the stapedial reflex to a speech spectrum noise (McCandless and Miller, 1972; McCandless, 1973). A narrow band noise centred around 500 Hz may be an alternative starting point. One must ensure however that the noise does not stray into the probe tone window of the impedance bridge as false reflexes (artefacts) may result. This reflex approach was advocated by McCandless – however, Northern (1978) has commented that it may not be of sufficient validity to be considered as a clinical procedure. It is, a method, however, that could be used as a starting point, particularly with uncooperative subjects. Unfortunately, many children do not exhibit reflexes due to the severity and/or pathology of deafness. Another approach is to use BSER audiometry and devise an intensity-amplitude function. This may not prove successful in more severe hearing-impairment (Kiessling, 1982).

Alternatively, the use of the Electroacoustic Approach to Hearing Aid Selection (Gengel *et al.*, 1971; Erber, 1971; Ross, 1975) may prove more fruitful. The method employed here involves use of an audiometer generating Narrow Band (NB) noise which is delivered to the ear via a high quality button earphone receiver connected to the child's earmould. This output channel from the audio-meter is often used together with an ear insert to facilitate masking in bone conduction audiometry. The signal level from the button receiver (dB SPL) must be measured in a 2 cc coupler, so that the audiometer attenuator dial readings equate with particular SPLs in the 2 cc coupler. This information is compared with the maximum output of the hearing aid when worn by the child, again as measured in a 2 cc coupler. As both measures will be affected by earmould and ear acoustics in the same manner the results may be directly compared.

To expand on the above:

1. The child must have his own earmoulds.
2. The button receiver is connected to the mould. If the mould is for a post-aural fitting then an adaptor will be required.
3. The NB noise should be set initially at 500 Hz (region where the maximum power of speech is located) and with an ascending method the child should be observed for his reactions to the increasing stimulus. (Increased in 5 dB steps, interrupted signals of 1 sec duration.)
4. Calibration charts should be available so that the attenuator dial of the audiometer is expressed in dB SPL developed in a 2 cc coupler when the earphone is linked to this coupler.

Two tables will be required, one for pocket aids and one for post-aural fittings – where the earphone connects to the 2 cc coupler via an adaptor and a standard length of plastic tubing (that is, as is used to connect a post-aural aid to a 2 cc coupler).
5. Having established an estimate of this LDL at one frequency repeat for 250, 1000 and 2000 Hz.
6. One may then proceed to measure the maximum power output (MPO) of a particular aid when worn by the child.

This is achieved by placing the aid on the child in the normal wearing position.

For pocket aids, the receiver should be connnected via the lead to a 2 cc coupler and sound level meter (held by an assistant). For post-aural aids the aid should be connected to the 2 cc coupler via the adaptor and plastic tube. The assistant will have to hold the sound level meter near the ear. The child should be positioned (perhaps on mother's knee) 1 m in front of a loudspeaker. The output of the aid should be monitored (dB SPL) for a 90 dB SPL input using NB noise at octave intervals 250 Hz to 2000 Hz. The use of the hand-held hearing aid tester (Jessops Acoustics) may prove valuable for this procedure.

7. A direct comparison between the child's LDL as expressed in dB SPL developed in a 2 cc coupler, and the MPO of the aid developed in a 2 cc coupler may now be made. The actual SPL in the child's ear canal will be unknown but this is unimportant with this approach.

As stated by Berger (1976) it is advisable to try and gradually build up a picture of tolerance limits over a wide range of frequencies (particularly 500-2000 Hz) so as to highlight any variations across frequency. This approach may take time and will inevitably be spread over a number of sessions. Some hearing-impaired children will show no observable signs of tolerance. This may be a function of the output capacity of the equipment and the degree of the impairment. However, despite such observations clinicians must work closely with parents and seek to obtain information on a child's reaction to everyday sounds when using hearing aids. A very useful check which we often make following aid fitting is to use the stimulus 'go' or 'ba' (Markides, 1980a) and observe the child as this is raised from a conversational level (65 dB SPL) to a level of very loud speech (90 dB SPL). Any signs of distress or reflex activity (APR) must be seen as an indication of too high an MPO from the hearing aid. We would concur with Byrne (1978) that the maximum power output (MPO) of a hearing aid should be set at least 30 dB above the child's threshold and 5 dB below the LDL. If the dynamic range is restricted to 25 dB or less, MPO should be set to a level equal to or just below the LDL. If a child has a much wider dynamic range than 40 dB then MPO may be set considerably below the LDL. Once a baseline on hearing threshold and possibly the upper tolerance limit has been established the question of suitable amplification must be considered.

The first question to resolve is what approach to use in arriving at the desired system. There are two possible approaches broadly defined under two headings: *selective* and *prescriptive*.

The *selective* or loaner model approach Zaner (1975) works on the principle whereby a number of possible aids (3 or 4) are chosen – issued in turn for a trial period (2 months) and compared. This approach is effectively the child version of an adult approach of Carhart (1946) where one applies specific comparative tests of discrimination ability with a number of aids. Doubt has been cast on the reliability of this method (Miller and Spring, 1956; Shore *et al.*, 1960).

As far as youngsters go the question clinicians must ask is: 'Can we determine "the aid" from observation – and what do we observe?'

A more practical approach is summarised by Zaner (1975) as 'finding audiological details you are confident about ... do the best job you can to match electroacoustically the needs of the youngster. Then put the hearing aid on and start working.' This approach and philosophy seems to be more akin to the procedure adopted in the UK. It is best described as a *prescriptive* procedure. (See Zelnick, 1982; Berger, 1976; Keith and Sininger, 1978; Lybarger, 1978 for a thorough discussion of both selective and prescriptive procedures.)

Prescription is, as a minimum, choosing a specific hearing aid for a particular loss on a deductive basis (Berger, 1976). The aim is one of issuing the child with an electroacoustic package that will provide optimum speech intelligibility. There have in fact been two main categories of prescription used in the provision of hearing aids for individuals. The first approach is concerned with the properties of the time averaged speech signal (that is, the intensity-frequency composition of speech and the relative importance of this spectral composition to speech intelligibility). The hearing aid parameters of gain, frequency range, and maximum output are selected so that the relevant components of the time averaged speech signal are reproduced at a comfortable level, while preserving as far as possible their relative sensation levels across frequency (Ross *et al.*, 1982). The second approach is predictive and is based on empirical findings related to the preferred gain settings of hearing-impaired subjects (mainly adults) across frequency in relation to their hearing-impairment as measured by conventional pure tone audiometry (Corell *et al.*, 1983).

The approach which seems most appropriate for application with the child user comes under the heading of the first category. However, we must add that a prescriptive approach based on a predictive formula (category two) may be necessary in cases where the audiological details are very limited. These will be expanded upon shortly.

The speech signal

The speech signal is a rapidly changing, wide ranging stimulus in time, frequency and intensity domains. The sounds of speech cover a frequency range of approximately 8000 Hz and have an intensity range of approximately 28 dB at each frequency. The intensity differences between the strongest and weakest components within the speech spectrum is approximately 50 dB. The stronger components are centred around 500 Hz and the overall intensity declines with an increase in frequency. Our ears are tuned to 'effectively amplify' these higher weaker components (see Chapter 1) resulting in the actual shape and sensation level at the eardrum being significantly different from that measured in the free field. Figures 8.1 and 8.2 graphically display the frequency-intensity composition of free-field conversational speech and the relative intensities of the component sounds of spoken English (Ballantyne, 1960). It may be seen that the more powerful speech sounds lie below 1000 Hz and are vowel-like in nature. The speech information above 1000 Hz is far weaker in intensity terms and contains consonants, higher vowel formats and transitions. These particular sounds are critical for good speech intelligibility. It is of interest to note that the frequency region up to 500 Hz contains 60 per cent of the power of speech, while the region up to 1000 Hz contains 90 per cent. Yet for normally hearing individuals with normal language development this power contributes only 5 per cent to intelligibility in relation to 500 Hz and 40 per cent to intelligibility in relation to 1000 Hz (Gerber, 1974). Taken another way, the frequency band between 500 and 4000 Hz contains 40 per cent of the power and contributes 94 per cent to intelligibility. It is very desirable therefore, when furnishing a hearing-impaired child with amplified speech, to ensure that every effort is made to facilitate effective amplification — particularly above 1000 Hz. Usually, there is little difficulty in providing sufficient amplification below this frequency — more often than not the danger is one of overemphasis, particularly below 500 Hz. While one cannot draw absolute conclusions from such studies on the importance of speech sounds and their influence on speech intelligibility for the hearing-impaired, one must nevertheless take note of the findings and strive to provide children with as wide a linguistic experience as is possible. The 30 dB range in intensity at each frequency between strongest and weakest components of speech serves as our target sensation level when aiding hearing-impaired children (Huntington, 1975).

Figure 8.1: The frequency components of English speech sounds.

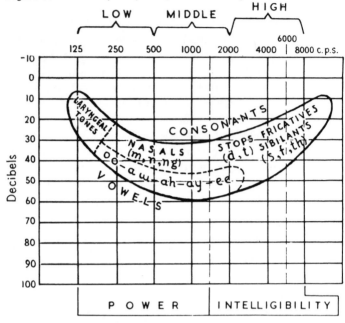

Source: after Ballantyne, with permission.

Figure 8.2: The relative intensities of English speech sounds.

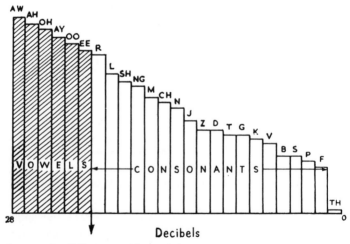

Source: after Ballantyne, with permission.

The Preliminary Considerations – Features of the Components of the Speech Signal Influencing Intelligibility

Although all details of the relationship may not be clear the pattern of amplified sound reaching the ear of a hearing-impaired child bears some relationship to speech intelligibility. The important electro-acoustic dimensions and particularly their interaction in specific instruments have not been absolutely defined but some knowledge has been obtained from studies carried out on adults and children.

The prescriptive approach whereby the clinician decides upon an electroacoustic package for the child will be a function of the available audiological information and a knowledge of the most salient perceptual cues in the auditory signal.

A number of studies have highlighted certain electroacoustic characteristics of the processed speech signal which have been shown to improve intelligibility for adults. The problem which has not been clearly resolved is whether these factors are as significant to congenitally deaf children who are using this signal to develop speech and discrimination ability, as has been found to be the case with adults who are recognising speech they already know. A number of authors working with very young hearing-impaired children appear to believe that such factors are indeed significant and work accordingly (Ross, 1975; Matkin, 1981; Rubin, 1975; McCandless, 1975).

Work by Danaher *et al.* (1973), Villchur (1973) and Sung *et al.* (1971) draw attention to the upward spread of masking and/or temporal masking effects resulting in poorer auditory discrimination of severely deaf subjects with a wide frequency range of residual hearing when an extended low frequency amplification system is employed (down to 100 Hz). The presence of a low frequency first formant interfered with the perception of higher frequency weaker second formant transitions. This type of system (VLF aid) was developed for those children with slash audiograms and research has indicated that such provision does often result in better development of basic receptive and expressive communication skills with such children (Ling, 1964; Rhis, 1980; Rowland, 1980; Matkin, 1981). Pitch, inflection and speech rhythms are reported as factors of importance. Success in our own department has been noted too. However, such systems must facilitate a favourable signal-to-noise ratio to be effective. What is perhaps most important in this context is that we must try to avoid overemphasis of the low frequencies, but without depriving the children of all experience of low frequencies.

A point of interest is what to do about severely deaf children who have residual hearing across to 4000 Hz. From the available findings it would seem sensible to consider fitting such children with a power aid having a conventional 300 Hz-4000 Hz response, provided that it can be demonstrated that useful residual hearing above 1 kHz is being utilised. It must be noted that the earmould can have a considerable influence here as was noted by Huntington (1979) and Nueva Espania (1980). Use of aided threshold measures is therefore valuable in exploring this matter.

Studies on extending the high frequency end of the spectrum have indicated an enhancement in discrimination ability although this has not been widely taken up by manufacturers (Watson, 1960; Olsen, 1971; Pascoe *et al.*, 1973; Triantos and McCandless, 1974). However, clinicians can themselves attempt to extend high frequency performance as described earlier (for example, earmould plumbing).

Watson's (1960) study on children does highlight the importance of high-fidelity amplification and emphasises the importance and benefits afforded by auditory training units and group hearing aid systems. It is disturbing to observe the apparent demise of auditory training units and group hearing aid systems particularly when the results of Watson (1960), and more recently Markides *et al.* (1980) are considered. We recommend the use of such systems with all our severely and profoundly hearing-impaired children.

Prescriptive Approaches

A considerable number of prescriptive approaches which lead to the determination of the required electroacoustic package (frequency response and maximum output) have appeared.

Basically these procedures require an input of information on factors such as auditory thresholds, dynamic range of hearing, preferred listening levels, loudness discomfort levels — and suggestions on a desired electroacoustic package appear at the output end based on the particular researcher's findings and hypothesis. The clinician then seeks to find a hearing aid to match the package.

The problem with young children is one of very limited information on which to operate. The aim of fitting is one of providing the child with an experience of language, that is, of the sounds of speech, and therefore the aim is to present speech at a level that is both comfortable and wide ranging in frequency content.

When a consideration of these various approaches to prescription is made, it is soon obvious that one is often functioning on a minimum of information with young children. Hence the need for seeing provision of hearing aids as an ongoing team effort.

It is important not to lose sight of the fact that prescriptive approaches have to be applied with some degree of compromise. The range of aids available are not infinite and the final prescription will be determined to some degree by what is available. The maximum power output (MPO) facility is not an issue of compromise, however. The road to follow in prescription will be a function of the information available and the ability of the child to participate in other electroacoustic measures. In cases where information on threshold is limited and the child is not going to be able to further the clinician's data base at that time, then a prescriptive approach based on a predictive procedure must be applied. In other words from an input of the child's known data base, the prescriptive procedure will indicate the desired 2cc coupler maximum gain performance of the hearing aid across frequency. Maximum gain is chosen because it is a readily obtainable parameter. It is to be anticipated that a child would not need to use a hearing aid at maximum gain setting. An additional 10dB gain factor is included in these procedures so as to take account of this point. It is important to note that the frequency response of a hearing aid when worn by a child will not be the same as indicated by the 2cc coupler. There will be significant differences between them which will vary as a function of frequency and the type of hearing aid employed (Dalsgaard and Jensen, 1976). The prescriptive methods of Byrne and Tonisson (1976) and Berger (1976) do attempt to take some account of real ear-2cc coupler differences – a different prescriptive formula being applied depending on the type of aid desired (that is, pocket or post-aural). However, while the 2cc coupler gain performance of the aid thought to be suitable will include a factor to take account of these differences it must be appreciated that this can be seen as nothing other than an approximation. This is a direct result of the known differences between individual real ears. This is why both of the above authors express the need for determination of the 'real ear' performance of the aid when fitted – obviously something that will take time with very young children.

An alternative 'formula' approach which was specifically developed for use with children is that of Powell and Tucker (1976). In this approach consideration is given not only to degree of loss but also to aetiology of deafness – the method indicating a desired output (dB SPL) from the hearing aid for a conversational speech level input.

It is perhaps worth noting the following points in relation to these 'paper-pencil' approaches to the required electroacoustic package. The information on hearing levels of the child (if measured free field) must be expressed relative to the normal threshold of hearing rather than in dB SPL. This can be achieved by simple subtraction of the normal unaided free field thresholds (for the test rig) from the child's unaided thresholds.

In cases where the data base is stronger and the child is able to co-operate in more detailed investigations, then the prescriptive approach, where a consideration of the long-term average speech spectrum and its relation to aided and unaided thresholds, should be made. The basic aim in this procedure, that has evolved from the work of Booth royd (1968), Gengel *et al*. (1971), Erber (1973), Ross (1975), Huntington (1975), Byrne and Tonisson (1976) and Nolan (1977) is to arrive at an aid fitting by consideration of the sensation level (SL) of speech across frequency. Sensation level (SL) is by definition the number of decibels that the stimulus exceeds threshold. For example:

Threshold (dB SPL)	= 85
Aided speech level (dB SPL)	= 100
Therefore sensation level	= 100 − 85 = 15 dB

The approach in this procedure is outlined as follows (recall that LDL measures will have already been investigated).

1. All measures are made free field and are recorded in dB SPL.
2. Unaided thresholds (for example, for warble tones) are recorded using either distraction or performance format.
3. A decision is taken as to type of aid to be fitted (that is, post-aural or pocket).
4. An aid is provisionally selected on the basis of 'paper-pencil' approach and fitted. With older children the child would be asked to adjust it to the most comfortable level. With youngsters the level should be set by the clinician. Aided thresholds are then measured for monaural listening.
5. The difference between aided and unaided thresholds is a measure of real ear gain of the aid.
6. The amplified level of the speech signal may now be estimated by addition of gain to the long-term average conversational speech spectrum signal (for example, Pascoe, 1978; Huntington, 1975).

7. A comparison of this amplified speech level with unaided thresholds provides a measure of speech sensation level across frequency.

8. A consideration of this level in relation to the child's dynamic range of hearing, the normal relative SL across frequency (Ross *et al.*, 1982), and of those factors in the spectrum that are important to speech intelligibility are vital when deciding whether the fitting is satisfactory. Manipulation of gain and/or tone controls may be necessary with youngsters.

9. We must ensure that the child is given as wide an exposure to sounds as speech as possible. The target sensation level should include consideration of the 30 dB intensity range of speech at each frequency and of course the child's dynamic range of hearing.

10. If the fitting is not satisfactory then an alternative aid must be assessed.

11. If the fitting is satisfactory then binaural aided thresholds would be applied. As the thresholds will improve under binaural listening (~3 dB; Byrne, 1981) manipulation of gain control may be considered necessary.

In the example shown in Table 8.1 it was concluded that aid A was unsuitable for the child on the grounds of too much low frequency amplification and totally inadequate gain in the frequencies above 1000 Hz. Aid B was an improvement in that the speech SL was more in line with that desired, that is, a closer match to the normal relative SL (Ross *et al.*, 1982), although performance at 4000 Hz was still relatively poor. This factor was related to the child's earmould bore diameter and in view of the ear size nothing could be done at the time to widen it. The aid output was such that there was sufficient room in the dynamic range of hearing to accommodate the amplification of raised speech sounds and environmental noise without danger of exceeding LDL. Output limitation was facilitated by peak clipping. It was considered that the child was being furnished with satisfactory amplification.

While the prescriptive approach, where a consideration of the long-term average speech spectrum and its relation to unaided and aided thresholds, is a technique that is applied in many centres throughout the world, it is worth noting that it is fraught with pitfalls.

One drawback of all approaches where consideration of a speech spectrum is concerned is that use is made of a long-term average speech spectrum (in 1/3 octave bands) (see Byrne, 1977). Individual speaker's long-term speech spectra can differ from the 'norm' and it would seem to be desirable to consider measuring the speech spectrum of the young child's parents — who will after all be the primary source of input early on in life — matching to this rather than the norm could then occur.

Table 8.1: Consideration of hearing aid provision in the light of the speech spectrum.

Aid A	Frequency (Hz)				
	250	500	1000	2000	4000
Mode					
unaided (dB SPL)	70	75	65	70	75
aided (dB SPL)	20	20	25	45	70
gain (dB)	50	55	40	25	5
speech input (dB SPL)	60	60	50	50	45
speech output (dB SPL)	110	115	90	75	50
sensation level (SL) (dB)	40	40	25	5	−25
LDL (dB SPL)	115	120	120	120	120
approx normal speech sensation level (SL) (dB)	50	60	55	60	60

Aid B	Frequency (Hz)				
Mode					
unaided (dB SPL)	70	75	65	70	75
aided (dB SPL)	40	40	25	20	30
gain (dB)	30	35	40	50	45
speech input (dB SPL)	60	60	50	50	45
speech output (dB SPL)	90	96	90	100	90
sensation level (dB)	20	20	35	30	15
LDL (dB SPL)	115	120	120	120	120
approx normal speech sensation level (SL) (dB)	50	60	55	60	60

Other Considerations Related to Hearing Aid Provision

Before the aided thresholds are applied it will be important to give due consideration to a number of matters.

Dynamic Range

The average intensity of conversational speech is 65 dB SPL and loud speech averages 75 dB SPL. Within each of these levels individual speech sounds have a range of approximately 28 dB. If children are to receive the range of speech sounds associated with normal and raised speech signals (on which older children probably set their aids) above their hearing thresholds, they will need a dynamic range of hearing of 40 dB. Such children should be able to use hearing aids with output limitation facilitated by peak clipping. If the dynamic range is reduced, it is advisable to consider a form of compression amplification so that excessive distortion as a result of clipping does not result and/or weaker speech sounds are not lost. Basically this approach attempts to squeeze the speech signal into the usable window of hearing — providing experiences of the weaker consonants while avoiding excessive overload from the more powerful vowels.

It is our belief that there are children with 'too narrow' a window of hearing using hearing aids with inappropriate maximum power output and inappropriate limitation systems. Such children 'set' the gain of their aids for comfort from the more powerful low frequency signals and as a result miss out on the higher frequency weaker sound information because gain is linear until MPO is reached. The use of aided versus unaided thresholds for narrow speech bands may highlight this problem (Christen and Byrne, 1980). Similar comments apply where over-amplification of the low frequency region occurs, because the child will set his aid to make such sounds comfortable and as a result will lose out on high frequency amplification.

Body Worn or Post-aural Type Amplification?

This question is certainly one that is controversial but really need not be if the position is considered carefully.

There are very real practical factors that influence hearing aid selection. As a point of information the advantages of post-aural fitting are a more natural sound field, with better performance in the mid/high frequency region of speech compared to a 2 cc coupler specification and hence an equivalent body aid (Byrne, 1976; Stacey, 1977; Dalsgaard and Jensen, 1976) while such factors such as clothes' rub, body worn weak spots of lead, receiver, microphone-controls susceptible to food-drink damage, localisation (Markides, 1978) and associated binaural fitting effects are additional benefits.

Contra-indications to post-aural fitting relate to the degree of loss and the effective usable gain of the aid, an extended good low frequency performance for very deaf slash audiogram children, and the practical problems of coupling post-aurals to very young children.

No one would argue that the goal is post-aural provision but the under lying philosophy must be one of efficient and effective amplification There is little point in having a blanket post-aural provision unless one can efficiently fit all the children.

Considerations relating to body worn or post aural provision should include:

(a) type and degree of loss
(b) age of child
(c) parental situation (should not be a problem if good counselling is available)
(d) flexibility of aid (remember this is an ongoing team effort which may warrant change)
(e) general level of functioning of child
(f) additional handicap
(g) earmould service.

The local earmould service is a primary consideration with young children. The problems of and reasons for inadequate earmould provision have been described.

Electroacoustic Properties of the Hearing Aid

There will generally be some 'choice' in which particular package to go for. One should therefore think carefully and preselect candidates on the following basis:

1. Service history.
2. Technician familiarity.
3. Child orientation.
4. Flexibility — for example, use with a radio aid?
5. Internal signal-to-noise ratio. This should be 30dB down on the primary signal; checked by measurement at the proposed 'use gain' level as described earlier. (Random noise level in test box must be negligible.)
6. Harmonic distortion; this ought to be at least 20dB down on the primary signal. Checked as described earlier.
7. Ease of replacement.
8. Reliability.

Examples of this may be:

a) A child X for whom a moderate gain post-aural aid was considered appropriate — the question of which one to choose. When two aids both produced similar speech SL. Consideration of (i) top front microphone, and (ii) numbered volume control *may* be significant factors.

b) a child Y for whom high power pocket aid was considered appropriate. Factors of (a) output limitation facility, (b) distortion effects, (c) service and replacement facilities, and (d) flexibility may be of primary importance.

What has to be faced up to is the fact that hearing aids are not designed for children. When selecting, for example, post-aural hearing aids from a 'pool' of aids a consideration of the size, thickness of the package and child orientation is of primary importance because if ignored it may lead to inefficient use of amplification. Basically slimmer post-aural aids are required for children. This will prevent helix distortion and the 'lop ear' effect (Rubin, 1975). Some form of standardisation on audio input leads is also necessary. Perhaps as a starting point a body of professionals, parents and older children should produce guidelines on the design of hearing aids for children. This has occurred in the USA (1973) although without much effect. However, such guidelines could be incorporated into specifications for future aids.

During the time that the clinician is considering the question of suitable amplification for a child thought must also be given to other factors which are of prime importance.

Binaural or Monaural Fitting?

The question of issuing a child with one or two hearing aids requires clarification. A considerable amount of research has been applied to this question (see Markides, 1977; Byrne, 1981; Yonovitz, 1974). Work has been carried out with adults and children and the results indicate that there are advantages in fitting two hearing aids in terms of better discrimination ability in noise (although this may be minimal in very poor conditions), localisation ability for both body and post-aural provision and binaural summation effects. It may be difficult to quantify a binaural advantage with infants but the procedure of fitting binaurally should be applied where practically possible. The possible problem of loss of localisation ability through lengthy delay in binaural fitting (Beggs and Foreman, 1980) and auditory deprivation effects (Webster and Webster, 1977) are noted by Byrne (1981) as additional good reasons for a binaural fitting.

There may be cases, however, where such a fitting is not desirable. Such situations will be deduced from observation of the patient or determined on initial examination.

One important point of note with respect to binaural amplification relates to the fact that by definition each ear is supplied with acoustic information by a transducer spatially separated from that supplying the other ear.

In order to capitalise on the advantages that binaural amplification has on localisation ability (see Markides, 1981) and hence develop and extend a child's acoustic environment it is desirable to ensure that the signals delivered to each ear are presented homolaterally.

The technique of criss-cross or contralateral routing of signal in order to increase usable gain before feedback should not be employed, because of the known deleterious effects on localisation ability. In other words contralateral routing of signals should not be seen as a means of overcoming inefficient earmould provision.

Acoustic Environment

It is important to determine what environment the child will be in during his working day. Such information could have a significant influence on hearing aid provision. Many studies have highlighted the effects of noise and reverberation on the performance of a subject with sensori-neural deafness. The effects on receptive linguistic competence are more marked than would be the case for normally hearing individuals.

John (1957) has recommended reverberation times of no more than 0·5 sec for education and work by Tillman *et al*. (1970), Gengel (1971) and Ross (1972) have highlighted the effects of background noise. A $20\,dB^{+}$ S/N ratio is desirable. This can be achieved in a lounge but certainly not in a nursery or play group situation. For these reasons the use of a radio hearing aid system should be considered.

Deterioration in Hearing

The question of deterioration in hearing as a result of high levels of amplification is open to debate (Markides, 1971). However, it seems unreasonable to deny a child an experience of language, at an age when he is at optimum for development, because this *may* result in further deterioration in hearing. After all what is the residual hearing for if it is not to provide linguistic experience? A closely monitored fitting with ongoing audiological observation is desirable for all children using hearing aids. If any indications of further deterioration are observed, investigations into the cause should be carried out.

Reilly *et al.* (1981) suggest that in any such cases an examination for temporary threshold shift as a result of amplification should be made. If found this should alert the clinician to the need for reducing the MPO of the system employed. Alternating a monaural fitting is also useful in such cases. It should be noted, however, that the progression in hearing loss is often not a direct result of use of the hearing aid.

Effective Fitting

It is inspiring for both professionals and parents to observe clear evidence of the effectiveness of amplification. This does not necessarily come from language development early on in the fitting, but, for example, in:

(i) the child clearly disliking having to take his aids out — must go to sleep in them;
(ii) the child very, very reluctant to remove aids for testing;
(iii) the child with a partial hearing problem who simply says 'all gone' when the aids are removed (Nolan, 1981).

These and other observations, such as understanding of little commands, a responsiveness to environmental sounds, and an improved awareness of the environment in general terms, are factors that clinicians in their ongoing management should be looking for in addition to the progress in expressive language.

Management Procedures

The provision and fitting of a hearing aid is only a starting point. Clinicians must not sit back for this is when the work really starts if they are going to be able to evaluate the success of the fitting and add to the knowledge of hearing aid provision and its association with linguistic development.

As a starting point all clinicians must convince the parents of the importance of efficient and effective amplification.

The use of tapes highlighting common faults has far more impact than simply talking in descriptive terms. Application of a confident, workmanlike yet supportive approach is desirable. Professionals must ensure that:

1. The parents are first and foremost aware of the necessity and importance of their child using a hearing aid.
2. They can after a period of training become competent in developing and applying fitting, checking and maintenance procedures with the child's aids.
3. They act quickly when action is needed to keep the system in a state of maximum effectiveness.

The professional should supply the parent with:

(a) a complete spare aid of the same type as is being used;
(b) a comprehensive stock of spares including batteries with changing guidelines, cords of child length, receivers of the required type (Nolan and Tucker, 1981; Shaw, 1983; Nolan, 1978, 1982; Nolan *et al.*, 1981);
(c) good earmoulds for the child (Nolan, 1978);
(d) a routine monthly specification check of the aid on a hearing aid test box;
(e) stetoclip or earmould for the parent.

As part of the peripatetic kit the professional should have access to:

(a) a portable test box;
(b) tapes of common faults on aids;
(c) a portable impedance bridge;
(d) facilities for providing parents with literature on fault finding procedures, explanation of the hearing aid, information on battery changing, etc.
(e) A log of the day-to-day use of the hearing aid compiled in conjunction with parents including details on faults and their remediation. Such information would be of great value in the long term to the management team.
(f) Developmental schedules as discussed elsewhere in the book are also very important.

The importance of knowing the condition of the child's conductive pathway cannot be overemphasised. Problems will arise with a child's receptive ability when there is a deterioration in hearing as a result of a conductive overlay. Steps must be taken to spot and organise immediate medical intervention. One component of the peripatetic teachers visiting kit should be a screening tympanometer particularly in view of the relatively high incidence of middle ear disorder in youngsters (20 per cent) (Porter, 1974).

It is perhaps worth while noting that such occurrences can be spotted with some children because acoustic feedback becomes a problem. This results from the stiffening of the conductive pathway which reflects more sound — and is not as may be mistakenly assumed due to an ineffecient earmould.

The ongoing evaluation of the child's linguistic development will involve tests of speech discrimination — the test being appropriate to the language level *not* necessarily chronological age. These are best applied with the child aided in conditions which approximate the 'real world' situation.

The use of regular video sessions at intervals of two to three months is also a very valuable exercise from the professional and parental viewpoint. This is one way whereby parents can 'see' progress. It also permits a detailed investigation to be made into the developing interaction between parent and child.

The effective management of a hearing-impaired child does require a very comprehensive child oriented service. If there is to be an improvement upon the situation that has been in evidence for many years according to Sanders (1982) and Ross and Tomassetti (1980) — 'that many children are not using their residual hearing effectively' — it is imperative for parents, professionals and the child to work effectively in close liaison.

References

Ballantyne, J. (1960) *Deafness*, Churchill, London

Beggs, W.D.A. and Foreman, D.L. (1980) 'Sound localisation and early binaural experience in the deaf', *British Journal of Audiology*, *14(2)*, 41

Berger, K.W. (1976) 'Prescription of hearing aids: A rationale', *Journal American Audiology Society*, *2(3)*, 71

Boothroyd, A. (1968) 'The selection of hearing aids for children'. PhD thesis, University of Manchester, Manchester

Byrne, D. (1976) 'Letter to editor', *British Journal of Audiology*, *10(2)*

Byrne, D. (1977) 'The speech spectrum — some aspects of its significance for hearing aid selection and evaluation', *British Journal of Audiology*, *11(2)*, 40

Byrne, D. (1978) 'Selection of hearing aids for severely deaf children', *British Journal of Audiology*, *12(1)*, 9

Byrne, D. (1981) 'Clinical issues and options in binaural hearing aid fitting', *Ear and Hearing*, *2(5)*, 187

Byrne, D. and Tonisson, W. (1976) 'Selecting the gain of hearing aids for persons with sensori-neural hearing impairments', *Scandinavian Audiology*, *5*, 51

Carhart, R. (1946) 'Tests for selection of hearing aids', *Laryngoscope*, *56*, 780

Christen, R. and Byrne, D. (1980) 'Preferred listening levels for bands of speech in relation to hearing aid selection', *Scandinavian Audiology*, *9*, 3

Corell, I., Ludvigsen, C. and Birk Nielsen, H. (1983) 'Experiences with computer aided hearing and fitting', *Scandinavian Audiology*, *12(3)*, 151

Dalsgaard, S.C. and Jensen, O. (1976) 'Measurement of insertion gain of hearing aids', *Journal of Audiological Technique*, *15*, 171

Danaher, E.M., Osberger, M.J. and Pickett, J.M. (1973) 'Discrimination of formant frequency transitions in synthetic vowels', *Journal of Speech and Hearing Research*, *16*, 439

Downs, T.H. and Doster, M. (1959) 'A hearing test program for pre-school children', *Rocky Mountain Medical Journal*, *56*, 1

Erber, J.P. (1973) 'Body baffle and real-ear effects in the selection of aids for deaf children', *Journal of Speech and Hearing Disorders*, *38*, 224

Gengel, R.W. (1971) 'Acceptable speech to noise ratios for aided speech discrimination by the hearing impaired', *Journal of Audiological Research*, *11*, 219

Gengel, R.W., Pascoe, D. and Shore, I. (1971) 'A frequency-response procedure for evaluating and selecting hearing aids for severely hearing-impaired children', *Journal of Speech and Hearing Disorders*, *36*, 341

Gerber, S. (1974) *Introductory Hearing Science*, W.B. Saunders & Co., Philadelphia

Grammatico, L.F. (1975) *Hearing Aids Current Developments and Concepts*, M. Rubin (ed.), University Park Press, Baltimore, p. 134

Hieber-Finitzo, T., Gerling, I.J., Matkin, N.D. and Cherow-Skalka, E. (1980) 'A sound effects recognition test for the pediatric audiological evaluation', *Ear and Hearing*, *1(5)*, 271

Huntington, A. (1975) 'Selecting hearing aids for young children', *British Journal of Audiology*, *9*, 75

Huntington, A. (1979) 'How near is the end of feedback?', *Journal of British Association of Teachers of the Deaf*, *3(4)*, 123

John, J.E.J. (1957) *Educational Guidance and the Deaf Child*, A.W.G. Ewing (ed.), University of Manchester Press, Manchester

Keith, R.W. and Sininger, L. (1978) 'New ideas in hearing aid fitting', *Hearing Instruments*, June 1978

Kiessling, J. (1982) 'Hearing aid selection by brainstem audiometry', *Scandinavian Audiology*, *11(4)*, 269

Ling, D. (1964) 'Implications of hearing aid amplification below 33 cps.', *Volta Review*, *66*, 723

Ling, A.H. (1977) *Schedules of Development in Audition, Speech, Language, Communication, for Hearing Impaired Infants and Their Parents*, Alexander Graham Bell Association for the Deaf, Washington, DC

Lybarger, S.F. (1978) 'Selective amplification – A review and evaluation', *Journal of American Audiology Society*, *3(6)*, 258

McCandless, G.A. and Miller, D.L. (1972) 'Loudness discomfort and hearing aids', *National Hearing Journal*, *25(7)*, 28

McCandless, G.A. (1973) 'Hearing aids and loudness discomfort'. Paper presented at Oticongress 3, Copenhagen, Denmark, p. 39

McCandless, G.A. (1975) 'Special considerations in evaluating children and the aging for hearing aids' in M. Rubin (ed.), *Hearing Aids – Current Developments and Concepts*, University Park Press, Baltimore, p. 171

Madell, J.R. (1975) In M. Rubin (ed.), *Hearing Aids – Current Developments and Concepts*, University Park Press, Baltimore, p. 130

Markides, A. (1971) 'Do hearing aids damage the user's residual hearing?', *Sound*, *5(4)*, 99

Markides, A. (1977) *Binaural Hearing Aids*, Academic Press, London

Markides, A. (1978) 'Localisation of speech through similar and dis-similar binaural hearing and listening modes', *British Journal of Audiology*, *12(3)*, 65

Markides, A. (1980a) 'Best listening levels for children', *Journal of British Assoc. of Teachers of the Deaf*, *4(6)*, 190

Markides, A. (1980b) 'The Manchester speechreading (lipreading) test' in I.G. Taylor and A. Markides (eds.), *Disorders of Auditory Function 111*, Academic Press, London

Markides, A. (1981) 'Effect of homolateral and contralateral routing of signals through body worn hearing aids on the localisation ability of hearing impaired people', *Journal of British Association of Teachers of the Deaf*, *5(3)*, 68

Markides, A., Huntington, A. and Kettlety, A. (1980) 'Comparative speech discrimination of hearing-impaired children achieved through infra-red, radio and conventional hearing aids', *Journal of British Assoc. of Teachers of the Deaf*, *4(1)*, 5

Matkin, N.D. (1969) 'Analysis of a recorded test for the measurement of hearing in children' in *Final Report Project No. 8 – 0156*, BEH Grant No. OEG-0-8-080156

Matkin, N.D. (1981) 'Hearing aids for children' in W.R. Hodgson and P.H. Skinner (eds.), *Hearing Aid Assessment and Use in Audiologic Habilitation*, 2nd edn, Williams and Wilkins, Baltimore, Ch. 9, p. 171

Miller, W.H. and Spring, A.J. (1956) 'Variability of discrimination scores in clinical hearing aid selection'. Paper presented at the American Speech and Hearing Association Meeting, Chicago

Nielsen, T.E. (1974) *Hearing Aid Characteristics and Fitting Techniques for Improved Speech Intelligibility in Noise*, Oticon Technical Library Series, Copenhagen

Nolan, M. (1977) 'The performance of a wide range of hearing aids', *Journal of British Assoc. of Teachers of the Deaf*, *13*, 108

Nolan, M. (1978) 'Subminiature receivers for use with DHSS call of contract body worn hearing aids', *Journal of the British Assoc. of Teachers of the Deaf*, *2(3)*, 98

Nolan, M. (1981) 'Hearing aid seminar – Selecting hearing aids for young children'. Department of Audiology and Education of the Deaf, University of Manchester, Manchester

Nolan, M. (1982) 'Earmoulds – modern developments. Implications for the profoundly deaf'. Paper presented at the XVI International Congress of Audiology, Helsinki, Finland

Nolan, M. and Tucker, I.G. (1981) *The Hearing Impaired Child and the Family*, Human Horizon Series, Souvenir Press, London

Nolan, M., McArthur, K., Tucker, I.G. and Fulbeck, C. (1981a) *Hearing Aids*, National Deaf Children's Society, London

Nolan, M., Tucker, I.G., McArthur, K. and Fulbeck, C. (1981b) *Testing the Hearing of Young Children*, National Deaf Children's Society, London

Northern, J. (1978) 'Hearing aids and acoustic impedance measurements', *Contemporary Audiology*, p. 1 (monograph)

Nueva Espania, H. (1980) 'The influence of earmould characteristics on the frequency response of a hearing aid'. Unpublished MEd dissertation, Department of Audiology, University of Manchester, Manchester

Olsen, W.O. (1971) 'The influence of harmonic and intermodulation distortion on speech intelligibility', *Scandinavian Audiology Supplement*, *1*, 109

Pascoe, D.P. (1978) 'An approach to hearing aid selection', *Hearing Instruments*, *29(36)*, 12

Pascoe, D.P., Miemoeller, A.F. and Miller J.D. (1973) 'Hearing aid design and evaluation for a presbycusic patient'. 86th Meeting of the Acoustic Society of America

Porter, T. (1974) 'Oto admittance measurements', *American Annals of the Deaf, 119(1)*, 47

Powell, C.A. and Tucker, I.G. (1976) 'A method of predicting the optimum listening levels of hearing impaired children', *Scandinavian Audiology, 5*, 167

Redell, R.C. and Calvert, D.R. (1969) 'Factors in screening hearing of the newborn', *Journal of Auditory Research, 3*, 278

Reilly, K., Owens, E., Uken, D., McClathchie, A.C. and Clarke, R. (1981) 'Progressive hearing loss in children: Hearing aids and other factors', *Journal of Speech and Hearing Disorders, 46(3)*, 328

Rhis, A. (1980) 'The evaluation of hearing aids for the education of children who are hard of hearing'. Paper presented at XVIII National Hearing Aid Congress, Grenoble, France

Ross, M. (1972) 'Classroom acoustics and speech intelligibility' in J. Katz (ed.), *Handbook of Clinical Audiology*, Williams and Wilkins, Baltimore, p. 756

Ross, M. (1975) 'Hearing aid selection for the preverbal hearing impaired child' in M. Pollack (ed.), *Amplification for the Hearing-impaired*, Grune and Stratton Publications, New York

Ross, M. and Tomassetti, C. (1980) 'Hearing aid selection for preverbal hearing impaired children' in M.C. Pollack (ed.), *Amplification for the Hearing Impaired*, Grune and Stratton, New York, p. 213

Ross, M., Brackett, D. and Maxon, A. (1982) *Hard of Hearing Children in Regular Schools*, Prentice-Hall, New Jersey

Rowland, R.C. (1980) 'Very low amplification – 1980 update', *Hearing Instruments, 31(6)*, 24

Rubin, M. (1975) 'Hearing aids for infants and toddlers' in M. Rubin (ed.) *Hearing Aids – Current Developments and Concepts*, University Park Press, Baltimore, p. 95

Sanders, D.A. (1982) *Aural Rehabilitation – a Management Model*, 2nd edn Prentice-Hall, Englewood Cliffs, New Jersey

Shaw, D.A.J. (1983) 'Battery use in hearing aids'. Unpublished MEd dissertation, Department of Audiology, University of Manchester, Manchester

Shore, I., Bilger, R.C. and Hirsh, I.J. (1960) 'Hearing aid evaluation: reliability of repeated measurements', *Journal of Speech and Hearing Disorders, 25*, 152

Stacey, J. St G. (1977) 'Letter to editor', *British Journal of Audiology, 11(2)*, 63

Sung, G.C., Sung, R.J. and Angellei, R.M. (1971) 'Effect of frequency response characteristics of hearing aids on speech intelligibility in noise', *Journal of Auditory Research, 11*, 318

Tillman, T.W., Carhart, R. and Olsen, W.O. (1970) 'Hearing aid efficiency in a competing speech situation', *Journal of Speech and Hearing Research, 13*, 789

Triantos, T.J. and McCandless, G.A. (1974) 'High frequency distortion', *Hearing Aid Journal, 27(9)*, 38

Villchur, E. (1973) 'Signal processing to improve speech intelligibility in perceptive deafness', *Journal of Acoustic Society of America, 53*, 1646

Watson, T.J. (1960) 'Some factors affecting the successful use of hearing aids by deaf children' in *The Modern Educational Treatment of Deafness*, Manchester University Press, Manchester

Webster, D. and Webster, M. (1977) 'Neonatal sound deprivation effects on brain stem auditory nuclei', *Archives of Otolaryngology, 103*, 392

Yonovitz, A. (1974) 'Binaural intelligibility'. Paper presented at the ASHA meeting, Nevada, Speech and Hearing Institute, Houston, Texas

Zaner, A. (1975) 'Hearing aids for infants and children: non-instrumental selection criteria' in M. Rubin (ed.), *Hearing Aids – Current Developments and Concepts*, University Park Press, Baltimore, p. 109
Zelnick, E. (1982) 'Hearing aid selection', *Hearing Aid Journal*, February 1982, 29

9   THE DEVELOPING HEARING—IMPAIRED CHILD

In Britain the main system of communication used in the habilitation of hearing-impaired children is oral language, the language of society at large. This seems eminently logical to the present writers when a major tenet of habilitation is to help the disabled person to achieve a level of functioning which is as nearly as possible restored to normal. This is not the wish of all, and some adult deaf pressure groups are vociferous in their demands that the natural language of deaf people is sign language and that being happy, secure and communicating within a deaf sub-culture is a more desirable goal than assimilation into a hearing, talking society. The British Deaf Association are such a group, who have actively promoted the use of manual communication. They have done this through advertising and by publishing papers which support their views in their publication, *British Deaf News* (for example, Brennan, 1976; Evans, 1979). There is undoubtedly a need for a small number of children to be taught with assistance from manual signs and there is a need for adequate training of teachers to carry out this function. However, the situation of children in some of the residential special schools learning only from each other is to be deplored and has resulted in their 'manual literacy' (Murphy, 1976) being of a very variable standard. Hopefully research will address itself more specifically to the questions of 'which children?', 'at what age or stage?' and 'what type of language?'

The controversy about the *form* of communication (oral or manual) is compounded by controversy about the *type* of communication (British sign language or English) which should be used to educate hearing-impaired children (Quigley and Kretschmer, 1982). This controversy has raged for centuries and deserves some illumination for the educational audiologist who has to apply his skills within particular educational milieux. It is probably simplest to present the discussion in terms of languages which relate to English, that is, Oral English and Manual or Signed English and the separate and distinct language, British Sign Language (BSL) which does not follow the grammar of English (see Stokoe, 1960; Friedman, 1977; Siple, 1978; Klima and Bellugi, 1979; and Brennan, 1981).

314

British Sign Language (BSL)[1]

This is a mode of visual communication incorporating the national or regional signs used in Britain within a specific structure, recognised as a language in its own right (BATOD, 1981). In all parts of the world there is still argument as to whether it has developed to the state where it can fulfil all the educational functions of spoken languages. It is worth noting that there is no body of literature in this language as there is no written form to it. Makaton (see Walker, 1978) is a downward extension of BSL used primarily with mentally-handicapped children, but also with some hearing-impaired children.

Manual English

Manual English is the term which encompasses the variety of systems that use signs, fingerspelling, or gestures separately or in combinations to represent English manually, keeping word order and proper syntactic form (Quigley and Kretschmer, 1982).

Signed English

A system for representing the English language grammatically in a manual form, based on British regional and national signs and two-handed fingerspelling.

Fingerspelling

This is a manual alphabet which can be used to represent precise English syntax. The 26 different hand positions form the 26 letters of the English alphabet. The combinations of hand positions enable the formation of words or sentences.

Cued Speech

This is a one-handed supplement to lip-reading devised by Cornett

[1] For British you can read American (ASL) or any of the national languages associated with the deaf.

(1967) to clarify the phonemes of language that are ambiguous or invisible in lip-reading.

Paget Gorman Systematic Sign Language

This system devised by Sir Richard Paget and developed by Pierre Gorman and Grace Paget is designed to give a simultaneous grammatical representation of Spoken English for use as an aid to the teaching of language. It uses constructed signs and hand positions which differ from those used in BSL.

Signing Exact English (SEE)

This uses natural and invented signs to make ASL conform to the structure of English. Gustason *et al.* (1975) have suggested that SEE is composed of 61 per cent ASL signs, 18 per cent modified ASL signs and 21 per cent newly invented signs.

Signs Supporting English

This is used to assist oral communication and consists of signs for key words which would be used at appropriate points during utterances.

Oral English

There are two main forms of this approach used with hearing-impaired children to encourage them to develop spoken communication in the same way as normally hearing subjects.

The Auditory/Visual Approach

This stresses speech and speech-reading (including lip-reading) and places great emphasis on the use of residual hearing by means of amplification and auditory training.

The Acoupedic (Pollack, 1970) or Auditory/Oral Approach (Tucker, 1982)

In this approach no special emphasis is put on speech-reading and the major emphasis is put on using the child's residual hearing by applying as effectively as possible appropriate amplification. Within the oral approach teachers in the United Kingdom delineate two types, the first being structured oralism (Ingall, 1980) where teaching of language consists of planning highly structured thought-out sequences and involving the application of systematic intervention. Structuring would be applied to all aspects of language acquisition and specific training of speech may or may not be used. Natural gesture would be used but no other manual component.

The second type is natural oralism (Harrison, 1980) where guidance of parents and later teaching uses the same approach as that with normal children where language use is informal, speech-reading is as required by the child and not cultivated and the assumption is that language is caught not taught (Northcott, 1981). Language learning is taking place throughout the child's waking hours. Parents learn quite naturally to tune their use of language to the child's language level and the child learns the rules of language without them being made explicit and without the need for force or the use of drills.

Combination of the Above Methods. There are also systems whereby oral methods are combined with fingerspelling. One such is the Rochester Method. The combined use of manual communication (signs and fingerspelling) and oral methods used in English word order is known as the *simultaneous method.* The 'novel' term currently being used, *total communication*, is nothing new and could include any or all of the systems above. It appears to be essentially another name for a simultaneous method. Denton (1970) 'defined' total communication as:

> the right of a deaf child to learn to use all forms of communication available to develop language competence. This includes the full spectrum, child derived gestures, speech formal sign, fingerspelling, speech-reading, reading, writing, as well as other methods which may be developed in the future. Every deaf child should also be provided with the opportunity to learn to use any remnant of residual hearing he may have by employing the best possible electronic equipment for amplifying sound.

The Conference of Executives of American Schools for the Deaf defined total communication as 'a philosophy incorporating appropriate aural, manual and oral modes of communication with and among hearing-impaired persons'. This has resulted in some argument as to whether total communication is a philosophy or a method. Certainly if it is to be regarded as a method then practitioners would be forced to rationalise the multi-modal concept for application with children. Stimulus overload and asynchrony would be real problems. There is little doubt that in some special schools, particularly residential special schools, an approach which combines manual communication with oral communication has been in use for many decades.

How Has the Controversy About Communication Methodology Arisen?

The arguments are usually circular. Oralism was introduced because of the concern at very low standards of achievement and poor levels of social integration using manual approaches. The arguments about achievement are now being used by supporters of manualism for a return to that methodology.

Perhaps it would be helpful here to use numbers of hearing-impaired children in an exercise designed to assess the extent of a methodology controversy. In the United Kingdom there are approximately 37,000 hearing-impaired children of whom about 4000 are in special schools. The tendency is for the more severely impaired children to be placed in special schools and few would argue that the 26,000 children who are in ordinary schools (not even in special classes attached to ordinary schools) need to be taught via anything but oral language with varying amounts of support from specialist teachers. The controversy lies, for the most part, within the special schools where a very small percentage of the overall number of children with impaired hearing are actually placed. However, in some areas it seems that an audiometric approach is being used to select children for a total communication approach. We strongly object to approaches other than those related to child function being used and early hearing levels are not, in our opinion, sufficient ground for selection between approaches, so the controversy which sometimes takes on the picture of a huge split in the education of hearing-impaired children is not so.

There is disagreement about which deaf children within this relatively small proportion actually require a manual system, or an oral plus manual system (simultaneous or total communication). Most workers fortunately now agree that the selection of an arbitrary audiometric cut-off point is inadequate so it is not a simple matter of saying 80 dB loss or 90 dB or 100 dB means that the child will require a manual or a simultaneous means of communication. The present authors have experience of mainstreaming five year olds with audiometric hearing losses in excess of 100 dB. This indicates to us that functional considerations are far more important than audiometric values. A child needs most of all to be stimulated with a consistent and rich version of the language in use in the home. Rawlings and Jensema (1977) indicate that in the USA only 3 per cent of deaf children have two deaf parents with an additional 6 per cent having one deaf parent, so the *fluent* natural language of the home in over 90 per cent of cases is oral English. There are also to our personal knowledge deaf parents who strongly wish their child to be given the opportunity to develop oral language and we have, with families such as this, arranged for enhanced levels of interaction with hearing members of the family, early normal nursery placement with additional support and have been heartened by the oral progress of the children. There is no doubt that some of these children will have substantially better speech quality than their parents — parents who often have less hearing loss than the children! On the other hand we have supported hearing-impaired parents when they have wished to rear their children using British Sign Language and have ensured that the children have had the benefit of the best hearing aids currently available.

There is also controversy about whether the communication methodologies can be mixed. The Total Communication supporters would argue that they can, stating that they are only providing *more* information to an information-deprived child. There seems little doubt to us, however, that there are great problems with the total communication methodology when it is applied to children who could, if properly stimulated, develop spoken language. One major difficulty is the rate of articulation. In order to carry temporal and other prosodic cues which greatly help language learning the speech needs to be at a normal rate with normal interaction. Workers (Bellugi and Fischer, 1972; Marmor and Petitto, 1979) have reported that the rate for speech is approximately twice the rate for signs alone. This means that those using manual signs either have to speak very much slower or they have to miss out parts. Cokely and Baker, reported by Nix (1983) have suggested that skilled hearing simultaneous communication users decrease their speaking rate by 25 per cent. 'They were still speaking much faster than they were signing and deleting some important information from the signed portion.' Total communication requires *total synchrony* and total synchrony of manual signs and spoken language would seem to be impossible. Even with total synchrony some would argue that it would be impossible for the child's brain to abstract what is relevant.

In an Office of Demographic Studies investigation in the USA (Jensema and Trybus, 1978) it was found that a bewildering variety of methods were being used under the guise of total communication and that there was little consistency between schools and even less between schools and the home. One of the fundamentals of language learning is consistency of input. Only if the input is consistent can the child 'crack the code' of language. The most serious criticism of total communication is that in many of its forms it actually encourages inconsistent input to the child. The Jensema and Trybus research also indicated that where speech use is high, signing or fingerspelling use is low and vice versa. Latimer (1983), a total communication supporter, was appalled at the inadequate use of residual hearing and lack of care and application of hearing aids in many total communication pro- grammes. As Van Uden (1983) suggested after visiting establishments using total communication 'There was nothing total about the approach, it was just another term for the old manual communication.'

Sutcliffe (1983) has highlighted the fact that there are problems of pressure groups trying to encourage the use of British Sign Language with spoken language. As had already been suggested BSL is a language separate from spoken English. 'It is NOT English and does not use English words on the lips with English syntax. It has its own gram- matical structure' (Sutcliffe, 1983). It is therefore not possible for educators to use residual hearing and speech-reading with BSL since the two are separate languages and it is not possible to use two different languages simultaneously. Sutcliffe further argues that deaf adults who only use BSL for their everyday communication have long since aban- doned hearing aids and speech-reading.

In contrast to the United States the 'deaf community' in Britain is small and getting smaller as decline in population and changes in educational practice, with greater levels of integration, lead to there being fewer schools. Dispersal of the hearing-impaired population in this way can only serve to reduce still further the core of people who form the 'deaf sub-culture'. Interestingly some of the objections to the closure of special schools are made on 'cultural' rather than educational grounds, the special schools being regarded as being centres of 'deaf culture'.

The present writers believe that if a system of manual communica- tion is to be used to support the learning of spoken language then it must at least follow the grammar of English. The decision to use manual assistance to oral English is a very important decision and should be a joint one of educators of the deaf and parents. The child should still be provided by the audiologist with the best possible amplification and oral stimulation of residual hearing should retain a very high priority.

The Progress of Hearing-impaired Children

Practically all of the research into aspects of educational development of hearing-impaired children has been carried out in schools for the deaf. Here the populations are easy to get at from a research point of view, as opposed to mainstreamed children who are widely dispersed throughout the educational system.

In the United Kingdom, and we believe in other parts of the world too, such research (for example, Conrad, 1976, 1977a, b, 1979) has painted a depressing picture of the progress of hearing-impaired children. Conrad (1979) has reported the average deaf school-leaver as having a reading age comparable with a nine-year-old normally hearing child and many of having barely intelligible speech. We do not wish to be complacent, in fact we are far from it. At times we feel that we will never have the basic requirements for helping the hearing-impaired to make the maximum possible progress on all fronts. It seems that so often factors external to the child such as delayed diagnosis, poor treatment in the terms of amplification and support compound his already severe handicap. Research such as that by Conrad and others who see the reported low levels of achievement as simply meaning that educationalists should make a blanket move to manual approaches from the earliest possible time is of great concern to us. To quote Conrad (1981) 'I see the case for the use of sign language from the *very earliest years* as overwhelming.' *We do not agree* for several, we think crucial, reasons. The research does not tell us which children should use manual approaches; it was carried out largely in special schools where the great majority of hearing-impaired children are educated in a version of the mainstreamed environment. Also historically, and obviously, many of the special schools have catered for the children with the greatest problems, be they low intelligence, severity of hearing loss, presence of additionally handicapping conditions and presence of social factors which are regarded as handicapping. There are also the other problems of delay in diagnosis, inadequate or inefficient, or inappropriate amplification. Also, traditionally, many of the residential special schools for the deaf have never been truly oral in their approach anyway. They have openly encouraged or allowed manual communication and sometimes by design and sometimes by resource deprivation have had a less than adequate approach to the use of amplification.

In the United States, where schools have always indulged in greater use of manual communication than in the United Kingdom, low reading achievement is also reported. Trybus and Karchmer (1977) have reported reading scores for a stratified, random sample of 6871 deaf students and found that the median reading score at 20 years of age was a grade equivalent of 4·5. Only a very small percentage of the best group (10 per cent) could read at levels of eighth grade or above.

It is also well worth noting that there are here (Clark, 1978) and in the United States schools where the achievements do not parallel the national data. In the Lane and Baker (1974) study of former students of the Central Institute for the Deaf they noted that within a four-year period the students increased 2·5 grades. This compared favourably with national data for normally hearing children. The authors attributed the higher reading skills to continuous education in the same school, maximum use of residual hearing and oral communication both at home and school. It has been suggested by some that ability and socio-economic selection is a factor in these establishments, but this would be refuted, at least by Clark (1978), for the Birkdale population.

Those who advocate a manual approach should also be aware of the fact that developing any language depends on exposure to a *fluent* and tuned version of that language within everyday contacts between the caregiver and the child. If in over 90 per cent of cases both parents are normally hearing then sign language will not be the language of the home and the child will therefore receive, at best, a less than fluent exposure in a sign language approach. It is also important to note that the 'overheard language', that is, that between adults and between other members of the family will not be sign language, but spoken language and the hearing-impaired child would therefore receive inconsistent exposure.

The hearing-impaired are not a homogeneous population and the present authors believe that blanket prescriptions for oral or manual education will not be likely to foster the greatest development in the child. The child's individual needs must be assessed in the light of *all* the factors we have mentioned above and whilst in the great majority of cases our view would be to advise the parents to adopt an auditory-oral approach with their young child, other factors such as the existence of additional handicaps would lead us to consider other possible management options.

The Hearing-impaired Child Developing Language

The work with families is rightfully called Parent Guidance not 'child guidance' because the teacher of the deaf could not possibly provide by herself the necessary stimulation for a hearing-impaired child to learn spoken language. Encouraging the parent to provide a rich language facilitating environment ensures that the child will be stimulated throughout his waking hours rather than just when a 'therapist' arrives for an hour. This has always been the view of the team who advise and support families at Manchester University. The question naturally arises 'what kind of linguistic environment is facilitating?' and 'how can we help parents to provide it?' We might add the further question of how it is possible to assess whether the child *is* progressing and that the language environment is, in fact, appropriate and facilitating. The remainder of this chapter addresses itself to those questions. We will consider what can be learned from normal language development, try to see if similar features exist in the environment of the hearing-impaired child and whether there are ways of enriching the environment in a linguistic sense. The close link between play and early language development will be considered and implications drawn for the management of hearing handicap.

Experience from Normally Hearing Children Learning Language

Research in the 1960s and 1970s described a specific style of speech used in addressing young children who were learning to talk. An interesting finding was that even children as young as five or six would use this special style when speaking to younger children. Speakers to young children tend to use shorter syntactically simpler sentences, slower delivery, smaller vocabulary than adult to adult speakers (Drach, 1969). Other workers (Phillips, 1973; Fraser and Roberts, 1975) have shown it to be more redundant, to use more concrete referents and less pronouns. Kobashigwa (1969) has shown it to be more repetitive. All in all the style of speech seems to be closely geared to the child's need to learn to identify the structural and functional elements in the language. Researchers would be very interested to know if it is possible to speed language acquisition and there have been many attempts to find out which strategies might possibly aid this. Results of research so far have been largely inconclusive, repetitions, praising 'good' or 'advanced' use (Howarth, 1977), the filling out of the child's incomplete sentences all seeming to make little difference to progress. It seems that parents do not actively 'teach' language. Mother acts largely in a 'response' mode being very attentive to child overture. Halliday (1969) suggests that 'the child knows what language is because he knows what language does'. Language is part of his personal interaction with his mother. It relates to events and things within his immediate environment.

Total amount of talk is not the most important feature of linguistic input although obviously a certain minimum exposure will be necessary. What is crucial is the amount of talk which links linguistic and non-linguistic events for the child. 'Flooding children with chatter in the "bright", "nursery school" manner is uneconomical at best; at worst it encourages children to ignore talk and simply let it wash over them' (Howarth, 1977). There is now plenty of evidence to suggest that mothers of normal children adjust the form of their spoken language appropriately to the language level of their children and that they do not require conscious effort to do this. Snow (1972), Phillips (1973), Fraser and Roberts (1975) have all shown that adults adjust the rate of speech, mean length of sentence, language complexity, vocabulary and repetitiveness when engaged in conversation with young children.

Much of this research on normal babies took as a starting point the behaviour of children at 18 months plus, when meaningful verbalisations are already appearing. However, it has been argued that during the first years of life the relation between maternal speech and social play between mother and child (which of course centres around objects in the environment) is crucial for learning about language. Schaffer *et al.* (1977) have pointed out that mothers take note of and elaborate not only their children's speech but also their non-verbal behaviour as well. They stress the importance of contextual back-up for children learning language. The environment, preverbally, is then clearly very important. A summary of what 'normal' interaction looks like follows below:

1. Speech is addressed directly to babies and this is facilitatory.
2. There is close emotional bond between child and caregiver and this stimulates 'desire' to communicate.
3. 'Motherese' is used − this involves features mentioned above such as simplification, repetition, voice quality (prosody including temporal features and intonation, etc.).
4. The mother/caregiver is naturally responsive to the child. She responds linguistically to almost anything the child does, for example, vocalising, crying.
5. There is action-oriented interaction − games which encourage 'anticipation' 'turn-taking' take place, for example, peek-a-boo, pat-a-cake, wind the bobbin up, etc.
6. The link between child overture and caregiver responses can be said

to be crucial. As an extreme example of this, when spoken to, the blind child averts the eyes rather than contacts with them. This has the effect of turning *off* rather than *on* the caregiver.

So what seems to be crucial is that caregivers and even young children intuitively know how to interact with young children. Another crucial feature is that in early interaction the caregiver EXPECTS the baby to be ultimately able to understand and is not in the least put out in the early stages when it does not. With parents of hearing-impaired children it may well be that it is these expectations which are damaged or destroyed when the child is diagnosed as having a hearing handicap. It is a prime responsibility for the educational audiologist and the teacher of the deaf to help the parent rebuild these expectations.

What Do We Know About Hearing-impaired Children Learning Language?

Tucker and Hughes (1984) have compared the interaction research of some of the major groups concerned with hearing handicap throughout the world. There appears to be some divergence in the conclusions of these research groups which should be considered. There is a view (Howarth and Wood, 1977) that hearing-impaired children are exposed to a 'deviant' language sample, deviant both structurally and functionally. This view of the bizarre nature of the child's language environment is worthy of consideration in reports of other workers in the same team (Gregory *et al*., 1979; Mogford *et al*., 1979; Gregory and Mogford, 1981; Gregory and Bishop, 1982). The main body of data on the hearing-impaired child's language environment reported in these papers was collected as part of a longitudinal project involving eight families. Two of these families were not included in the reporting because the children were regarded as too severely hearing-impaired and at least one of the remaining six children had a very minor hearing loss and could have developed some spoken language without the use of amplification.

The hearing-impaired group were compared at 18 months with a group of six normally hearing children and again at 24 months with a different group of six normally hearing children. It is worthy of note that the children were matched for chronological age. To summarise the aspects of the language environment which are stated by this group to be different for hearing-impaired children it is necessary to consider the form, function and conversational features of the mother's speech. The main structural variable which was considered to be different was that of language complexity. The functional variables where differences were observed included use of declaratives, imperatives, self-repetition and the moulding and shaping of the hearing-impaired child's words. Conversational differences included responsiveness to child overture, turn-taking, joint reference and anticipation games. In reporting these differences there are certain inconsistencies within the data which are not accounted for by the authors. Also research by other workers contradicts these findings in several important ways.

The research group found, as had Fraser and Roberts (1975) and Phillips (1973) that the mothers of hearing children of 24 months used significantly more complex language with their children than did those mothers with children of 18 months on measures of language complexity. Interestingly, Phillips found little difference between 8 and 18 months, perhaps indicating a lack of tuning at this stage. Both authors noted, particularly, differences beyond 18 months. In the study by Gregory *et al.* (1979), mothers' speech to the hearing-impaired children differed little at 18 months except for the use of repetition, but at 24 months there was still greater use of repetition and there were also significant differences in the total number of utterances and mean length of utterance, mothers of hearing-impaired children making fewer and shorter utterances. The mothers of the hearing-impaired children also used fewer declaratives and more imperatives and made less use of the child's vocalisations than the mothers of normally hearing children at 24 months. They concluded that whilst the literature on the language development of hearing-impaired children suggests that they need to be talked to more and more notice needs to be taken of their utterances, it would appear that they are talked to less and that compared to hearing children less notice is taken of their overtures.

Further aspects of the language environment where differences were noted were difficulties in turn-taking, in establishing joint reference and complete absence of anticipation games. They also conclude that mothers of hearing-impaired children indulge in much single word teaching. Gregory and Mogford (1981) state that turn-taking may be difficult to establish with hearing-impaired children, but the only evidence presented to support this statement is that there are more vocal clashes for hearing-impaired child/mother dyads than hearing child/mother dyads. If the only evidence of difficulty in establishing turn-taking is vocal clash, then it would seem to the present authors that the conclusion is not supported by relevant evidence, vocal clash being an unsophisticated measure of interactional synchrony. They also state that joint reference may be more difficult to establish, arguing that normally hearing children have significantly more nominals in their vocabulary than hearing-impaired children because nominals arise from a joint focus of attention for mother and child. It seems to the present authors again that evidence is scant and that such conclusions should not be drawn from the data presented. A more likely reason for fewer nominals being present in the first words of hearing-impaired children is that their first words reflect the language in the environment of a child who is significantly older when he is learning his first words. It is therefore quite reasonable to expect that the hearing-impaired child, who may be two or two-and-a-half-years old when he says his first words, may use more personal social words such as 'please' and 'thank you', etc. than general nominals.

Gregory and Mogford (1981) also report that mothers indulge in much single word teaching, words from the child being deliberately elicited and trained rather than in the case of normally hearing children, arising from the interaction. One certainly wonders if the parents in that study were told (asked) to teach words or to indulge in practices which induce that sort of behaviour. One area that concerns us is the use of word counts and first word analysis where parents provide the information rather than it being obtained from video or audio tapes directly. Nothing is more stressful to parents of hearing-impaired children than to be continually asked 'Does he have any words yet?' – or 'Any more words?' and other workers have, in their research, avoided this tactic. It can, in stressed parents, lead to the very thing that one would wish to avoid, a distorted language environment of single word teaching. However there is a contradiction in that Gregory and Mogford report that there are less rather than more general nominals in the first words of hearing-impaired children. This fact is difficult to reconcile with their observation that mothers concentrate on single word teaching. One would have thought a concentration on 'word teaching' would have led to increased use of nominals rather than less use.

Finally, it is also stated in their work that mothers of hearing-impaired children do not indulge in anticipation games. 'We know that mothers of deaf children do not play these games' (Gregory and Mogford, 1981). The present authors would totally disagree with this generalisation and the statement is not even supported in their own data, when earlier in the same chapter they write 'the words that occur for more than one deaf child that do not occur for the hearing group at all are "look", "sit-down", "*peepbo*", etc.'

Tucker (1980) has reported, using cross-sectional data on 19 severely hearing-impaired subjects (hearing losses greater than 50dB) that the decline in complexity of mothers' language is reversed beyond 30 months at the time when the child's own language is showing signs of development and mothers therefore have something to which to tune. As workers interested in language development in the hearing-impaired move further and further back into the preverbal stage they would do well to recognise some of the characteristics of parents at around the time of diagnosis of a severe handicap in their child.

As we are all aware, mothers of normally hearing children expect their children to learn to communicate but for many parents of hearing-impaired children these expectations are shattered at diagnosis. 'Is it worth talking at all if he cannot hear?' Others lapse into the approach reported earlier of gross over-exaggeration use of single words and word teaching. Some are even advised to do this since special training, other than training as a teacher of the deaf, is not demanded of those who advise parents. Parents can be advised and supported to provide a natural and normal language environment for their child, but this does require an adviser who can distinguish the common reactions to deafness which may produce bizarre language use.

A longitudinal part of the study mentioned above and reported by Tucker (1981) investigated nine hearing-impaired children for 24 months after diagnosis. This research showed little growth in the language complexity of mothers to the sample overall, but in several subjects whose receptive and expressive language was showing rapid development, complexity of mothers' language (as measured by Type Token Ratio (TTR) and Mean Length of Sentence (MLS)) showed substantial increase in the 24 months post-diagnosis, thus providing support for a tuning hypothesis. When Tucker considered the number of single word utterances used by mothers this proved to be 6·9 per cent of the total number of parental utterances. There seems, therefore, to be no support in this sample for the argument that mothers of hearing-impaired children 'over-use' single words, thus providing an impoverished language sample for the child to imitate. Also the single words were, as far as one could tell, linguistically appropriate, being aimed at gaining attention or used in response, for example, 'no' or 'yes', or in games where a feature of the game was to say 'go' or 'stop'. The aim of the support team at Manchester is to encourage the mother to talk to her child as she did before the diagnosis was made. It may be the case that some mothers are inappropriately advised being asked simply to 'speak more' and in some cases to teach words directly. The biggest fault is impatience – impatience for the child to talk without a corresponding concentration on the sort of linguistic environment which is best able to get the child talking. Mere talk is not enough. More situations where joint activity and joint attention can take place are far more important than labelling objects or activities. Parents need to be advised of this fact.

When Tucker analysed vocal clash in his longitudinal sample he found (for six video tapes per subject for nine subjects in a two-year period) that vocal clash dropped from 19·7 per cent to 11·2 per cent this when total number of vocalisations or verbalisations rose from a mean of 223 for the first tape to 475 for tape six. There is clearly a need for more detailed research of this issue since vocal clash will depend on synchrony, but also on total number of vocalisations and type of activity. It seems from Tucker's sample that the hearing-impaired children were increasingly successful at avoiding clash as they developed over the two-year period.

Howarth (1977) studied teachers' language to young hearing-impaired children. Forty-six teacher-pupil dyads were tape recorded in a play/ conversation situation. The results of analysis of the adult language sample showed that the teachers modified their speech in terms of simplicity and redundancy according to the language level of the child (as measured by his Mean Length of Utterance) rather than according to his age. The complexity of their language (as measured by MLU and TTR) increased as the child's language competence increased.

Hughes and Howarth (1980) and Hughes (1981, 1983) reported on a cross-sectional study involving 60 mother-child dyads including 30 normally hearing children and 30 hearing-impaired children. The study described the interaction between mothers and young hearing-impaired children and compared it with the interaction observed between the mothers and normally hearing children. The children were matched for sex, socio-economic background and receptive language level. These matching criterion were chosen in the light of Howarth's (1977) findings and those of Cross (1977) who found the normally hearing child's receptive language level an even more significant determinant of mothers' speech adjustments than his MLU. More than 20 features of the mothers' speech were analysed, including structural, functional, interactive and conversational style measures. The results mirrored those of Cross (1977) for most of the variables — and the numerical values were very similar to those she reported for her normally hearing sample. The results were similar to those of Gregory *et al.* (1979) for the feature of maternal repetition only. Hughes found, like Gregory *et al.*, that mothers of hearing-impaired children used a significantly higher proportion of self-repetition than mothers of normally hearing children, whatever the child's language level.

On all the other comparable variables the results contradict those of Gregory *et al.* and on many features which Gregory *et al.* did not examine, most of the results showed similarity rather than difference between the two groups of mothers.

There was no significant difference in the total number of utterances addressed to the hearing-impaired children compared with the total number used to the normally hearing children. The reduction in input to the hearing-impaired children which Gregory *et al.* note was certainly not the case for this sample. A comparison of MLU, TTR and other complexity measures also revealed similarity so the author's suggestion, that Gregory's *et al.* method of comparing groups of similar chronological age may have produced the differences she observed for these features, seems likely in the light of the results from Hughes' study (1981, 1983).

Various measures of how much mother attended to the child's utterances, including the percentage of expansion or extension of a child's utterance, also gave very similar figures for both groups in Hughes' study. These measures also contradict the conclusion of Gregory *et al.* that less notice is taken of the hearing-impaired child's utterances. The overall picture from Hughes' study was one of similarity between mothers speech to hearing-impaired and normally hearing children of similar linguistic levels. Further statistical analysis of the data showed that mothers of hearing-impaired children, like mothers of normally hearing children were able to 'tune' their language to the level of their child and intuitively increase the complexity of their input as the child progresses with his language skills.

However, although the trends were the same, the correlations overall were weaker for the hearing-impaired group – showing that the mother found it more difficult to 'tune' accurately to the child's level, probably because of the reduced or confusing feedback from the child. Greater variability within samples shows the warning light to researchers. It highlights the danger of drawing firm conclusions from small samples. Recent work at the pre-verbal stage (Chadderton, 1983) investigating child initiation behaviours has shown overwhelmingly that his sample of mothers were alive and alert to child overtures and were very responsive. Anderson (1979) in the United States studied, longitudinally, three hearing-impaired children. She was interested in evidence of speakers' sensitivity to the partners in the choice of vocabulary, utterance forms, topics and expectations for turn-taking. She studied mothers' strategies for passing turns and was also interested in strategies for repairing the back and forth sequence when it breaks down. Her general conclusions regarding mothers' speech to hearing-impaired children were that maternal speech content reflected developmental changes in infants' cognitive and motor skills. This suggests tuning and supports the Manchester data. All researchers would agree with Anderson's finding that mothers repeat and reformulate utterances. Finally Anderson noted that the speech was oriented to the goal of the child taking a turn in the conversation.

Anderson compared her findings with what was known from research on conversations with young normally hearing children. She found that a percentage of questions, commands, etc. were very similar to those reported for mothers of normally hearing children by Snow (1977) in a survey of six major studies of maternal language.

Cross *et al.* (1980) have considered the interaction of young hearing-impaired children with their mothers. The framework of their research reflects the earlier work by Cross (1977) with normally hearing children. Their major interest in observing parent child interaction was in order to resolve the issue of what determines parental speech adjustments. By using groups of normal and hearing-impaired children they hoped to shed light on the following hypothesis.

1. That mothers tune to the communicative and particularly receptive maturity of the child (Cross, 1977).
2. That mothers tune to the 'conversation' ability of the child (Snow, 1977).
3. That mothers are influenced by many factors including age, cognitive ability, conversational co-operation, etc. (Newport *et al.*, 1977).

They selected two groups of hearing-impaired children of different ages and cognitive ability to be compared with a group of hearing two-year-olds who were equated in age with the younger hearing-impaired group in spontaneous language ability with the older hearing-impaired group. This permitted the child variables of age, spontaneous speech and receptive language to be investigated separately as contributors to aspects of maternal speech style. The complexity of their analysis measures and methods of data presentation make direct comparisons with the other research reports difficult, but overall they support the view that in terms of mothers' language complexity, age is not the major determinant but receptive language level is. Cross *et al.* conclude that 'for a number of features maternal speech to matched normally hearing and deaf children. . . is quite dissimilar' and they resolve the issue of determinants of maternal speech by opting for a multi-factor account. This allows them to explain certain adjustments being related to child hearing loss *per se*. However, they strongly qualify the multi factor account by stating that receptive feedback must be given a primary role and also that once the child has acquired some competence in speech and comprehension it is necessary to provide a major determining role for psycholinguistic feedback from these two sources.

The present authors believe the weight of evidence would support the following conclusions:

1. In respect of comparisons between hearing and hearing-impaired for language interaction age is largely irrelevant in any sense which can be helpful in terms of establishing what is an appropriate language data base.
2. The hearing-impaired are not a homogeneous population and many variables within and external to the child will affect his language development. Researchers are wise not to make exaggerated claims for what 'the deaf' can and cannot do on the basis of small-scale studies.
3. Tucker and Hughes (1984) have argued that more detailed audiological information is required than is currently being presented in interaction research papers.
4. The weight of evidence would support the position that parents of hearing-impaired children *can* tune their language input to the receptive language level of the child.

What Can Parents of Hearing-impaired Children Do to Facilitate Language Learning?

The present authors think it would be unwise to merely teach the tricks of interaction to parents since if they can gain an understanding of all the principles involved then they can expand and develop their own initiations and responses.

Responsiveness. This is widely recognised as a crucial feature of facilitatory interaction.

(i) It applies in both directions. It is particularly important to show parents of a hearing-impaired child his response.

(ii) Parents should be able to recognise initiation from the child and respond to it. Video tapes of early interaction are most valuable here.

(iii) Parents need to be *contingent* on the infant. This involves doing predictable things that relate to the infant's behaviour and development.

Routine Behaviour. Routinisation is a non-contingent teaching area. Mum sets out to teach the child something because she thinks *he should know it*. Obviously they can be adapted to particular behavioural or developmental signals. As an example the mother may wait until the child shows some interest in books before starting to have regular 'book reading' sessions. However, the parent in these situations is making conscious efforts to 'teach'. Examples of routinisation might be anticipation games such as 'peek-book' or language related to routine events such as bathtime or the training of personal social words such as please, thank you, etc.

Turn-taking. In normal subjects turn-taking is a very early behaviour. Trevarthen (1974, 1977) and others have shown that babies from two months are capable of taking an active role in interaction with their mothers. When the baby takes the initiative the mother becomes subdued and responsive. There are many behavioural aspects of these communication overtures including facial expression, gesture and eye contact. They include also the sounds made by child and mother and this aspect of turn-taking will need to develop after the fitting of appropriate aids. Being responsive to child overture is a major component of the facilitatory environment and as Chadderton (1983) has shown there is no reason why mothers of hearing-impaired children should be different here. Mothers would be advised not to drown the child in chatter but allow him 'his turn'. After all he needs the practice.

It would seem that CONTINGENCY and ROUTINES are two (of possibly many) crucial dimensions of a facilitatory input. It would be too easy in respect of parents of hearing-impaired children, to interpret this as meaning that parents should expand the child's utterances, or look at what the child is looking at and focus talk on that (this is called 'joint reference' in the literature), or use short sentences. What is perhaps more meaningful is to encourage and convince parents that their child has communication potential. We can be positive about this on the basis of the child's ability to use his residual hearing and other perceptual skills. No single play or language strategy is as important as the fact that parents use language in context-bound situations that the child sees as predictable and respectable.

Reception Precedes Production. It is very important for parents of hearing-handicapped children to understand that in language acquisition reception takes place before production. (The child understands before and more than he can say.) What the child learns is then applied to his production of language. However, parents should be aware that reception and production are interactive since the child will be providing himself with auditory feedback — talking to himself if you like — in order to build up the appropriate patterns in his brain. So a child's microphone is every bit as useful for him to hear himself talking as it is to hear others. As the child starts to recognise sounds, parents will feel rewarded for their efforts, particularly when the first words start to flow. Children learn words because the things they represent are appealing to them at the time and there is always the danger that parents will overemphasise the *teaching* of words at this time. Even if parents are successful in getting a child to say a particular word it is unlikely to appear again spontaneously in his vocabulary or at least it will not appear until he has heard it many more times and he decides the time is right to transfer it from his passive to his active vocabulary. Parents need to concentrate on giving the child the opportunity to receive spoken language and leave him to organise his own production.

When the child reaches the stage of seeing that words can be strung together he has reached a very important milestone. He has started to understand the *structure* of language. There are two elements in his speech which have syntactic connection, for example, 'All-gone cup'. What is interesting is that such two word sentences do not occur in adult speech in the same way. He has constructed his own unit of language from his experience. The two words encompass a 'meaning' for that child at that time. At this point the child will be greatly encouraged by the parents feedback to him. His statement 'Bye-bye Teddy' might be followed by mum saying 'Where's Teddy gone.' This repeats part of his utterance (to reinforce it) and gives new information for his brain to work on. This leads on to the stage where the child uses what some people have called telegraphic speech and says such sentences as 'Mummy rabbit garden'. These sentences are rather like the telegrams we send and just as susceptible to confusion. Key words carry the message. In the child's utterances we often need clues about the situation in order to understand what is meant.

Another interesting stage is where children perceive the general rule for tense changes and we hear sentences like 'Iain waked up', 'The house is saled'. The child will almost certainly have heard 'wake up' and 'sold' but has perceived the rule that to change past tense we usually add 'ed' and is applying this to his language use. The same applies to plurality where we hear the child saying 'mouses' instead of 'mice'. What is of great interest to us is that researchers are reporting the same happening for hearing-impaired children (for example, Howarth, 1977), thus providing further support for the notion that hearing-impaired children act positively on the language input in constructing their own grammar. The present authors would argue that the language of hearing-impaired children suffers delays related to an absence of early stimulation, but that once started and providing sufficient stimulation is given, it follows a very similar pattern to the language development of normally hearing children.

Children begin to acquire language because very early on they realise that speech is a way of operating on the world to control and manipulate it. From the language input the child must start to abstract the acoustic features such as stress, rhythm and intonation and it is likely that normal users of the same language will process these speech sounds differently. This will be of no consequence so long as the individual devises a method which helps him to recognise all the distinctions which the language 'English' demands. Hearing-impaired children can use their remaining hearing to make these distinctions just as a colour blind person can learn to accommodate the fact that they cannot distinguish between the colour of the traffic lights.

Help From and Some Problems With Lip-reading

As far as hearing-impaired children are concerned we would want to provide a similar kind of stimulating environment to the one which seems to be so successful for hearing children. The normally hearing child receives most of his linguistic information auditorily with a little support from vision, with information carried by non-verbal aspects such as facial expression, lip movements, gesture, etc. A lot is claimed for lip-reading and undoubtedly skills are developed in this direction, but there is no doubt that taken as the major component of reception it is unreliable and imprecise. Two-thirds of the sounds that make up the English language are invisible or else are ambiguous visually. Many are greatly dependent on voicing and nasality for their intelligibility. Since these features are not visible various groups such as p, b, m; t, d, n; s, z are liable to frequent confusion. Many other consonants — k, g, y — are made far back in the mouth and are totally invisible. Another feature which adds to the difficulty of lip-reading is that speech is very rapid and impermanent.

Ross *et al.* (1982) argues that there is no strong evidence that lip-reading can be taught. Conrad (1977a) has argued that the hearing impaired are no better at it than normally hearing subjects. Shepard *et al.* (1977) has suggested that the ability to speech-read is related to the speed at which the visually received signal can be converted into neural information and transmitted to the brain. He showed a high correlation (0·93) between the latency of a visually evoked response and speech-reading ability. There is a distinct possibility that lip-reading is one of the many skills which rely heavily on innate capacity and are not very amenable to training. Lip-reading will support a child in his attempts to build a communication system *at a level which he prescribes* and our newest evidence would suggest that there is possibly less of a role for lip-reading with hearing-impaired children than was formerly thought to be the case. We are most definitely noticing with young hearing-impaired children fitted with modern high powered hearing aids that they are paying much less visual attention to their mothers. We believe they are building language auditorily and they are using vision for the same purposes as normally hearing children, that is, to maintain contact in the interaction situation, to signal to mum that she should say something, to make sure that she is paying attention and so on. In our view there is no point in insisting on visual attention before speaking, but there is every point in speaking if the child looks, and the interpretation is that he requires information. There is some evidence to suggest that continually attempting to draw visual attention actually results, on many occasions, in the breakdown of interaction. An increase in the number of child looks at mother's face takes place between one-year-old (23·8 in ten minutes) and two-year-old (54·9 in ten minutes) normally hearing children (Schaffer *et al.*, 1977) whilst mean length of glance remains very stable at 1·32 seconds at 1 year and 1·39 seconds at 2 years. If these glances at mother's face are the 'opportunities' to 'lip-read' (we say opportunities because the child could be looking directly at the eyes not the lips), then data on developing hearing-impaired children would be very useful. Tucker (1983) reported a longitudinal sample of nine severely hearing-impaired children and found that mean length of glance was 1·1 seconds over a period of two years from diagnosis and that numbers of glances showed a mean of 23 glances at diagnosis and a mean of 62 glances after two years of use of aids. Tucker (1980) had also looked at the synchrony of visual regard of the child with mother's talk and found that 68·4 per cent of child periods of visual regard, which were synchronous with the mother's talking, started *before* the talking started. For only a very small percentage of mothers' talking time was the child actually looking so lip-reading opportunity was very limited. It will be interesting to study patterns of child visual regard as they gain more experience and knowledge of spoken language. In the first two years of *use of hearing aids* their visual regard patterns are very similar to those reported for the first *two years of life* of normally hearing children.

In conclusion if we stress lip-reading we stress the least efficient means of receiving language and there is the great danger of audition being relegated to a merely supportive role to the visual (Pollack, 1970). Visual cues are important, indeed the evidence is strong that auditory visual reception is superior to that of audition and vision, but the child himself must 'specify' the amount of vision information he personally requires.

The Importance of Play in Early Language Development

'Play is the freely chosen and natural activity of children undertaken as an end unto itself' (Garvey, 1979). This is one of many definitions of play. The important role of play in language development has been stressed by Garvey (1979) and McCune-Nicolich and Carroll (1981). Training studies have demonstrated a relationship between enhanced play and improved performances on measures of social and cognitive functioning. Peer interactive play has been shown to be related to increasing social language competency (Freyberg, 1973).

Surprisingly there has been little research carried out to investigate play behaviour in hearing-impaired children. This seems odd in view of its close relationship with language development and the hearing-impaired child's difficulties in learning language. Lovell *et al.* (1968) and Higginbotham *et al.* (1980) have suggested that children with communication handicaps will have reduced social contacts which in turn will lead to reduced opportunity to participate in social play, although the present authors would argue that this need not be so. Darbyshire (1977) has added to this argument the view that hearing-impaired children will find it increasingly difficult to participate in age-appropriate play.

Bruner and Sherwood (1976) contend that play goes beyond just the practice of simple learned skills. They argue that it is a form of variation seeking, where the child increases his repertoire of responses to the environment. This could well help him later on in problem solving situations. Many researchers see language and play as two aspects of a more generalised cognitive function, with play and language both reflecting the child's developing symbolic ability. They see play and language developing in parallel and some recent researchers (Garvey and Hogan, 1973) have shown that play episodes between infant and caregiver facilitate language acquisition by providing a familiar non-verbal context on which language can be elaborated.

Stages of development of symbolic play have been researched and workers have usually highlighted difficulties related to an inability to engage appropriately in play forms requiring responsive communication contexts. Deficits in play experience are seen as affecting language development because the child is denied the vital experience with symbolism and social interaction. Where the development of symbolic play forms part of developmental testing it is generally assumed to be normal in hearing-impaired children until they reach 3 years (Sheridan, 1960; Lowe and Costello, 1976).

Gregory and Mogford (1982), as part of a larger study of the development of communication skills in hearing-impaired children of 15-30 months, investigated the development of symbolic play using the Lowe and Costello Symbolic Play Test. This was carried out at three monthly intervals. Mothers were also interviewed on their child's make-believe play and a video tape was made of the child playing freely with a given set of toys.

The results on the Lowe and Costello test showed the hearing impaired group, on average, were functioning at a slightly higher level than that reported for normals and in the interview the mothers reported the presence of make-believe behaviours. However, Gregory and Mogford reported that in terms of percentage of time spent in various play types the hearing-impaired as a group were less likely to display symbolic play behaviour than normals. The major differences they argued were at the age of 2½ years with normally hearing subjects displaying more appropriate play while the hearing-impaired displayed more inappropriate and prompted play.

Gregory and Mogford suggested that the hearing-impaired were:

(i) more stimulus bound;
(ii) more easily distracted;
(iii) less likely to plan and sequence their play;

They argued, tentatively, that this was because:

(i) the hearing-impaired children were retarded in symbolic functioning as language was required to help symbolism develop;

(ii) symbolic play requires the ability to plan but to plan one needs language;

(iii) hearing-impaired children have a different structural configuration of their world so play does not develop in the same way;

(iv) the ability to play symbolically is learnt but when there are communication difficulties the necessary interaction for learning does not occur.

Darbyshire's (1977) study of 45, 3-8-year-old hearing-impaired children reported a lack of appropriate social play skills and a greater level of egocentric play. Games were reported as providing the most difficulty because they required co-operation and association. Higginbotham and Baker (1981), using a scale which combined social and cognitive play ratings, found that the hearing-impaired children displayed more non-interactive constructive play and less co-operative and dramatic play than normals. The hearing-impaired preferred solitary constructive and associative dramatic play whilst normally hearing children preferred dramatic play activities requiring organised group participation.

The overall picture reported in the literature (Kosaner, 1983) is that the hearing-impaired face increasing difficulty in maintaining normal play patterns as the play of normals becomes more and more socially interactive. It is also claimed above that reduced amounts and complexity of dramatic play reflect a deficit in symbolic functioning related to poor linguistic development.

Kosaner (1983) in her own study used and extended Higginbotham's *et al.* (1980) Social Participation, Cognitive Play and Non-playful Activity Classifications. The extension was to the cognitive categories and was devised to give a more detailed assessment of symbolic play and simple game behaviour. Fifteen severely/profoundly hearing-impaired children were studied. Mean age was 76 months (range 72-84 months). The results of this carefully controlled study indicated that the cognitive play patterns of this group of children were *not* deviant but slightly retarded with age. Their characteristic level of social participation was very positively interactive. Significant correlations were found between time spent in socio-symbolic play and verbal competence and between length of listening experience and degree of social participation.

The present authors would agree that environmental features play an enormous part in the early development of hearing-impaired children and that whilst the application of amplification and appropriate advice and family support are so variable we can expect great variation in studies into play behaviour. We need studies which are longitudinal and which take place on children who have been reared in as facilitating an environment as possible, so that we can get nearer to what is the real extent of the problem of deafness.

The parents provide the first few years of this environment and Jeffree and McConkey (1976) in their book *Let Me Speak* have shown how a parent can facilitate language acquisition through play and games. So play is important, children are highly motivated to do it, parents can and should give a rich variety of types of play, the child plays before he talks, play leads to turn-taking and turn-taking is one of the crucial elements of communication.

Parents of hearing-impaired children should be encouraged to set aside time each day to play with the child. This should be a time when other activities are not distracting. There should be a wide variety of construction toys, exploratory toys and toys which aid the growth of symbolism and involve the child in as many of the 'domestic' areas where language interaction is possible (Nolan and Tucker, 1981). There should be definite encouragement to invite other children in and to encourage the hearing-impaired children to return visits. As well as what we call 'contrived' play the child should have access to a rich variety of play materials with which he can engage in solitary or group play. Mothers should also engage in singing games with the child, particularly the ones where actions are involved, since this encourages the child to take turns and the child is highly motivated to vocalise and ultimately verbalise in time with mum.

Interaction Measures in Monitoring Progress of Hearing-impaired Children

Video recordings of children interacting with their caregivers have been shown by several researchers to provide a realistic display of mother/ infant communicative behaviour (Brazelton *et al.*, 1975; Trevarthen, 1977; Stern *et al.*, 1977; Als *et al.*, 1979). Indeed other than using video recordings in the early stages it would be impossible to undertake in-depth communicative analysis. The authors will, however, describe shortly an 'on line' interaction procedure whereby it is possible to observe specific behaviours using a small team of observers.

The present authors have used, for both research and monitoring procedures, the recording arrangement shown in Figure 9.1. Here the

Figure 9.1: The arrangements for filming mother-child dyads.

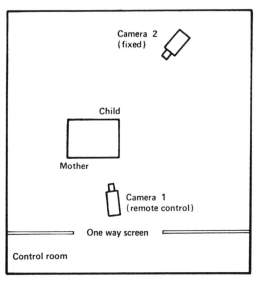

child plays with table top toys with his caregiver.

A simpler arrangement using only one camera is possible and again the infant is filmed full-face over mother's shoulder and a large wall mounted vertical mirror placed behind the child allows a view of the mothers face. Trevarthen (1977) has described this technique. We have found it extremely helpful to have the 'control room' in an adjacent room. This enables observation, but means that the interaction is not interfered with. In our experience, young children are not distracted by cameras but by people standing behind cameras.

Those interested in the early development of hearing-impaired children would wish to analyse the linguistic environment provided by the parent and much analysis of the type mentioned earlier can take place from a transcription of all parental verbalisations in, say, a 15 or 20 minute face-to-face interaction session. For transcription work it is helpful if there is a separate audio recording of the interaction, and for close analysis of, say, non-verbal aspects of the interaction it is helpful if the video has a frame freeze and variable speed viewing capability.

Below are details on the linguistic analysis possible from transcriptions of mothers' speech together with definitions of the measures.

The Analysis of Spoken Language

Demands

Verbal (V). This is a demand which explicitly requires the child to respond verbally — perhaps imitating a model, for example, 'say all gone'.

Non-verbal (NV). A demand where the response is specifically non-verbal, for example, 'You hold it.'

Attention (Att). Where the child's attention is demanded, for example, 'Look, see, watch.'

Questions

Type (a) Closed. The question is closed in the sense that it requires a Yes/No answer but it also requests confirmation, for example, 'Is that the red ball?' It is child initiated.

Type (b) Closed. This question does not require further information. The speaker is not requesting confirmation, but agreement or not, for example, 'Is this the only horse in the jigsaw?' It is parent initiated.

Type (c) Open. Mainly Wh- questions, that is, those for which there is no criterion of rightness or wrongness, for example, 'What's this?'

Statements

These give information or may describe an action, for example, 'This is a red man.' They are not demands nor are they questions.

Feedback

This can be positive or negative and can be feedback to a verbal or non-verbal stimulus, for example, POSITIVE 'Yes, that's right.' Or, NEGA-TIVE 'No, he doesn't do that.'

Tags

Usually attached to statements, for example, 'Isn't it?' 'Aren't we?'

Unclassified Utterances (Unc)

Interrupted, unclear or inaudible utterances.

Type Token Ratio

In a thousand word sample the type token ratio (TTR) is the number of different words as a proportion of the total number of words.

Repetitions

Partial. Ratio of the number of repetitions of one or more major units within an utterance (for example, repetition of the subject phrase or a subordinate clause) or of an entire utterance without a verb, to the total number of utterances.

Complete. Ratio of the number of complete repetitions of sentences (that is, utterances which contain both subject and verb) to the total number of utterances (within three utterances of the original).

SE Utterances. Ratio of the number of repetitions of the meaning of a previous utterance which did not include repetition of any of its grammatical units, to the number of utterances (paraphrase or paraphrase with a new idea added).

Expansions (EP)

An expansion of any preceding child utterance that corrected the child's grammar — that is, built up the child's utterance into a well formed simple sentence by adding words or functions (percentage per 100 utterances).

Extensions (ET)

An expansion of any preceding child utterance which also adds a new idea.

Mean Length of Sentence (MLS)

Sentences analysed as follows:

> FUNCTIONALLY COMPLETE — 'Because I said so.'
> GRAMMATICALLY COMPLETE — 'Here is the ball, Emma.'
> Incomplete — where parents use sentences interrupted by the other speaker.

Number of morphemes per sentence will be entered and means calculated. NB: A morpheme is the minimum distinctive unit of grammar. It is a decision of the researcher to include Mmm's and ah's, etc. (but only where they constitute an utterance) but to discount animal noises, etc.

For example, birth/day   =   2 morphemes
                 an/other   =   2   ″

$$\text{sense/less} \quad = \quad 2 \text{ morphemes}$$
$$\text{ing/ed/plurals} = \quad 2 \qquad ''$$

Proportion of Single Word Utterances (PSWU)

Proportion of Long Utterances (PLU)

Many workers use six or more morphemes for this.

Morphemes per Minute (MPM)

This gives a picture of rate of talk.

It will be seen that the measures in Table 9.2 contain:

(a) Structural analysis with such measures as mean length of sentence (MLS), proportion of single word utterances (PSWU), type token ratio (TTR).
(b) Functional analysis, where the parent's language is coded accordingly to the effect intended or otherwise, which the utterance has within the interaction (for example, statements, demands, questions, feedback).
(c) Interactive analysis can be included where the communicative aspects of language are stressed, particularly whether utterances have a response or an initiating purpose in the interaction. For example:

'Get daddy an ashtray please.'

This is a 'demand' (initiating).

'No, yellow' (after child says blue).

This is a statement (response vocal).

Another interactive category might be expansions and extensions where this is measured as a percentage of the occasions when it was possible to expand or extend the child's utterance. It should be a time consuming but relatively easy task to indicate the categories as a percentage of the total number of utterances.

The features are not very precise but it should be possible to pick out the mother who is presenting a very restricted language sample with a large percentage of single words or the mother who is completely dominating in the interaction and does not allow the child the chance to initiate or give him the chance to respond when she has initiated.

With appropriate video recorder facilities it is also possible to count the child glances at mother and retrospectively calculate mean length of glance. Young children glance frequently at mother's face to initiate, to seek approval, to watch for communication cues. A very low number of glances in relation to the levels reported earlier by Schaffer *et al.* (1977) and for hearing-impaired children by Tucker (1983) would be odd especially if related to gaze avoidance.

If the child has a developed communication system then the above format can be applied to his contribution to the interaction. If he is at the pre-verbal stage it is possible to ascribe communicative categories to his behaviour (see Brinker and Goldbart, 1979 and Table 9.1; Tronick *et al.*, 1980; and for a case study approach on two hearing-impaired children, Nienhuys and Tikotin, 1983).

Table 9.1: Scale for assessing child vocalisations.

U   Unclear. Non-verbal utterances from which no clear meaning can be inferred from gesture or context, or for which no meaning seemed intended by child, babbling which is not I or P. Utterance itself was intended, but no meaning in the communication situation seemed intended.

I   Imperatives. Non-verbal vocalisations which are intended to produce a particular effect such as a change of situation, obtaining an object, getting an adult's attention. Intonation serves as a cue to the imperious nature of the utterance.

D   Declaratives. Non-verbal vocalisations that state the existence of something. Purpose is to state rather than request something. Declarative must involve reference to some state of affairs or some object. Intonation helps define declarative (Look, give me that, do this).

P   Performatives. A non-verbal vocalisation which accompanies an action and is part of action; for example, the child has just completed building a tower, clasps her hands and says, 'yay'; for example, the child pushes car along making 'broom broom' noise.

Source: after Brinker and Goldbart, 1979

Obviously measures of this type require careful definition and also reliability study to ensure that they are being applied efficiently.

An 'On-line' Scheme for Observing Interaction

The play arrangement is as described above and investigators are situated in the viewing room. A ten minute spell is studied, each observer having his own single task.

Observer 1. Counts the number of glances at mother's face and comments on the length of glance and any instances of glance avoidance.

Observer 2. Records child *vocalisations*, if possible specifying vowel, consonant, or vowel/consonant combinations and comments on voice quality and intonation. Records child *verbalisations* writing down if possible the whole utterances. If some words are unintelligible or missed then the number of words or utterances spoken is marked so that a grand total of communication attempts can be scored.

Observer 3. Records the child's non-verbal communicative behaviour indicating whether it is (a) an initiation or (b) a response. Whenever possible the observer will write down the event and what surrounds it.

Observers 4 and 5. These record as follows:

(1) The number of maternal turns in the conversation. They are 'turns' not utterances so must be separated by some form of child turn non-vocal or verbal.
(2) The number of maternal responses to child overtures are recorded. These are definitely responses to child initiation or topic setting and not just responses to what the child says.

Observer 6. Records the number of child initiations (where the child sets a new topic in the communication) noting what the child did or said, and where possible indicating whether the initiation was non-verbal, vocal or verbal or a combination of these.

All observers are instructed to mark areas of uncertainty (with time clock reading if possible) and it is then possible to review the ten minutes to look at these areas of uncertainty.

The data is scored and entered on a sheet as shown in Table 9.2.

Obviously this technique relies on a large supply of trained observers, but where this is possible it greatly speeds the business of producing reportable and useful information. As an example mothers of hearing impaired children have been reported as less responsive to child overture. We have certainly not found this, in fact we have found the opposite but the above methodology produces a direct count of responses so a percentage responsiveness is easy to calculate. When a full retrospective transcription is made the assessment can be made of mother's 'tuning' to the child's receptive language and also the normality of her speech in terms of rate, range of functions and amount of talk can be assessed.

Table 9.2: Score sheet parent/child interaction.

Subject	Age
Date	Total
Obs.(1)	Child looks ....
Obs.(2)	Child vocalisation ....
	Child verbalisations ....
	MLU ....
	Max. LU ....
	No. of SWU ....
	No. of unclear ....
Obs.(3)	Child non-verbal turns ....
	Responses ....
	Initiations ....
Obs.(4 & 5)	Mother's turns ....
	Mother's responses to child overtures ....
Obs.(6)	Child initiations ....

In conclusion we must say that before the interaction measures are carried out, tests of aid function are undertaken and this would include 'on the child' as well as 'coupler' measures.

References

Als, H., Tronick, E. and Brazelton, T.B. (1979) 'Analysis of face-to-face interaction in infant adult dyads' in M.E. Lamb, S.J. Soumi and C.R. Stephenson (eds.), *The Study of Social Interaction: Methodological Problems*, University of Wisconsin Press, Wisconsin

Anderson, B.J. (1979) 'Parents' strategies for achieving conversational interactions with their young hearing-impaired children' in A. Simmons-Martin and D.R. Calvert (eds.), *Parent-Infant Intervention*, Grune and Stratton, New York

BATOD (1981) 'Methodology in education of hearing-impaired children', *J. Brit. Assn. Teachers of the Deaf, 5(5)* (8-9 Mag.)

Bellugi, U. and Fischer, S. (1972) 'A comparison of sign language and spoken language: rate and grammatical mechanisms', *Cognition,* 1, 173-200

Brazelton, T.B., Tronick, E., Adamson, L., Als, H. and Wise, S. (1975) 'Early mother-infant reciprocity' in M.A. Hofer (ed.), *Parent-Infant Interaction*, Ciba, London

Brennan, M. (1976) 'Can deaf children acquire language?' *Supplement to British Deaf News*, February 1976

Brennan, M. (1981) 'Grammatical processes in British sign language' in B. Woll, J. Kyle and M. Deuchar (eds.), *Perspectives on Sign Language and Deafness*, Croom Helm, London

Brinker, R. and Goldbart, J. (1979) 'Developments in research: the language programme' in J. Hogg (ed.), *A Report on the Work of the Anson House Pre-*

school Project for Mentally Handicapped Children and Their Families, Dr Barnados, London

Bruner, J.S. and Sherwood, V. (1976) 'Peekaboo and the learning of rule structures in play' in J.S. Bruner, A. Jolly and K. Sylva (eds.), *Play*, 2nd edn, Penguin, London

Chadderton, J. (1983) 'Child initiations and mothers' responses in joint enterprise interactive play'. Unpublished MEd thesis, University of Manchester, Manchester

Clark, M.H. (1978) 'Preparation of deaf children for hearing society', *J. Brit. Assn. Teachers of the Deaf*, *2(5)*, 146-54

Conrad, R. (1976) 'Towards a definition of oral success'. Paper given at the RNID/NCTD Education Meeting, Harrogate

Conrad, R. (1977a) 'Lipreading by deaf and hearing children', *British Journal of Educational Psychology*, *47*, 60-5

Conrad, R. (1977b) 'The reading ability of deaf school leavers', *British Journal of Educational Psychology*, *47*, 138-48

Conrad, R. (1979) *The Deaf School Child: Language and Cognitive Function*, Harper and Row, London

Conrad, R. (1981) 'Sign language in education: some consequent problems' in B. Woll, J. Kyle, and M. Deucher (eds.), *Perspectives on British Sign Language and Deafness*, Croom Helm, London

Cornett, O. (1967) 'Cued speech', *Amer. Annals of the Deaf*, *112*, 3-13

Cross, T.G. (1977) 'Mothers' speech adjustments: The contribution of selected child listener variables' in C.E. Snow and C.A. Ferguson (eds.), *Talking to Children*, Cambridge University Press, Cambridge

Cross, T.G., Johnson-Morris, J.E. and Nienhuys, T.G. (1980) 'Linguistic feedback and maternal speech: comparisons of mothers addressing hearing and hearing-impaired children', *First Language*, *1*, 163-9

Darbyshire, J. (1977) 'Play patterns in young children with impaired hearing', *Volta Review*, *79(1)*, 19-26

Denton, D. (1970) *Remarks in Support of System of Total Communication for Deaf Children*, Communication Symposium, Maryland School for the Deaf, Frederick, Maryland

Drach, K. (1969) *The Language of the Parent: A Pilot Study, Working Paper 14*, Language and Behaviour Research Laboratory, University of California, Berkeley

Evans, L. (1979) 'Psycholinguistic strategy for deaf children – the integration of oral and manual media', *Supplement to British Deaf News*, Feb. 1979

Fraser, C. and Roberts, N. (1975) 'Mothers speech to children at four different ages', *Journal of Psycholinguistic Research*, *4*, 9-16

Freyberg, J.T. (1973) 'Increasing the imaginative play of urban disadvantaged kindergarten children through systematic training' in J.L. Slinger (ed.), *The Child's World of Make-Believe*, Academic Press, London

Friedmann, L. (1977) *On the Other Hand*, Academic Press, New York

Garvey, C. (1979) *Play*, 2nd edn, Fontana/Open Books, Glasgow

Garvey, C. and Hogan, R. (1973) 'Social speech and social interaction: egocentrism revisited', *Child Development*, *44*, 562-8

Gregory, S.M. and Bishop, J.A. (1982) 'The language development of deaf children during their first term at school'. Paper presented at the Child Language Seminar, London, March 1982

Gregory, S.M., Mogford, K. and Bishop, J.A. (1979) 'Mothers' speech to young hearing-impaired children', *J. Brit. Assn. Teachers of the Deaf*, *3(2)*, 42-3

Gregory, S.M. and Mogford, K. (1981) 'Early language development in deaf children' in B. Woll, J. Kyle and Deuchar, M. (eds.), *In Perspectives on British*

Sign Language, Croom Helm, London

Gregory, S.M. and Mogford, K. (1982) 'The development of symbolic play in young deaf children'. Unpublished Paper, Department of Psychology, University of Nottingham

Gustason, G., Pfetzing, D. and Zawolkow, E. (1975) *Signing Exact English*, Modern Signs Press, Rossmor, California

Halliday, M.A.K. (1969) 'Relevant models of language', *Educational Review*, *22(1)*, 26-7

Harrison, D.R. (1980) 'Natural oralism – a description', *J. Brit. Assn. Teachers of the Deaf*, *4(4)* (8-11 Mag.)

Higginbotham, D.J. and Baker, B.M. (1981) 'Social participation and cognitive play differences in hearing-impaired and normally hearing pre-schoolers', *Volta Review*, *83(2)*, 135-48

Higginbotham, D.J., Baker, B.M. and Neill, R.D. (1980) 'Assessing the social participation and cognitive play abilities of hearing-impaired pre-schoolers', *Volta Review*, *82(3)*, 42-54

Howarth, J.N. (1977) *The Development of Spoken Language*. Report of the Proceedings of the Conference on Diagnosis and Early Management of the Deaf Child. University of Manchester, March 1977

Howarth, C.I. and Wood, D.J. (1977) 'A research programme into the intellectual abilities of deaf children', *J. Brit. Assn. Teachers of the Deaf*, *1(1)*, 5-12

Hughes, M.E. and Howarth, J.N. (1980) *Verbal Interaction Between Mothers and Their Young Hearing-impaired Children*, Proceedings of the International Congress on Education of the Deaf, Hamburg, 1980, vol. II, pp. 527-32

Hughes, M.E. (1981) 'Verbal interaction between mothers and their young hearing-impaired children'. Unpublished MEd thesis, University of Manchester

Hughes, M.E. (1983) 'Verbal interaction between mothers and their young hearing-impaired children', *J. Brit. Assn. Teachers of the Deaf*, *7(1)*, 18-23

Ingall, B.I. (1980) 'A structured oral programme', *J. Brit. Assn. Teachers of the Deaf*, *4(4)* (5-8 Mag.)

Jeffree, D. and McConkey, R. (1976) 'An observation scheme for recording children's imaginative doll play', *J. Child Psychol. and Psychiat.*, *17*, 189-97

Klima, E. and Bellugi, U. (1979) *The Signs of Language*, Harvard University Press, Cambridge, Mass.

Jensema, C. and Trybus, R. (1978) *Communication Patterns and Educational Achievement of Hearing-Impaired Students*, Series T, no. 2, Gallaudet College, Office of Demographic Studies, Washington, DC

Kobashigwa, B. (1969) *Repetitions in a Mother's Speech to Her Child, Working Paper 14*, Language and Behaviour Research Laboratory, University of California, Berkeley

Kosaner, J.M. (1983) 'Social and cognitive play levels in hearing-impaired children'. Unpublished MEd thesis, University of Manchester

Lane, H. and Baker, D. (1974) 'Reading achievement of the deaf: another look', *Volta Review*, *76*, 489-99

Latimer, G. (1983) 'T.C. or not T.C? – that is the question', *J. Brit. Assn. Teachers of the Deaf*, *7(4)*, 99-101

Lovell, K., Hoyle, H.W. and Siddall, M.Q. (1968) 'A study of some aspects of the play and language of young children with delayed speech', *J. Child Psychol. and Psychiat*, *9*, 41-50

Lowe, M. and Costello, A. (1976) *Manual for the Symbolic Play Test*, NFER, London

Marmor, G. and Petitto, L. (1979) 'Simultaneous communication in the classroom: how well is English grammar represented?' in W. Stokoe (ed.), *Sign Language Studies*, Linstok Press, Silver Spring, Maryland

McCune-Nicolich, L. and Carroll, S. (1981) 'Development of symbolic play: implications for the language specialist', *Topics in Language Disorders*, *2(1)*, 1-15

Mogford, K., Gregory, S. and Keay, S. (1979) 'Picture book reading with mother: A comparison of hearing-impaired and hearing children at 18 and 24 months', *J. Brit. Assn. Teachers of the Deaf*, *3(2)*, 43-5

Murphy, K.P. (1976) 'Communication for hearing-handicapped people in the United Kingdom and the Republic of Ireland' in H.J. Dyer (ed.), *Communication for the Hearing Handicapped: An International Perspective*, University Park Press, Baltimore

Newport, E.L., Gleitman, L. and Gleitman, H. (1977) 'Mother I'd rather do it myself: some effects and non-effects of maternal speech style' in C.E. Snow and C.A. Ferguson (eds.), *Talking to Children: Language Input and Acquisition*, Cambridge University Press, Cambridge

Nienhuys, T.G. and Tikotin, J.A. (1983) 'Pre-speech communication in hearing and hearing-impaired children', *J. Brit. Assn. Teachers of the Deaf*, *7(6)*

Nix, G.W. (1983) 'How total is total communication', *J. Brit. Assn. Teachers of the Deaf*, *7(6)*

Nolan, M. and Tucker, I.G. (1981) *The Hearing-Impaired Child and The Family*, Souvenir Press, London

Northcott, W. (1981) 'Freedom through speech: every child's right', *Volta Review*, *83(3)*, 162-81

Phillips, J.R. (1973) 'Syntax and vocabulary of mothers' speech to young children: age and sex comparisons', *Child Development*, *44*, 182-5

Pollack, D. (1970) *Educational Audiology for the Limited Hearing Infant*, Charles C. Thomas, Springfield, Ill.

Quigley, S.P. and Kretschmer, R.E. (1982) *The Education of Deaf Children: Issues, Theory and Practice*, Edward Arnold, London

Rawlings, B. and Jensema, C. (1977) *Two Studies of the Families of Hearing-impaired Children*, series R, no. 5, Office of Demographic Studies, Gallaudet College, Washington, DC

Ross, M., Brackett, D. and Maxon, A. (1982) *Hard of Hearing Children in Regular Schools*, Prentice Hall, Englewood Cliffs, NJ

Schaffer, H.R., Collis, G.M. and Parsons, G. (1977) 'Vocal interchange and visual regard in verbal and pre-verbal children' in H.R. Schaffer (ed.), *Studies in Mother Infant Interaction*, Academic Press, London

Shepard, D.C., Delavergne, R.W., Frueh, F.X. and Clobridge, C. (1977) 'Visual-neural correlate of speechreading ability in normal-hearing adults', *J. Speech and Hearing Res.*, *20*, 752-65

Sheridan, M.D. (1960) *The Development Progress of Infants and Young Children*, Reports on Public Health and Medical Subjects, no. 102

Siple, P. (1978) (ed.), *Understanding Language through Sign Language Research*, Academic Press, New York

Snow, C.E. (1972) 'Mothers' speech to children learning language', *Child Development*, *43*, 549-65

Snow, C.E. (1977) 'The development of conversation between mothers and babies', *J. Child Language*, *4*, 1-22

Stern, D., Beebe, B., Jaffe, J. and Bennett, S.L. (1977) 'The infant's stimulus world during social interaction: a study of caregiving behaviours with particular reference to repetition and timing' in H.R. Schaffer (ed.), *Studies in Mother-Infant Interaction*, Academic Press, London

Stokoe, W. (1960) 'Sign language structure: an outline of the visual communication systems of the American deaf', *Studies in Linguistics, Occasional Paper no. 8* (reissued), Gallaudet College Press, Washington, DC

Sutcliffe, B. (1983) 'Total communication or total confusion?', *J. Brit. Assn. Teachers of the Deaf*, *7(5)*, 134-6

Trevarthen, C. (1974) 'Conversations with a two-month-old', *New Scientist*, *62*, 171, 230-5

Trevarthen, C. (1977) 'Descriptive analyses of infant communicative behaviours' in H.R. Schaffer (ed.), *Studies in Mother-Infant Interaction*, Academic Press, London

Tronick, E., Als, H. and Brazelton, T.B. (1980) 'Monadic phases: a structural descriptive analysis of infant-mother face-to-face interaction', *Merrill-Palmer Quarterly*, *26(1)*, 3-24

Trybus, R. and Karchmer, M. (1977) 'School achievement scores of hearing-impaired children: national data on achievement status and growth patterns', *American Annals of the Deaf Directory of Programs and Services*, *122*, 62-9

Tucker, I.G. (1980) 'Some linguistic aspects of the guidance of parents of hearing-impaired children', *J. Brit. Assn. Teachers of the Deaf*, *4(3)*, 74-6

Tucker, I.G. (1981) 'The implications for parent guidance of recent research into parent-child interaction'. Proceedings of the Conference of Heads of Schools and Services for Hearing-impaired Children, University of Manchester, Manchester

Tucker, I.G. (1982) *The Auditory/Oral Approach to Language Development: Research Issues*, Conference of the British Society of Audiology, Dublin, March 1982

Tucker, I.G. (1983) 'The visual regard for mother of a group of hearing-impaired children reared using the auditory/oral approach, compared with a group of normally hearing children', *J. Brit. Assn. Teachers of the Deaf*, *7(1)*, 8-12

Tucker, I.G. and Hughes, M.E. (1984) 'The Language Environment of the Hearing-Impaired Child: Conflicts and Consensus in Current Research' (in press)

Uden, A.M.J. van (1983) Personal communication

Walker, M. (1978) 'Makaton Vocabulary' in *Ways and Means*, Globe Education Ltd, Basingstoke

Wood, D.J. and Howarth, C.I. (1982) 'Psychological and educational consequences of pre-lingual severe/profound deafness', personal communication

EDUCATIONAL PROVISION AND PLACEMENT

Special Schools

Traditionally, hearing-impaired children have been separated from their hearing peers and educated in residential special schools. However, the movement over many years has been towards day instead of residential, towards special classes instead of special schools and towards mainstreaming where the child is placed with his ordinary hearing peers and given supportive teaching by a specialist teacher of the hearing-impaired. Either this or he is withdrawn on occasions to a base within the school where this additional teaching can be provided. It would be useful if the newcomer to this field looked at the provision as a broadly based service rather than as a special school or class because it would be hoped that education authorities, within the limitations of their size, are providing a whole range of options for the varying educational needs of hearing-impaired children. Special schools and classes are options within a 'service'.

The reaction against special schools has been partly because people feel that educational achievement can be greater where the demands of integrating with normal children are higher. It has also been a belief that aspirations tend to be higher in ordinary schools rather than merely a belief that there were dangers from the institutionalisation effects of residential placement in special schools. Undoubtedly there were fears for the emotional and personality development of children who were separated from their families for long periods, but as fewer and fewer children under the age of five attended residential schools these fears have lessened. There is no doubt that there has been a strong reaction from parents against being separated from their very young children. Most researchers are now agreed that the institutionalising effects of separation are most severe in the first three or four years of life.

In Britain the first residential special school for hearing-impaired children was opened in Edinburgh in 1760 by Thomas Braidwood and this was followed by the opening of schools in London and Birmingham, the one in Birmingham being started by Braidwood's nephew, Watson.

Schools for the deaf in the United States were influenced by work taking place in Europe. A member of the Braidwood family, John Braidwood, set up a small school for the deaf in Cobbs, Virginia (Rae,

1851). Shortly after Thomas Hopkins Gallaudet studied under the Braidwoods in England and also in France. He established a school in West Hartford, Connecticut. It seems likely that the school in Connecticut was modelled on the school founded by Abbé Charles Michel de L'Epée in Paris in 1750. This was the first permanently established school for hearing-impaired children and Gallaudet trained there under Abbé Roche Ambroise Sicard, de L'Epée's successor.

Table 10.1: Hearing-impaired children in England and Wales, 1981.

	Survey figure	Corrected estimate
1. In special schools for the deaf or partially-hearing	3,722	4,144
2. In special units attached to ordinary schools	3,782	4,211
3. In ordinary schools	23,072	25,690
4. Children under 5 years, not attending special school	2,138	2,380
5. In full-time further education, with support from a qualified teacher of the deaf	505	562

Source: after Powell, 1984.

It may seem that day placement is a relatively modern development, but this is not so, since the first day schools were established before 1900 and, throughout the history of education of hearing-impaired children, there have been many successful efforts to educate children with their hearing peers. However, this movement has now increased quite markedly and supportive legislation both in Britain and the USA is likely to foster further development in this direction (see Table 10.1).

In the United Kingdom only 23 of 96 Local Education Authorities (LEAs) maintain special schools. The number of special schools has been declining in recent years and it is likely to decline still further with falling pupil numbers and an increased level of mainstreaming. However, there remains a need for special schools for those children who require the highest levels of specialist teaching (see Table 10.2).

Table 10.2: Special schools in 1981 in England and Wales.

Schools		Maintained (LEA)[a]	non-maintained[b]	Independent[c]	Total
Deaf	Day	8	—	—	
	Residential	7	5	6	26
Partially-hearing	Day	1	—	—	
	Residential	2	2	—	5
Deaf and partially-hearing	Day	8	—	—	
		7	6	—	21
	Total	33	13	6	52

Notes: a. Maintained schools funded and maintained entirely by an LEA; b. non-maintained schools funded and maintained by charities administered by Boards of governors and trustees. Costs are met from fees charged for each pupil. Supportive grants from central Government are often given towards approved capital expenditure. These schools are non-profit making; c. Independent schools funded and maintained privately by individuals or groups. Income is from fees and profits may be made.

Source: after Powell, 1984.

The educational picture in the United States has been outlined by Oyer (1976) and the authors have adapted his data for presentation in Table 10.3. Readers will see the much larger percentage of children being educated in special schools as opposed to special classes or integrated settings. One would imagine that in the intervening years since such data were collected that, as in the United Kingdom, the number of special classes and children in integrated settings has been the area of greatest growth.

As readers will see from Table 10.2 the schools in the United Kingdom are designated deaf or partially-hearing, but placement decisions would be based on a functional assessment of the child rather than solely looking at levels of hearing on the audiogram. It is clearly possible to see very severely hearing-impaired children in partially-hearing establishments if their level of functioning makes this the most appropriate placement.

Special schools both here and in the USA have the logistical advantage of being able to provide sophisticated support services, often employing specialist audiologists, psychologists, etc. whereas the more diffuse mainstream services are sometimes unable to do this. It is our view that provision should be made on a 'Service for hearing-impaired'

Table 10.3: Educational provision in the United States.

Type of educational establishment				Number
Special schools	(A)	Residential	(Public)	63
		"	(Private)	12
	(B)	Day	(Public)	65
		"	(Private)	22
Day classes			(Private)	61
Programmes for children in ordinary schools				525

The numbers of children involved in 1973 were:

(a)	Deaf and hard of hearing:	41,109
(b)	Number being educated in residential special schools:	18,705
(c)	Number being educated in day special schools:	2,960
(d)	Number being educated in special classes:	12,662
(e)	Number being educated in integrated settings:	4,358

basis and specialists provided as in the larger schools.

Some residential special schools are also taking in pupils who have severe handicaps additional to deafness, indeed in this country some schools have wholly gone over to catering for the needs of such children. These children, formerly, would have had little or no chance of a stimulating educational environment.

Types of Mainstreamed Provision

Mainstreaming, the practice of educating hearing-impaired children alongside their normally hearing peers is widespread in Britain and the USA. Britain mainstreams more children with hearing losses greater than 50dB than any other European country (52·1 per cent), with Denmark (43·8 per cent), Italy (50·1 per cent) and Ireland (34·5 per cent) being the other European countries mainstreaming substantial numbers of hearing-impaired children.

There are many variants of mainstreaming and McGee (1976) has outlined what would seem to be most of the options available to the educators of the hearing-impaired. If mainstreaming is mentioned in literature on hearing-impaired children it should include the degree of interaction it allows between hearing-impaired and hearing pupils. The options are:

1. Complete integration or mainstreaming within the ordinary class without any supportive help.
2. Mainstreaming with varying levels of individual support.
3. Basing the child in a resource room or base unit and integrating him on a part-time basis into the ordinary class. The subjects he integrates for can also vary.
4. Team teaching of the ordinary teacher and a teacher of the deaf of an integrated class into which is placed one or more hearing-impaired children.
5. Reversed mainstreaming where normally hearing pupils become part of a class of hearing-impaired pupils. This is less common in the United Kingdom, but seems to be done more frequently at the nursery end where the educators of the hearing-impaired rate very highly the influence of ordinary children and set up a nursery to attract in ordinary children to mix with the hearing-impaired. Nursery places are difficult to find in many areas and this seems to be a successful route to integration of such children.
6. Self-contained classes or units from which pupils go to ordinary classes for one or more specific academic subjects.
7. Self-contained classes or units from which pupils go to ordinary classes for one or more non-academic activities.
8. Completely self-contained classes or units with little or no contact with normally hearing peers.

All British teachers of the deaf are also certified to teach normally hearing children, so another option suggested by Quigley and Kretschmer (1982), that of putting a teacher of the deaf in charge of an ordinary class into which are integrated one or more hearing-impaired children, is open. The present authors have not heard of this option being used in the United Kingdom. For an excellent, and more detailed account of mainstreaming rationale and practice, readers are referred to Nix (1976).

Special Classes in Ordinary Schools – Partially-hearing Units

The partially-hearing unit (PHU) is to be found in most LEAs, although Powell (1984) has suggested that this title is somewhat misleading since many such units now contain children with severe or profound hearing losses. This is an expanding area of provision there being 413 such units in England in 1980 staffed by between 650 and 700 teachers of the deaf or about 36 per cent of the specialist teacher force. The units cater for just over half the total number of children placed in either a special school or special unit (Powell, 1984). Most units employ only a small number of teachers, and some, particularly those for younger children, also have classroom assistants.

When PHUs first came into being they tended to cater for the less severely hearing-impaired children who had good spoken language, but now the units have both wide age ranges and cater for a wider range of hearing loss. It is only natural therefore that class teaching, as in schools for the deaf, has given way to much greater emphasis on individual or very small group educational programming and also that the levels and extent of integration with the normally hearing children varies widely. Some may only be integrated for less academic areas such as physical education, art and craft, etc. whilst others are assigned to a regular class and only receive extra help within that class or are occasionally withdrawn to the resource base to receive intensive specialist help.

The Peripatetic Teaching Service

In Britain this is also called the 'Advisory' teaching service, or the 'Visiting' teacher service and covers support for the families of pre-school hearing-impaired children and those placed in mainstream without a special resource unit. In the USA this teacher would be called an 'Itinerant' teacher. The difficulty in ascribing them a firm single name highlights the variety of roles they fulfil, from counselling and guiding parents of very young hearing-impaired children, to advising teachers of ordinary children who have a hearing-impaired child in their class, to visiting the hearing-impaired child in the ordinary school to carry out remedial micro-teaching. For some of them there are other tasks as well, such as participating in multi-disciplinary diagnostic teams, providing short courses for all kinds of interested and involved personnel, supporting students in further and higher education and supporting hearing-impaired children in other types of schools, for example, schools for the mentally or physically handicapped. This has been a major growth area of special education for hearing-impaired children with 4 such teachers in the United Kingdom in 1958, 259 in 1972 and about 500 at the present time.

Provision for Pre-school Hearing-impaired Children

Quigley and Kretschmer (1982) have suggested that in the USA, whilst an extensive system of education exists for hearing-impaired children from five years to eighteen years plus, there is perhaps a significant gap from birth to about three or four years. In our view, and that of

Quigley and Kretschmer, these pre-school years are the most important years in the child's life for the development of language and communication skills.

In the USA the first systematic programmes of pre-school intervention began with the establishment of the charitably funded John Tracy Clinic in Los Angeles in 1943. John Tracy is a clinic based and correspondence organisation providing free help to families of hearing-impaired children anywhere in the world. The John Tracy Clinic has expanded since its first meetings as a tiny parents' group, but the focus has remained the same; *not* what the medical people can do to help; *not* what the educators and schools can do to help, but a concentration on what the parents themselves can do to help their child. There are demonstration homes, a four-year demonstration nursery programme, summer school sessions and as mentioned above the world famous correspondence courses for the parents of hearing-impaired children and also one for parents of children who are both hearing and visually impaired. The clinic also, in conjunction with the University of Southern California, prepares teachers for work with pre-school age children and work with parents. Clinics such as John Tracy are not usually part of the public education system in the USA. In contrast, in Britain educational guidance and counselling are offered by the majority of local education authorities to parents of hearing-impaired children. This service is provided by peripatetic teachers in the families' home and/or in clinic bases. In addition major national centres such as the Department of Audiology and Education of the Deaf at Manchester University and the Nuffield Speech and Hearing Centre in London offer a wide range of specialised services in assessment and early management, including individual and group guidance. The Ealing Centre attached to Nuffield offers week-long residential courses to parents and their hearing-impaired children. Manchester University's Department of Audiology and Education of the Deaf is Britain's major training centre for Audiologists (Medical, Scientific and Educational) and teachers of the hearing-impaired. It also pioneered the work in guidance of parents of hearing-impaired children (Ewing and Ewing, 1938, 1947). Parents and their children are seen by the guidance and counselling team immediately following diagnosis and this support is ongoing right into the school system. A multi-disciplinary support team is provided within the Department. The work with families is given very high priority within the Department and there are good grounds for strengthening, both numerically and in terms of quality and training, this service throughout the country.

Legislation Affecting Provision and Placement

In the last decade there has been a wide ranging review of Special Education in England. The Government set up a committee under the Chairmanship of Warnock. This reported in 1978 – 'Special Educational Needs', The Warnock Report – and resulted in the Government bringing forward a new Education Act in 1981. Section 1 of the Act gave effect to the principle that handicapped children, who were formerly classified into specific categories of handicap should now be provided for on the basis of their individual special educational needs. It also established that children with special needs in terms of educational provision are to be 'educated in ordinary schools, so far as it is reasonably practical, and are to associate in the activities of the school with other children'. There seems little doubt that in conforming with provisions of the Act there will tend to be a reduction in the number of special schools and greater emphasis on mainstreaming.

Section 4 of the Act places LEAs under a duty to attempt to identify children with special educational needs and where it is deemed appropriate to prepare a 'statement' of special educational need. (The LEA must inform the parents of their intention to make an assessment.) Parents have the right to be given information about the assessment procedure, to contribute their own statement and to appeal to the Secretary of State if the LEA decide after assessment not to determine the special educational provision to be made for their child. The Statement is drawn up under the following headings:

1. Introduction – details of the child and parents.
2. Special educational needs.
3. Special educational provision.
4. Appropriate school or other provision.
5. Additional non-educational provision.

The appendices provide the information on which the statement is based:

A. Parental representations.
B. Parental evidence.
C. Educational advice.
D. Medical advice.
E. Psychological advice.
F. Other advice obtained by the education authority.

Parents can demand that an assessment be made and LEAs can only refuse if they regard it as a request that no parent acting reasonably would make. Parents again can appeal and LEAs are informed that the Secretary of State will normally expect LEAs to comply with such requests. The Act is also important in so far as it places a duty on health authorities to inform both parents and LEAs if it believes a child has or is likely to have special educational needs. The health authority is also required to give the parents an opportunity to discuss this opinion prior to bringing the child to the attention of the LEA.

The Act's emphasis on *need* rather than *category* should be a step forward in encouraging a flexible set of arrangements for the education of hearing handicapped children.

In the United States recent changes have been strongly influenced by two important court cases: *Pennsylvania Association for Retarded Citizens* v. *Commonwealth of Pennsylvania* (1971) and *Mills* v. *Board of Education* (1972). These cases found in favour of the plaintiffs and established that all retarded children had the right to a free and appropriate public education within the 'least restrictive environments'. This has been widely interpreted as being educated within the ordinary public school system and there has been tremendous pressure towards mainstreaming.

In (1975) the US Congress enacted Public Law 94-142 which mandates that the education of all handicapped school-aged children is the responsibility of the state and local school educational agencies and all handicapped children are to be educated in what is the least restrictive environment for the child. Each district was thus obliged to draw up a plan consistent with the mandate, a plan which contained a full range of options. Arrangements were also made to provide for non-biased testing and placement and for the preparation of Individual Educational Programmes (IEPs).

Clearly legislation like that in Britain and the USA will have far reaching effects on the education of hearing-impaired children right into the twenty-first century.

Educational Factors Affecting Hearing-impaired Child Placement Decisions

When a child is being considered for educational placement it is important to look at the problem from as many angles as possible. Throughout these considerations the present authors would make the assumption that parents would be involved, consulted and actually contributing to the placement decision. In our view the following areas merit consideration: (1) philosophy related areas; (2) school related areas; and (3) child related areas.

Philosophy

The prevailing philosophy has been much influenced by the growing number of severely and profoundly hearing-impaired children who have been so successful in developing language skills that they have been capable of education in a normal environment. This has been resultant on many factors including improvements in the technology of hearing aids, in some areas earlier diagnosis, better parent training and improvements in our knowledge of the language learning process. Education Acts have given weight to the pressure for the 'integration' of hearing-impaired children into the ordinary school. Being educated with normal children is, for many people involved with handicapped children, synonymous with the term integration. If this is indeed what integration is about then for hearing-impaired children the trends have been in this direction since the formation of the first partially-hearing units in the late 1940s, and the appointments of the first peripatetic teachers in the late 1950s. Those factors involved with the *physical* integration of hearing-impaired children into the normal educational system are illustrated in Table 10.4 and Table 10.5.

Table 10.4: Number of peripatetic teachers.

Year	1959	1969	1971	1972	1973	1975	1976	1977	1981
Peripatetic teachers	4	200	212	259	283	363	461	469	501

Table 10.5: Number of partially-hearing units.

Year	1966	1967	1968	1971	1976	1977	1980
Number of units	162	173	191	212	454	463	413

The rapid development of these forms of educational provision through the 1960s and 1970s is clear. It can also be seen that placement of hearing-impaired children in special schools has changed correspondingly.

There has been a decline in the number of children placed in schools for the deaf, and an increase in those placed in schools for partially-hearing children and in partially-hearing units (Nolan and Tucker, 1981).

Along with these trends, however, is a growing tendency for more multiply handicapped children to be placed in schools for the deaf, which is to some extent disguising the rapid fall in numbers of deaf children in the special schools.

The movement in the direction of more normal educational environments for hearing-impaired children is not uniform with some authorities still very rigidly placing children in special schools, but the movement is gaining momentum. It is based on the assumption that hearing-impaired children can learn to talk and that they will do it best where the environment is naturally oral and the motivation to achieve good oral standards is high. It is also felt that normal social relationships develop best if they are started early. We do detect a new attitude of flexibility in the teaching profession and this is what is required if the best interests of hearing-impaired children are to be served. There is a need for a wide variety of educational provision in view of the lack of homogeneity in the population of hearing-impaired children. Selection for that provision should be on the basis of satisfying the child's individual educational needs (see Northcott, 1981 for a very persuasive argument for a flexible needs based approach to the hearing-impaired child).

It may be thought that integration means 'sameness', but integration first implies differences between individuals (Lynas, 1980), since if there were no differences there would be no need to integrate. It also implies bringing together or unifying these different individuals. Differences as far as hearing-impaired children are concerned are not once-and-for-all differences. They lie on a continuum and may have differing impacts on the child's life at different stages. For example, if a school-age child has a minor hearing loss only, it may not even be detected, or if it is it may be regarded as insignificant. Yet at the language learning stage even a minor loss can have a marked impact on the rate of language development. This highlights the fact that assessment of special need cannot be a once and forever assessment. Needs will require frequent up-dating.

There is also a problem in that terminology such as partially-hearing, severely and profoundly deaf mean different things to different people. The British Association of Teachers of the Deaf have regularised their terminology (if not the title of their own Association) to use the less stigmatising term, hearing-impaired, for all children with hearing difficulties. The United Kingdom statutory definitions of deaf children are — 'Pupils with impaired hearing who require education by methods suitable for pupils with little or no naturally acquired speech or language' (HMSO, 1962); and for partially-hearing children — 'Pupils with impaired hearing whose development of speech and language even if retarded is following a normal pattern and who require for their education special arrangements or facilities though not necessarily all the educational methods used for deaf pupils' (HMSO, 1962). These clearly no longer serve the needs of the teaching profession. The Association felt that 'deaf' and partially-hearing can often lead to confusion since a child can on an audiogram evaluation be profoundly deaf, but if looked at functionally be partially-hearing and so on. It was felt that there was a need for simple definitions which could be scientifically applied and would be useful particularly for published material on hearing-impaired children. The Association chose to prefix hearing-impaired by slightly (children whose average hearing loss, 250 Hz to 4 kHz regardless of age onset, does not exceed 40 dB HL), moderately (children whose average hearing loss, regardless of age of onset, is from 41-70 dBHL), severely (children whose average hearing loss is from 71-95 dBHL and those with a greater loss who acquired their hearing-impairment after the age of 18 months), profoundly (children who were born with or who acquired, before the age of 18 months, an average hearing loss of 96 dB or greater (BATOD, 1981). This sort of classification does at least have some scientific basis and is useful for publications but it is not very useful for placement decisions and most professionals are classifying children on a functional basis, according to what the child can do: the absolute level of any child's hearing loss is not being seen as important as how he is using that remaining hearing to aid his development. His responses will depend on many things, including the age at which he was diagnosed, whether or not he has additional handicaps, his intelligence and personality, the fitting and use made of amplification, the support and stimulation from his family and the quality and effectiveness of early counselling and guidance.

A cascade approach to provision has been suggested by Reynolds (1962), Deno (1970) and others and a variant of these approaches would seem to be ideal. Deno's model with its seven categories ranging from regular classes with or without supportive services to homebound, hospital or residential settings with total separation from the mainstream would be worthy of consideration. The model advocates placing the majority of children in ordinary classes, and if special settings are required the model would aim to return the children to the ordinary class as soon as is feasible. The Deno cascade model was not designed specifically for hearing-impaired children but would seem to be transferable to that handicap. For a model of early education of hearing-impaired children readers are referred to the Massachusetts early education model designed by David Luterman (Hein and Bishop, 1979). The cascade is seen as providing a hierarchy of least to most restriction in educational environment with the constant provision for a return to less restriction. The superior provision in the cascade is the one which best meets the individual child's educational needs at that time.

Consideration of Children for Mainstream Placement – Factors Relating to the School

Education in Britain has always allowed a large measure of freedom to headteachers to develop their own philosophy and practices. Also the individual teacher in the classroom enjoys substantial freedom to develop a personal teaching style within the constraints laid down by school policy. Lynas (1980) has outlined some of the significant dimensions along which schools vary:

1. Size – some schools cater for over 2,000 pupils, others for less than 100.
2. Organisation – there are many ways of organising the pupils, for example, vertical grouping (when more than one age group is in one class) team teaching, streaming by ability, subject teaching, etc.
3. Buildings – vary in nature, shape, size and layout, for example open-plan, separate classrooms.
4. Declared philosophy – schools differ in their ethos, their emphasis of aims, for example, firm discipline, high standards, individual care, all round development are examples of possible aims.
5. Atmosphere – schools have noticeable atmospheres, for example, friendly, intimate, purposeful, industrious, casual, *laissez-faire*, authoritarian.
6. Population – schools cater for different social and ethnic categories of pupils, for example, working class, middle class, Black immigrant, Asian or any mixture of these.
7. Noise – different levels of noise exist in schools according to the prevailing acoustic conditions, but also according to what level of pupil noise will be tolerated by the teaching staff.

Lynas (1980) wisely asks us to consider carefully what sort of environment would be suitable for particular hearing-impaired children. High noise levels greatly affect the reception of personal aids, a school with many problem children may find it difficult to integrate a hearing-impaired child, a small friendly, caring environment may, for a particular child, be better than a large diffuse comprehensive school. Those involved in placing hearing-impaired children would certainly need to be perceptive enough to spot these school features and to be able to identify the one best suited to the child.

Factors Relating to the Teacher and Teacher Style

The hearing-impaired child interacting with teacher and class peers will be confronted by a great variety of situations which vary considerably in their difficulty for him. When the child is engaged with his table group he may find it easier to follow context and content than when, say, he is involved in a whole class discussion where there are many speaker changes. He may find certain subjects more difficult than others, for example, English more difficult than Maths when the teacher adopts a group teaching style for the former and an individual style for the latter. There is no doubt that hearing-impaired children benefit in many ways from contact in groups with their hearing peers, but it is important to realise that some teachers reject this teaching/learning style in favour of practically all whole class work. When group co-operative projects are not encouraged then the hearing-impaired child misses much, he misses the help of the other children in clearly formulating what is required of them, the social aspects of co-operating and sharing, the opportunity to be led and be part of the team and also on occasions to be the leader. This can affect the adaptation of the hearing-impaired child to the class — it can increase a possibly already existing feeling of isolation.

Teachers also vary widely in other facets of their style, for example, rate of speaking, clarity and manner of presentation. Technique varies in the amount the teacher talks before checking that the children have followed and understood, the way they summarise and encapsulate the main messages of the lesson and in their reactions to child contributions.

The hearing-impaired child is helped greatly by careful use of the blackboard or overhead projector, by reformulation of questions to give more clues and particularly by the 'reflection' technique of the teacher repeating the answer of another pupil so that the hearing-impaired child can hear, aided possibly by a radio transmitter, what the correct, or incorrect answer was.

Lynas (1980) has suggested a way of conceptualising the various levels of acceptance shown by ordinary teachers who have a hearing-impaired child in their class. It shows a continuum of positive discrimination from:

1. No positive discrimination — teacher accepts the child providing it can cope with only 'normal' attention.
2. Limited positive discrimination — teacher accepts the hearing-impaired child as only one of a variety of children with special needs, for example, the slow learners or those with reading difficulties. This teacher would not offer specialist help, but would be prepared to make minor changes to technique such as facing the child when speaking and sitting him near the front of the class.
3. Considerable positive discrimination — teacher will make carefully thought out changes to teaching style in order to help the hearing-impaired child. She may adjust her speaking rate and articulation in order to improve clarity, use the blackboard or overhead projector to clarify terms or to provide summaries of work covered. She will ensure that the hearing-impaired child is appropriately positioned, use reflection techniques and assign times to check that the child has followed the lesson. She may become so skilled that she anticipates many of the 'difficult' areas and pre-empts them by preparatory work.
4. Excessive positive discrimination — this teacher Lynas calls the 'big production' teacher. She makes concessions at the expense of the rest of the class, spends considerable individual time with the child, makes the rest of the class wait and in some cases actually alienates the class from this privileged person the hearing-impaired child. She gives effusive praise for the child's only modest achievements.

Apart from possibly number 4, all of the levels on the continuum could be useful to a hearing-impaired child providing it was the right child for the right level of favourable discrimination or providing that what was lacking in the teacher of ordinary children could be made up by specialist input from the teacher of the deaf.

Factors Relating to the Child Himself

Before a child is mainstreamed it is essential that he is closely scrutinised from as many angles as possible. Simmonds-Martin (1976) has suggested that the disparity between the child's chronological age and his linguistic age should not exceed one year. Others suggest that it should not exceed two years. Most authors agree that it should be close to chronological age. The present authors believe that rather than looking at absolutes such as present language age it can often be more meaningful to monitor from diagnosis and then look at the rate of change of language age. In this way a more realistic picture of the child's capability for mainstreaming emerges. Simmonds-Martin also suggests scrutiny of communication skills, verbal intelligence, academic skills and social and emotional maturity.

In terms of communication skills measure should be made of the intelligibility of his speech, his ability to communicate in the relatively high signal-to-noise ratios which pertain in most primary school classrooms, and some assessment of his ability to follow the teacher and his peers.

Simmonds-Martin (1976) has suggested the dangers of forcing the child to operate at a cognitive level which is above his ability and she adds that even in the early years in the primary school the load can be very heavy.

The child should be able to handle the curriculum of the receiving school. Failure in this area can result in damage to self-image. Simmonds-Martin stresses the development of reading skills without the commonly reported 'plateau' of reading ability at about a reading age of seven to eight years. Others would argue that mainstreaming would or should have taken place before the child has actually had the chance to develop his reading skills and Lane and Baker (1974) suggest that properly placed children do not suffer a plateau in their reading ability.

The immature child finds difficulty in mainstreaming whereas the socially adaptable tend to make good mainstreamers. Simmonds-Martin urges caution: 'Start the child in a programme where he can succeed, gain in confidence rather than fail and withdraw in defeat.' The whole of her world famous parent programme at the Central Institute for the Deaf in St Louis, Missouri, is geared to the aims of getting parents to 'know their own child' and 'setting realistic goals'. We too are convinced that if we inform, educate and work *with* parents then disputes about the most appropriate placement will rarely arise. Parents will have seen the variety of places where their child could be educated, they will have a fairly accurate appraisal of their child's capabilities and know which placement will suit him best at that particular time in his educational career.

Successful mainstreaming depends on many things. It depends on early detection, supportive parents who have been well trained, it depends on appropriate aid fitting with correct levels of gain being used. The child must be a 'waking hours' hearing-aid user. He must be socially well adjusted with a well formed personality, gregarious and willing to persist in his attempts to communicate. It is a great help if his linguistic and academic skills are close to those of his peers and if he is average or better in intelligence. Add to these factors the support of a range of professionals and you have the ideal candidate for mainstreaming. If some of these factors are not present it does not mean that mainstreaming is not possible but the type of mainstreaming may change and even greater care in placement and support arrangements will be required.

Advising Ordinary School Teachers of the Problems of Hearing-impairment

In the view of the present authors, specialists in the educational management of hearing-impaired children should have a well formulated programme of advice for the ordinary teacher. This should be a long-term programme, not a 'crash' course, since there is a real danger of frightening teachers with too much special knowledge all at once. There is a possibility that such teachers will see the hearing handicapped child as 'too special' for me.

Over a period of time we would hope that the teachers would learn about the following areas (some of which are covered in more detail in other chapters of this book):

1. The practical operation of hearing aid systems and their limitations in certain educational environments, particularly noisy ones. Even if the educational audiologist is prescribing gain settings, tone settings, type of aid used, etc. it will be the classroom teacher who will make the daily aid efficiency checks and monitor aid use. The specialist will be the 'troubleshooter' for the major breakdowns, but the classroom teacher should be capable of making simple repairs by substitution.
2. The areas of the child's progress which deafness may have affected and which may require the teachers special attention. For example, the child may need to be taught the everyday customs and courtesies which ordinary children pick up incidentally. The teacher will need to be aware of, and look for, the symptoms of social isolation.
3. The teacher will need help in planning the child's learning experience. (In the USA preparation of the IEP – Individualised Educational Programme.) This will mean being able to describe the student's performance in the various areas of the curriculum and to set academic goals. They may also need help on the use of audio-visual aids and strategies for integrating their use into the teaching programme. This

might include greater use of video-taped material, slides and overhead projection transparencies.

4. There will need to be joint discussion and appraisal of the level and type of involvement of the specialist teachers and also of the extent of contact between the handicapped and non-handicapped pupils.

5. The teacher will need to be taught the teaching techniques which aid the hearing handicapped, for example, repetition, rephrasing, paraphrasing, 'reflection', positioning of teacher *vis à vis* students, control of teacher movement, etc.

6. At a more leisurely pace the teacher could learn about the causes of deafness including conductive losses which are, of course, very common in the ordinary primary school.

7. Finally there will need to be joint discussion on the form of methodology and the extent of special evaluation of the pupil's progress.

Ongoing Audiological and Educational Assessment

It is not feasible, nor appropriate, in an introductory text such as this to describe in detail all aspects of assessment. However, in many United Kingdom authorities the educational audiologist is the professional who carries out such evaluation of the educational development of the hearing-impaired child and assesses his audiological status. He may also collate the information drawn from other specialists such as psychologists or speech pathologist and therapists. This makes it essential that we at least draw attention to the major areas of investigation.

Audiological. It would be hoped that the following pattern of audiological reassessment would be carried out in any service for hearing-impaired children:

(1) Hearing aid checks daily by parents and the regular class, or special class teacher. This check would be basic, covering need for replacements of battery, cord, etc. and an indication of the aids' ability to achieve the output requirements set by the audiologist.

(2) A full specification check should be carried out monthly by the educational audiologist and fresh impressions for new earmoulds taken if required.

(3) There should be a monthly tympanometry check to monitor middle ear condition. This would be carried out by the educational audiologist with a direct line of referral to the otologist for any necessary medical or surgical treatment. Tucker (1972) has shown in an all-age school for hearing-impaired children that a substantial (19 per

cent) of children may at any one time have abnormal middle ear function in addition to their sensori-neural loss. See also Ross (1976) who reported 50 per cent abnormal middle ear function in a new programme for hearing-impaired children.

(4) Six-monthly, or at least annually, complete audiological review. This should include pure-tone testing air and bone, with masking if necessary, tympanometry and stapedius reflex tests, and speech tests of hearing at an appropriate level of sophistication for the child. There should also be a re-evaluation of the provision for the child's amplification needs, checking whether he still has the most appropriate aids for his hearing problem, and whether a radio system should be called into use. This check should bear in mind our philosophy that consistency of sound experience is all important, so aids should only be changed if it is felt the new system will offer *substantial* advantage. It is well worth keeping a cumulative audiogram to ensure that any deterioration (or improvement) in hearing level is immediately spotted. Markides (1971) has reported that in spite of much debate there is no strong evidence that high levels of amplification are damaging the residual hearing of severely hearing-impaired children, but close monitoring is important.

Academic. The educational audiologist should receive an annual report from the host school on the various subjects studied by the pupil. He may also collate these findings in the special school setting.

Speech and Language. This is obviously an area of great interest and will require special annual monitoring. The results of speech and language evaluation serve 'to provide specific guidelines for remedial work and as a base line against which the results of training can be compared' (Ling, 1976). Ling is critical of the dearth of literature on speech evaluation of the hearing-impaired child and that other workers have taken for granted that teachers are always familiar with the extent of the child's speech skills. He suggests that in this area teachers are responsible for three evaluation tasks:

1. Oral-peripheral structures and function, facial structure, lip movement, the jaw and teeth, the tongue, diadochokinetic rate, the hard palate, the soft palate and the larynx.
2. Phonological speech evaluation.
3. Phonetic level evaluation.

He suggests that these measures be carried out on a 50 representative utterance sample collected in good acoustic conditions and tape recorded for analysis. In an appendix to his text Ling provides model forms for carrying out and recording the analysis. Particularly with young children there is something to be said for the use of video records. This greatly improves the chances of accurate transcription and analysis. Tucker (1980a, 1980b) has shown the value of this form from the point of view of both analysing child language and for investigating the linguistic environment provided by parents.

Language evaluation is confused by language methodology since some children are taught using an oral approach and others using one of a variety of manual approaches.

It is common to investigate language either by (a) studies based on secondary language skills, reading and writing, or (b) by evaluation of written compositions according to parts of speech used, sentence complexity and quantity of language used. Other investigators have approached the language acquisition area by studying (c) word association abilities or the use of word classes and syntax.

Bellugi and Klima's (1972) results indicated that a child's sign vocabulary covered the full range of concepts expressed by the hearing child. Schlesinger and Meadow (1972) reported parallel development of sign language and verbal language. Perhaps the most exciting development in recent years has been the growing body of research based on 'language interaction' measures. These measures have been carried out in both home and laboratory (Tucker, 1980b; Hughes, 1983; Anderson, 1979; Gregory *et al.*, 1979), and at school with the class teacher (Huntington and Watton, 1981, 1982). This methodology attempts in many cases to assess the language as used in a relatively 'free' situation (say playing with table-top toys) as opposed to the more formal standardised tests such as the Reynell Developmental Language Scale (Reynell, 1977) which is widely used in the United Kingdom with hearing-impaired children to assess both comprehension and expressive language. Clearly interaction is a fruitful area for research but there is already sufficient methodology to encourage its use in assessment, and methodology is discussed in more detail in Chapter 9.

Reading. Audiologists should be aware that reading depends on a well developed internalised language system which in turn depends on the infant being exposed to a wealth of meaningful interaction experience. Reading will not make up for or replace this need for a developed communication system. Reading is the basis for developing many academic skills and for the transmission of knowledge but it cannot exist prior to the existence of the oral or manual communication system.

There are a great many skills involved in reading and because of this there are a wide range of tests of reading skills. Those involved in ongoing assessments of reading skill will require a multi-purpose test and then access to tests which attempt to provide more detail about a specific reading skill which may be giving the child difficulty. Pumfrey (1977) has outlined criteria for selection of reading tests as follows:

1. *Content*

Is the content valid for my purpose? (For example, does it test the skill in which I am interested, such as 'ability to read regular three-letter words; to read accurately, or to understand instructions of a particular type'?)

Is the test reliable in the way important for my purpose?

Is the test intended for the group with which I am concerned?

Is the material appropriate to the children's background?

2. *Form*

What type of administration best suits my purpose? (For example individual or group? oral or silent? timed or untimed? multiple choice or constructed response? power or speed?)

3. *Marking and Interpreting*

How are the results presented? (For example, will they be in terms of raw scores, reading ages, percentiles or quotients?)

Will I be able to relate these results to my purpose?

How long does it take to administer, score and interpret?

How can the results best be recorded?

Has the test been given to the children before?

If so, when and will this affect my interpretation?

Are the norms of the test up to date?

Is it important if they are not?

4. *Availability*

Am I qualified to use the test?

Is the test already available in the school or in the area?

Is it part of the reading assessment programme of the school or the local education authority?

Is the test 'open' or 'restricted'?

5. *Cost*

Is the test material expendable or reusable?

What is the cost per pupil of administering the test?

Is the expenditure incurred in both time and money justified?

As has already been mentioned the average levels of reading skill of hearing-impaired children are low and it has been claimed by some that reading tests for ordinary children actually overestimate the hearing-impaired child's ability. Studies of particular areas of the reading task, particularly syntax (Quigley *et al.*, 1977), but including word analysis, vocabulary and inferencing ability, tend to show that the hearing-impaired child has difficulty. Quigley *et al.* concluded that there was a need for further research which concentrated on modifying reading materials at the early stages and on developing a greater understanding of the psychological processes involved in hearing-impaired children's learning to read. Others are resigned to the fact that production of 'special' materials for such a small group would not be feasible and that teachers need to use currently available materials to greater effect. Redgate and Palmer (1972) investigated whether the initial teaching alphabet (ita) enabled hearing-impaired children to more easily grasp reading skills, but found that their traditional orthography (to) group was outstripping the ita group by the time of the transition from ita to to. The research also found, as have other studies, that there is a high correlation between reading attainments and other measures of language ability. Many teachers of hearing-impaired children use the language of the child to construct his first reading material and when the child moves on to a scheme they ensure that it is one with finely graded stages and wealth of supplementary material. At later stages the supplementary reading can be selected by teachers using readability procedures such as 'Cloze', Taylor (1953) and formulae such as those of Dale and Chall quoted by Gilliland (1972). McNally and Murray (1962) have investigated and identified 200 key words in everyday reading matter and note that only 21 of these are nouns. The teacher of the hearing-impaired has to work very hard in order to ensure that the sight of many of these words evokes responses in hearing-impaired children. Many companies now sell support materials relating to basic words. Undoubtedly further research will extend our knowledge of the hearing-impaired child's difficulties and may prompt the production of specialised teaching material.

Perhaps the best sources of critical reviews of reading tests are the Buros' (1938-72) Mental Measurement Year Books. These books contain references to, and critical reviews by, specially selected reviewers of tests of all types. The seventh Buros yearbook (1972) also contains a list of the major test publishers and suppliers. It is well worth consulting sources such as this since the reviewers often point to weaknesses that the more unsuspecting reader of the manual could overlook. Educationalists involved in testing reading skills should be aware that using one test once merely gives a single 'static picture of a dynamic process' (Pumfrey, 1977), therefore it is felt to be much more important to build up cumulative records and Zintz (1970) has developed individual progress records for use at various stages in the teaching of reading. An inevitable weakness of publications such as the Mental Measurement Yearbooks is that they soon become out of date. Pumfrey (1976) in part meets this criticism of the Buros' series in so far as British reading tests are concerned.

Psychological Tests. It is highly likely that the educational psychologists will be involved with the hearing-impaired child soon after diagnosis. He would certainly be involved at the time of preparing the IEP in the United States or the Statement of Special Needs in the United Kingdom.

In order properly to plan for the child's future it is important that an estimate of his cognitive ability is made. It will be obvious to all that merely reporting a full-scale verbal and performance intelligence test will penalise the hearing-impaired child. These scores should be presented separately and the verbal part of the test should not be reported as the child's verbal intelligence quotient. The performance score is the best estimate of the child's intelligence.

Psychologists frequently choose to use the Wechsler Intelligence Scale for Children (WISC-R) because it separates verbal and performance portions. The Hiskey Nebraska Test of Learning Aptitude was specially designed for use with hearing-impaired subjects and provides norms for both normally hearing and hearing-impaired children. Boyle (1977) has provided a comprehensive review and analysis of psychological tests commonly used with hearing-impaired children including any necessary modifications.

Psychologists need to keep a very watchful eye for specific perceptual and language disorders in the hearing-impaired child. They may not be common in the overall hearing-impaired population, but when present can result in severe retardation.

Social Adjustment. Those who have hearing-impaired children in their care need to monitor the social adjustment and social integration of such children (especially handicapped children) placed in ordinary schools.

An important recent study by Cameron (1979) attempted:

1. To compare the degree of social acceptance of hearing-impaired and normally hearing children in the same classes and the perceptiveness of both groups in estimating their own relative social status with those classes.
2. To compare the interactive behaviour of hearing-impaired children with normally hearing children in the same class.

Her sample was 20 hearing-impaired primary school age children who were fully mainstreamed, 20 who were attending partially hearing units and 1,037 normally hearing children in the same classes. The tests used were:

(a) Moreno Peer Nomination Scale (Moreno, 1934). This is a forced choice social acceptance scale. 'You are going to the zoo in a coach tomorrow, who would you most like to sit next to?' being the sort of choice put to the child (see also Bronfenbrenner, 1944).
(b) A socio-empathy scale (to determine social status, social acceptance and socio-empathy) (Bruininks *et al.*, 1974).
(c) A Classroom Observation Schedule modelled on the Personal Record of School Experiences (PROSE) (Medley, 1973). This was used to collect data on behavioural interactions of the hearing-impaired children and an equal-sized same sex sample of non-handicapped children randomly selected from the same classes.

From Cameron's data analysis she concluded that:

1. The hearing-impaired children in ordinary classes, particularly those integrating on a partial basis were not as socially accepted as non-handicapped children within the class.
2. The hearing-impaired children were not rejected by their peers, but occupied a position of neutrality, whereby other children were happy to accept them but 'chose' them less frequently as preferred companions.
3. The hearing-impaired children were more perceptive of their attained peer status within their classroom groups than the non-handicapped children.
4. The children from PHUs 'identified' with their unit groups rather than the ordinary classes in which they integrated on a partial basis.
5. The hearing-impaired children equally with the non-handicapped children were strongly influenced by what they perceived to be their teacher's expectations for them, in judging their own academic status

in the class and in estimating that of others (see also Pidgeon, 1970; Burstall, 1970; Nash, 1973).

6. The hearing-impaired children differed significantly from the non-handicapped children in their total interactive behaviour of interacting with teacher, with other pupils and not interacting at all.

7. The behavioural interactions of the hearing-impaired children did not differ significantly from their non-handicapped classmates except that

  (i) Teachers initiated and sustained contact with the hearing-impaired children significantly more often. (Positive discrimination!)

  (ii) Hearing-impaired children had significantly more non-verbal interactions than the controls.

8. The hearing-impaired children were non-involved and distracted from their work significantly more often than the controls.

Cameron noted the varying degrees of success at integration but concluded that all of the children were achieving a measure of 'functional integration' as described by the Warnock Committee Report (HMSO, 1978).

It is vital that hearing-impaired children are not 'isolates' within the classroom community and those responsible for their placement and monitoring should undertake measures such as those used by Cameron and others to indicate the child's level of integration and social acceptance.

Readers are referred to other sociometric studies which have been carried out with hearing-impaired children. Bonney (1943) was one of the first to show that children who are 'different' were treated with great kindness and sympathy, but were not chosen as friends by their peers. Studies by Justman and Maskowitz (1957), Elser (1959), Force (1956) all showed that their hearing-impaired samples were not as socially acceptable as their normally hearing peers. Shears and Jensema (1969) conclude that a visible handicap (for example, a hearing aid) may actually reduce awkwardness between handicapped and 'normal' peers but they also observed that if a person's handicap involved interference with communication, the strain of engaging in conversation could provide negative social interaction between handicapped and non-handicapped. Results from a Moreno peer acceptance scale used in the Kennedy *et al.* (1976) study showed that children with severe to profound hearing losses scored higher than their normally hearing peers and higher than those with a less severe loss. One could speculate that the additional attention afforded by the teacher to the severely handicapped children possibly encouraged the children, in a wish to 'please' the teacher, to befriend them. There are of course other possible explanations but generally the research in this area would indicate fairly positively that hearing-impaired children stand a good chance of being received warmly in ordinary schools.

Medley and Mitzel (1963), Flanders (1966) and Boyer and Simon (1968) have contributed significantly to the methodology of assessing classroom interaction. The work of Huntington and Watton (1981, 1982), using Flander's techniques on hearing-impaired children is worthy of note. They have drawn attention to features in teaching style which are likely to be facilitative for the hearing-impaired child learning language.

References

Anderson, B.J. (1979) 'Parents strategies for achieving conversational interactions with their young hearing-impaired children' in A. Simmonds-Martin and D.R. Calvert (eds.), *Parent Infant Intervention*, Grune and Stratton, New York

BATOD (1981) 'Audiological definitions and forms for recording audiometric information – NEC', *J. Brit. Assn. Teachers of the Deaf*, *5(3)*, 83-7

Bellugi, U. and Klima, E. (1972) 'The roots of language in the sign talk of the deaf', *Psych. Today*, *6*, 60-7

Bonney, M.E. (1943) 'The relative stability of social, intellectual and academic status in grades 2 to 4 and the inter-relationships between these various forms of growth', *Journal of Educational Psychology*, vol. XXXIV, 88-102

Boyer, G.E. and Simon, A. (eds.) (1968) *Mirrors for Behaviour*, II, Research for Better Schools Inc., Philadelphia

Boyle, P. (1977) 'Psychology in hearing loss in children' in B. Jaffe (ed.), University Park Press, Baltimore

Bronfenbrenner, U. (1944) 'A constant frame of reference for sociometric research: Part 2 experimental inference', *Sociometry*, *111*, 40-5

Bruininks, R., Rynders, J. and Gross, J. (1974) 'Sociometric acceptance of mildly retarded pupils in resource rooms and regular classrooms', *Amer. J. Mental Deficiency*, *70(4)*, 135-47

Buros, O.K. (ed.) (1938-1972) *Mental Measurement Yearbooks*, Gryphon Press, New Jersey

Buros, O.K. (ed.) (1972) *The Seventh Mental Measurement Yearbook*, Gryphon Press, New Jersey

Burstall, C. (1970) 'French in the primary school: some early findings', *J. of Curric. Studies*, *2(1)*, 48-58

Cameron, M.K. (Sr) (1979) 'Social status and behavioural interactions of hearing-impaired children in ordinary schools'. Unpublished MEd thesis, Manchester University, Manchester

Deno, E. (1970) 'Special education as developmental capital', *Exceptional Children*, *37(3)*, 229-37

Elser, R. (1959) 'The social position of hearing-impaired children in the regular grades', *Exceptional Children*, *25*, 305-9

Ewing, I.R. and Ewing, A.W.G. (1938) *Handicap of Deafness*, London, Longmans Green and Co.

Ewing, I.R. and Ewing A.W.G. (1947) *Opportunity and the Deaf Child*, University of London Press, London

Flanders, N.A. (1966) *Interaction Analysis in the Classroom: A Manual for Observers*, School of Education, University of Michigan, Michigan

Force, D.G. (1956) 'Social status of physically handicapped children', *Exceptional Children*, *23*, 132-4

Gilliland, J. (1972) 'The assessment of readability: an overview' in A. Melnik and J. Merritt (eds.), *The Reading Curriculum*, University of London Press, London

Gregory, S., Mogford, K. and Bishop, J. (1979) 'Mothers speech to young hearing-impaired children', *J. Brit. Assn. Teachers of the Deaf*, *3(2)*, 42-3

Hein, R. and Bishop, M.E. (1979) 'Models and processes of mainstreaming' in M.E. Bishop (ed.), *Mainstreaming*, A.G. Bell Association for the Deaf Inc., Washington, DC

HMSO (1962) *Handicapped Pupils and Special Schools Ammending Regulations 1962*, Statutory Instrument No. 2073

HMSO (1978) *Report of the Committee of Enquiry into the Education of Handicapped Children and Young People*, Cmnd. No. 7212 Special Educational Needs – The Warnock Report

Hughes, M.H. (1983) 'Verbal interaction between mothers and their young hearing-impaired children', *J. Brit. Assn. Teachers of the Deaf*, *7(1)*, 18-22

Huntington, A. and Watton, F. (1981) 'Language and interaction in the classroom (Part 1: teacher talk)', *J. Brit. Assn. Teachers of the Deaf*, *5(6)*, 162-73

Huntington, A. and Watton, F. (1982) 'Language and interaction in the classroom (Part 2: pupil talk)', *J. Brit. Assn. Teachers of the Deaf*, *6(1)*, 18-21

Justman, J. and Maskowitz, L. (1957) *The Integration of Deaf Children in a Hearing Class*, publication no. 4, Bureau of Education Research, Board of Education, New York

Kennedy, P., Northcott, W., McCauley, R. and Williams, S. (1976) 'Longitudinal sociometric and cross-sectional data on mainstreaming hearing-impaired children: implications for pre-school programming', *Volta Review*, *78(2)*, 71-8

Lane, H.S. and Baker, D. (1974) 'Achievement of the deaf: another look', *Volta Review*, *76*, 489-99

Ling, D. (1976) *Speech and the Hearing-impaired Child: Theory and Practice*, A.G. Bell Association for the Deaf Inc., Washington, DC

Lynas, W. (1980) 'The hearing-impaired child in the ordinary school', *J. Brit. Assn. Teachers of the Deaf*, *4(2)*, 49-57

Markides, A. (1971) 'Do hearing aids damage the user's residual hearing', *Sound*, *5(4)*, 99

McGee, D.I. (1976) 'Mainstreaming problems and procedures' in G.W. Nix, (ed.), *Mainstream Education for Hearing-Impaired Children and Youth*, Grune and Stratton, New York

McNally, J. and Murray, W. (1962) *Key Words to Literacy*, Schoolmaster Publishing Co., London

Medley, D.M. and Mitzel, H.E. (1963) 'Measuring classroom behaviour by systematic observation' in N.L. Gage (ed.), *Handbook of Research on Teaching*, Rand and McNally, Chicago

Medley, D.M. (1973) 'The personal record of school experiences (PROSE)' in E.G. Boyer, A. Simon and G. Karafin (eds.), *Measures of Maturation: An*

Anthology of Early Childhood Observation Instruments, vol. 2, Research for Better Schools Inc., Philadelphia

Mills *v.* Board of Education of District of Columbia (1972) 348F Supp 866, 968, 875 (DDC)

Moreno, J.W. (1934) *Who Shall Survive?* Nervous and Mental Disease Publishing Co., Washington, DC

Nash, R. (1973) *Classrooms Observed*, Routledge and Kegan Paul, London

Nix, G.W. (ed.) (1976) *Mainstream Education for Hearing-Impaired Children and Youth*, Grune and Stratton, New York

Nolan, M. and Tucker, I.G. (1981) *The Hearing-Impaired Child and the Family*, Souvenir Press, London

Northcott, W.H. (1981) 'Freedom through speech: every child's right', *Volta Review, 83(3)*, 162-81

Oyer, H.J. (ed.) (1976) *Communication for the hearing Handicapped: An International Perspective*, University Park Press, Baltimore

Pennsylvania Association for Retarded Citizens (PARC) *v.* Commonwealth of Pennsylvania (1971, 1972) 334F Supp. 1256 (E.D. Pa) 343F Supp 279, 282, 296. (E.D. Pa)

Pidgeon, D.A. (1970) *Expectation and Pupil Performance,* NFER, London

Powell, C.A. (1984) *Education in England, Overview*, in press

Pumfrey, P.D. (1976) *Reading: Tests and Assessment Techniques*, Hodder and Stoughton, London

Pumfrey, P.D. (1977) *Measuring Reading Abilities*, Hodder and Stoughton, London

Quigley, S., Power, D. and Steinkamp, M. (1977) 'The language structure of deaf children', *Volta Review, 79*, 73-84

Quigley, S. and Kretschmer, R.E. (1982) *The Education of Deaf Children: Issues, Theory and Practice*, Edward Arnold, London

Rae, L. (1851) 'Thomas Braidwood', *Amer. Annals of the Deaf, 3*, 255-6

Redgate, G.W. and Palmer, J. (1972) *Teaching of Reading to Deaf Children*, Research Report, Dept. of Audiology and Education of the Deaf, University of Manchester, Manchester

Reynell, J. (1977) *Reynell Developmental Language Scales* (Revised), NFER, London

Reynolds, M.C. (1962) 'A framework for considering some issues on special education', *Exceptional Children, 28*, 367-70

Ross, M. (1976) 'Model educational cascade for hearing-impaired children' in G.W. Nix (ed.), *Mainstream Education for Hearing-Impaired children and Youth*, Grune and Stratton, New York

Schlesinger, H. and Meadow, K. (1972) *Sound and Sign: Childhood Deafness and Mental Health*, University of California Press, Berkeley, California

Shears, L.M. and Jensema, C.J. (1969) 'Social acceptability of anomalous persons', *Exceptional Children, 36(2)*, 91-6

Simmonds-Martin, A. (1976) 'The Central Institute for the Deaf Demonstration Home Program' in G.W. Nix (ed.), *Mainstream Education for Hearing-impaired Children and Youth*, Grune and Stratton, New York

Taylor, W.L. (1953) 'Cloze procedure: a new tool for measuring readability', *Journalism Quarterly, 30*, 415-33

Tucker, I.G. (1972) 'The hearing for speech of a sample of partially hearing children', *J. of the Soc. of Teachers of the Deaf, 13*

Tucker, I.G. (1980a) 'Some linguistic aspects of the guidance of parents of hearing-impaired children', *J. Brit. Assn. Teachers of the Deaf, 4(3)*, 74-6

Tucker, I.G. (1980b) *Some Linguistic and Paralinguistic aspects of Parent Child Interaction.* Proceedings of the International Congress on the Education of the Deaf, Hamburg, June

Zintz, M.V. (1970) *The Reading Process: The Teacher and the Learner*, W.C. Brown, Iowa

There is a good deal of argument about the prevalence of additional handicaps in hearing-impaired children. It also seems likely that certain additional handicaps remain undetected or are diagnosed very late adding markedly to the effects on the child's development. Bond (1982) has suggested that 'Unfortunately in our enthusiasm to understand "deafness" and in efforts to "normalise" the hearing-impaired, it is possible to overlook additional or exogenous factors which contribute to the problems of the hearing-impaired.' He also wonders if the true extent of hearing-impairment has been discovered in other populations, for example, anywhere where there is a tendency to focus on one handicap (physical/mental, etc.) and overlook others. As an example he reports that the congenitally hearing-impaired child is about 1000 times more likely to go blind compared with normally hearing children, there being approximately 4-8 per cent who are likely to suffer from Usher's syndrome or other conditions which cause visual deterioration. In Usher's syndrome there is progressive deterioration of vision through retinitis pigmentosa.

Nance (1976) has reported more than 50 different genetic syndromes which are known to be associated with hearing-impairment. Some of these are extremely rare conditions. Nance further suggests that:

(a) Approximately 84 per cent of all the genetic cases of deafness are transmitted as a recessive trait.

(b) Approximately 14 per cent of genetic cases are transmitted as a dominant trait.

(c) Approximately 2 per cent of genetic cases are transmitted by a gene on the X chromosome. In this case the males are affected and females are usually normal.

What would seem vital to us would be that every effort is made to determine the causation of deafness. Every child referred to the Department of Audiology at Manchester University and found to be hearing-impaired is investigated for causation. A protocol of investigation for both hereditary and environmental conditions is pursued and this is followed by routine monitoring throughout the child's early years and on into the school system.

Vernon (1969), as a result of a major survey of 1,468 hearing-impaired children, has shown a significant correlation between deafness and additional physical handicaps (see Table 11.1).

It is interesting to see the lower frequency of additional conditions in the hereditary group.

Aetiology and Deafness

(1) Hereditary

There are varying accounts of the proportion of deafness caused by heredity. They range from 11·5 per cent (Miller, 1965) to 60 per cent (Brill, 1961). Vernon (1969) reports a heredity percentage of 5·4 per cent in his study along with 30·4 per cent unknown. Taylor *et al.* (1973) and (1975) have shown that most if not all of carefully investigated 'unknowns' were likely to be cases of hereditary deafness associated with an autosomal recessive factor. In such cases the parents are normal but both carry the recessive gene for deafness and a proportion (about 1 in 4) of the children are affected by deafness. In Taylor's own study (Taylor, 1981) it could be regarded that 38 per cent of the meticulously examined sample were hereditarily hearing-impaired. In Vernon's (1969) sample the hereditary group was characterised as having a minimum of other physical anomalies (see Table 11.1). He considered this group to have 6.5 per cent multiply handicapped children, but their hearing losses tended to be among the most profound (mean 88 dB HL). There is evidence of additionally handicapping conditions of genetic origin, such as Usher's syndrome and Down's syndrome, about which more will be reported shortly.

Some Syndromes Associated with Deafness

(a) Klippel-Fiel Syndrome. This is one of the familial dominant disorders with poor penetrance and variable expression. The bony labyrinth is normal, but there is degeneration of the organ of corti, atrophy of the stria vascularis, abnormalities of the tectorial membrane and spiral ganglion and evidence of saccular changes. In addition there is fusion of some or all of the cervical vertebrae (neck) which gives the impression that the head is sitting straight on the shoulders. Club foot and cleft palate can also be present. The hearing-impairment can range from mildly conductive to profoundly sensori-neural.

Table 11.1: Prevalence of physical anomalies in the five major aetiologies of deafness

Aetiological group	Cerebral palsy and/or hemiplegias		Mental retardation (IQ below 70)		Aphasoid disorder		Visual defects		Orthopaedic defects (excluding cerebral palsy)		Seizures	
	N[a]	Per cent[b]	N	Per cent	N	Per cent	N	Per cent	N	Per cent	N	Per cent
Hereditary	79	0.0	62	0.0	63	1.5	63	20.6	63	1.5	63	0.0
Meningitic	92	9.7	92	14.1	92	16.3	87	5.7	92	5.4	92	3.2
Premature	113	17.6	115	16.5	113	36.2	113	28.3	101	8.9	113	1.7
Rubella	104	3.8	98	8.1	105	21.9	104	29.8	104	4.8	104	0.0
Rh factor	45	51.1	39	5.1	35	22.8	45	24.4	45	2.2	45	6.6

Note: a. N = total sample for which data were available; b. per cent = percentage of each N with defect.

Source: after Vernon, 1969.

(b) Treacher Collins Syndrome. This is an autosomal dominant condition with high penetrance and variable expression. It is one of the mandibulo-facial dysostoses and is recognised by these deformities of the facial bones. There is underdevelopment of the lower jaw and some facial bones, the pinnae can be deformed and there can be atresia of the auditory meatus. A poorly developed middle ear and cleft palate are also common. The hearing-impairment is usually of the conductive type, but sensori-neural loss is not unknown.

(c) Waardenburg's Syndrome. This is an autosomal dominant condition with variable penetrance. The condition is characterised by a white forelock. A prominent fold of skin at the inner angles of the eyes gives the impression of a broad nasal bridge and wide set eyes. Hearing-impairment is of the congenital sensori-neural type and is often very severe. It can be unilateral, bilateral and also progressive.

(d) Usher's Syndrome. This is a recessive condition where sensori-neural deafness is associated with retinitis pigmentosa. There is a progressive degeneration of vision. The deafness is congenital so the child who is already hearing-impaired becomes progressively visually-impaired. Night blindness is an early noticeable effect.

(e) Pendred's Syndrome. This is a recessive condition associated with goitre. It is thought that the goitre and deafness are independent manifestations of the same recessive defect. There is an abnormal metabolism of iodine. Some workers have estimated that as much as 10 per cent of recessive sensori-neural hearing loss can be ascribed to this defect.

(f) Jervell and Lange-Nielson's Syndrome. This is a relatively recently reported syndrome which is recessive in nature and includes congenital functional heart disease and profound sensori-neural deafness. Death usually occurs in childhood.

(2) Meningitis

Meningitis is the leading post-natal cause of deafness. It begins as an infection of the membranes which surround the brain. Meningitis can be divided into two main types, those accompanied or not accompanied by a purulent exudate. When the exudate is present this is diagnosed as suppurative, pyrogenic or purulent meningitis and it is this form of the disease which is a frequent cause of hearing-impairment.

Tuberculous meningitis is an example of non-suppurative or aseptic meningitis. Taylor (1981) reports no tuberculous meningitis in his sample, suggesting that improved socio-economic conditions, a vigorous vaccination programme and a less toxic chemotherapy regime as being the prime reasons for this. 'Mycin' drugs — strepto, kano, neo — are often toxic to auditory nerves.

Meningitis is most common in children with about half the cases occurring in those under 5 years of age. Many are below 2½ years of age with premature infants and newborns being particularly affected. Many forms of meningitis (for example, meningococcal, streptococcal or staphylococci, pneumococcal) were almost inevitably fatal but modern microbial therapy has greatly reduced the level of fatality to about 20 per cent.

The pathological effects of the disease are wide ranging as one would expect. The major ones are hydrocephalus, monoplegia, deafness, cortical blindness, hemiplegia, mental retardation, convulsions, aphasia, brain damage, paralysis and learning disorders (De Graff and Creger, 1963); the same authors, reporting the work of Myhan and Richardson, suggested that 32-43 per cent of those having meningococcal or hemophilus influenzae have major central nervous system pathologies. MacKay (1964), studying 47 cases of neonatal meningitis, found that of 19 survivors 63 per cent had serious complications.

Meningitis damages hearing both centrally and peripherally. Centrally the complications tend to be especially serious including central auditory perceptual problems and brain damage. The build-up of purulent exudate, and the severe inflamation of the vestibular and cochlea mechanisms causes peripheral sensori-neural deafness.

Modern treatment means that very young patients, who would formerly have died are now frequently saved. Unlike the older meningitic survivors these children will need to learn their language with a damaged hearing mechanism as opposed to conserving already acquired language. Additional neuro-physiological sequelae will greatly add to the difficulty of this task.

(3) Rubella

Maternal rubella is the leading prenatal cause of deafness but it is difficult to be sure of prevalence because research methods vary considerably. Some surveys use control groups, others do not: the occurrence of abortions, stillbirths and low birth weight are not always included in the data: estimates of gestational age are made by different methods and few studies follow up the children into childhood. This is a most important factor since many defects do not become apparent until later childhood. If we compare the research reviews of Michaels and Mellin (1960) Sallomi (1966) and Cockburn (1969) we see that all are agreed that after the first 16 weeks of pregnancy there is little or no evidence of damage to the foetus, except in hearing impairment. For the first twelve weeks the overall incidence of defects is estimated at 25 per cent by Michaels and Mellin, 31 per cent by Sallomi, 28 per cent by Cockburn. These figures are close to those of a large scale Ministry of Health Study in 1960 which found an incidence of 31 per cent (15 per cent major defects and 16 per cent minor defects). The overall incidence, however, conceals the sharp difference between the first and third months. Michaels and Mellin conclude that the incidence in the first month averages 47 per cent, in the second month 22 per cent, and in the third month 7 per cent, while Sallomi's review of studies quotes 61 per cent, 26 per cent, and 8 per cent respectively. Estimates of stillbirths and spontaneous abortions are harder to make and vary more widely. Reanalysing the findings of relevant studies Sallomi concludes *that after rubella in the first 8 weeks of pregnancy, the chance of having a normal infant is only 35·8 per cent.*

An interesting development reported by Taylor (1981) was the marked absence of the significant other disabilities usually associated with congenital rubella infection in his research sample. Reported sequelae such as congenital heart disease, visual defect, mental subnormality, blood dyscrasias and viraemia continuing long after birth were common in previously reported studies. Taylor suggests that the absence of the other congenital abnormalities is indicative of a trend of increasing therapeutic abortion. Early abortion is eliminating those children who might otherwise have had multiple disabilities. Even so of his 1981 sample 30 per cent were deafened by rubella.

A vigorous vaccination programme is under way to ensure that potential child bearing females are protected against the disease. Rubella has little effect on the adult other than a mild rash and a sore throat, but the virus, which enters the body through the nose or mouth, is carried in the mother's bloodstream to the embryo, where it attacks the rapidly multiplying cells. Here the damage is substantial. It is vital that the greatest possible encouragement is given to teenage girls to be vaccinated and here the educational audiologist can be influential in informing the teenage population of the risks of *not* being vaccinated.

Investigations have suggested that approximately 5 per cent of vaccinated girls *fail* to produce rubella antibodies indicating that they are not protected. This vaccination failure rate seems to be consistent and is minimised by proper storage of the vaccine and by accurate reconstitution and administration. It has been suggested that host factors may also play a part in the failure to produce antibodies and this may arise if the subject has had gammaglobulin, blood transfusion or other live viral vaccines just before vaccination. These subjects require re-vaccination.

Although some individuals with low levels of antibodies after vaccination will have them boosted by sub-clinical reinfection of exposure to *wild* rubella, it is interesting to note that there will be numbers of vaccinated girls who will believe, wrongly, that they have been protected. It would seem sensible to have a rubella antibody screening programme among women who present for contraceptive advice.

(4) Rhesus Incompatibility

This was a highly significant but now declining and hopefully soon to be eradicated cause of deafness. This problem is regarded as being among the perinatal causes of problems for the baby. Perinatal as a term is ill-defined but is usually taken to cover a period of about a week including a period prior to birth, the birth itself and a short period immediately after birth. Among the reported causes of deafness at this time are toxaemia, anoxia, prematurity, birth injury and neonatal jaundice.

The rhesus factor is present on the red blood cells of approximately 85 per cent of Europeans. These subjects are called Rh-positive and the remainder Rh-negative. If an Rh-negative mother is carrying an Rh-positive baby the Rh-factor (antigen) may pass from the child's blood into the mother's circulation. Antibodies to the Rh-factor are formed and pass between the mother and her unborn child. The concentration remains low in first pregnancy but increases gradually with each subsequent pregnancy. When it reaches a certain level the antigen and antibody react and the child's red blood cells are destroyed and there is a build-up of bilirubin (bile pigment) in the child's bloodstream. Whilst the baby is still connected up to the mother her liver disposes of the bilirubin but after birth the child's immature liver is unable to cope and its concentration in his circulation rises causing a yellow staining of the skin (jaundice). If the child's blood is not replaced within a few hours the pigment may enter the brain where it stains nerve cells (a. kernicterus) possibly including the cochlea nuclei. This causes deafness and possibly other central nervous disorders including those of the extrapyramidal system such as cerebral palsy. Motor disorders of the athetoid type, mental retardation, epilepsy and behaviour disorders are other sequelae recorded in the literature. A high incidence of brain damage relating to the rhesus factor is reported by Vernon (1969).

An awareness of the need to replace blood undoubtedly improved matters and Taylor (1981) noted complete absence of Rh factor deafness in his study ascribing this to better neonatal care, exchange transfusions and especially the introduction of a vaccine for rhesus incompatibility (anti-D). Taylor further suggests that providing a degree of vigilance is maintained there is no reason why the rhesus factor should return as a significant cause of deafness.

(5) Asphyxia

Birth asphyxia is a known important aetiological factor which may lead to subsequent brain damage in the neonate (De Souza, 1981). Sensori-neural deafness may also occur in some children with a history of low birth weight, birth asphyxia and neonatal jaundice (Dinnage, 1972; Fraser, 1976). Three recent studies (Scott, 1976; Thomson *et al.*, 1977; De Souza *et al.*, 1981) have examined the outcome of survivors of severe birth asphyxia. The infants selected in these three studies had cardiac arrest at birth and no other vital signs, or delayed onset of spontaneous regular respiration, greater than 20 minutes (Scott, 1976); 5½ to 60 minutes (Thomson *et al.*, 1977); greater than 10 minutes (De Souza *et al.*, 1981). Most of the children were full term although there were some pre-term babies and some small for dates babies as well. In relation to hearing impairment both Thomson *et al.* (1977) (23 babies) and De Souza *et al.* (1981) (26 babies) reported one case of bilateral sensori-neural deafness. Both children were reported as receiving 'normal education' and had made 'average progress'. It has been suggested (De Souza, 1981) that acute circulatory failure due to birth asphyxia may predispose to sensori-neural deafness. An association between perinatal cardiac arrest and sensori-neural deafness has in fact been reported (Steiner and Neligan, 1975). Further, as in the case of postnatal apnoea, damage to the inferior colliculus as a result of birth asphyxia may produce a sensori-neural deafness.

(6) Prematurity

It has been known for a considerable time that the very low birth weight baby (VLBW) who survives the neonatal period has an increased risk of suffering sensori-neural hearing loss. The reported incidence ranges from 4 per cent to 18 per cent, this in comparison with an expected incidence of 0·5 per cent in the general childhood population (Hope *et al.*, 1981). The fact that the reported incidence varies widely between studies is likely to be a result of differing selection and categorisation criteria of the children and of course the rapid changes that have been made in neonatal care techniques. A number of agents have been cited in the aetiological considerations relating to sensori-neural hearing loss (SNHL). Some of these arise in the post-natal period and may therefore be susceptible to neonatal management (Hope *et al.*, 1981). Incubator noise, antibiotic therapy, kernicterus, and hypoxia resulting from apnoea episodes in the early days of life have all been considered 'factors of effect'. In addition, there is also a known high incidence of conductive hearing loss in such children (Balkany *et al.*, 1978) resulting from chronic serous otitis media. Hope *et al.* (1981) who reported on a study of 366 VLBW children of whom 9 per cent had sensori-neural hearing loss stated that: 'the commonest cause of SNHL in our VLBW population may be hypoxic damage to the inferior colliculus at a particularly vulnerable stage of its development'. This hypoxic damage was considered as resulting from repeated episodes of apnoea in the early years and weeks of life. Hope *et al.* (1981) also commented that the factors of severe neonatal apnoea and decreasing birthweight were the most powerful independent predictors as to the likelihood of SNHL in such children.

Deafness and Mental Retardation

Many workers have shown the close association between hearing loss and mental handicap and have reported a higher incidence of deafness in the mentally handicapped population than in normal population (Lloyd, 1970).

There is a higher probability of hearing disorders in Down's syndrome, which is characterised by a tendency for upper respiratory tract infection, including sinuses and middle ears, an abnormally shaped skull and small ear canals (Yannet, 1964; Hilson, 1966). In older children and adults several studies have confirmed this (Rigrodsky *et al.*, 1961; McIntire *et al.*, 1965; Glovsky, 1966; Fulton and Lloyd, 1968; Brooks *et al.*, 1972; Davies and Penniceard, 1980). Furthermore, the latter two studies have drawn attention to a progressive high frequency sensori-neural loss, possibly resulting from premature ageing.

Workers in the Department of Audiology and in the Hester Adrian Research Centre into Mental Handicap at Manchester University investigated babies to see if the findings on older children and adults were related. They considered that in babies, in whom it is considered that there are more upper respiratory tract infections and heavy catarrh problems, deafness would be greater. Down's children are notably delayed in speech and language and yet the extent to which this might be due to auditory deprivation rather than difficulties with central processing or slow growth is unclear. There is a marked possibility that even a slight hearing-impairment in the early years of life when language is emerging may be critically damaging. It may be possible for children with normal ability to use their ability to compensate for an element of sensory deprivation. The intellectually impaired child may be unable to do so and it may be the case that the combination of sensory impairment and mental handicap is *cumulative* and results in an even greater disability than the sum of the separate deficiences would suggest. In the study, Cunningham and McArthur (1979) on 24 Down's babies aged 9 to 32 months tested using the methods, including impedance, described in Chapter 2, all failed. One child had a profound loss, one a very severe and four a severe loss. The majority of the losses were conductive in nature although five were mixed and one wholly sensori-neural. The tests were repeated on three occasions in the spring, summer and winter and only in three cases in summer did the hearing return to normal. This indicates that even the conductive conditions, which were actively treated both medically and surgically, were most reluctant to resolve. Several of the children were subsequently fitted with hearing aids to aid linguistic stimulation. It is our strongly held view that all Down's children should bypass routine health visitor screening to be seen at specialist audiology centres. It would also be very useful if audiological service were attached to the provision for mentally handicapped children, within regions, to ensure ongoing monitoring.

It is also commonly thought that mentally retarded subjects are untestable by conventional methods. In many cases this is not so. Nolan *et al.* (1980) using the techniques described earlier on 53 subjects in an adult training centre found 25 subjects (47·1 per cent) to have abnormal hearing and only seven subjects (13·0 per cent) were considered difficult to test. Clearly the ability to use objective measures such as impedance techniques, brain stem evoked responses and electrocochleography should aid satisfactory assessment in the very difficult cases.

If the Nolan group as a whole is subdivided into Down's and non-Down's subjects, the sample constituted 25 per cent Down's, 75 per cent non-Down's. The incidence of hearing loss in the Down's subjects was 69 per cent. Middle ear dysfunction was seen in 69 per cent of Down's subjects. The incidence of hearing loss in the non-Down's subjects was 40 per cent. However, it should be noted that 15 per cent of the non-Down's subjects were unclassified. It is particularly interesting to note that only 26·6 per cent of the non-Down's subjects assessed by the impedance bridge showed abnormal middle ear function. The results indicate that the incidence of hearing disorders in Down's subjects is higher than in non-Down's cases. This observation on middle ear dysfunction in Down's subjects is supported by the study of Cunningham and McArthur (1979) already reported, and the work of Brooks *et al.* (1972) working with Down's children and adults, who found 60 per cent of the 100 patients studied had abnormal middle ear function while only 17·5 per cent of a non-Down's control group showed middle ear dysfunction. Furthermore, the incidence of sensorineural loss was three times higher in Down's than in non-Down's individuals.

The results of the speech discrimination tests applied in the Nolan *et al.* study indicated that words presented at normal voice levels may be misheard by trainees with hearing losses because of loss of essential acoustic cues. This, they thought, led to a depression in the scores achieved on verbally applied tests such as the English Picture Vocabulary Test. It is important, in view of the high incidence of hearing loss, that any user of such tests should be aware of the possibility of hearing loss and ensure that the auditory function of the subject is determined.

Problems of Diagnosis of Deafness Where the Patient has Additional Handicaps

It is first of all important to point out that the numbers of such children are small relative to the size of the multiply handicapped population. Initially only minor changes to the standard test procedures may be required. For example, in a severely physically handicapped child of distraction age it may be possible to accept eye movement where head turns are impossible. It may be that a test designed for younger children such as the distraction test or performance test can be used with older multiply handicapped patients who are unable to undertake pure tone audiometry. Free field testing such as this in a play situation may be the only way to achieve a variety of frequency specific hearing levels. Visual Reinforcement Audiometry (VRA) (Thompson *et al.*, 1979) has been shown to have application with mentally retarded hearing-impaired subjects.

However it may be the case that it is impossible for the patient to co-operate in any of the standard behavioural tests and the clinician may then need to use techniques such as behavioural observation audiometry (BOA) described by Kershman and Napier (1982) and others where a variety of meaningful pre-recorded stimuli are played to the child and an observational schedule used to assess his response, looking for such things as quieting, eye movement, etc.

It is vital with this methodology to assess pre-stimulus behaviour for comparison with post-stimulation response. It is also vital to ensure that the signal levels and frequency specificity are carefully controlled and monitored.

Objective tests which are available to the audiologist can help to provide more information about the patient's hearing levels. The impedance bridge will indicate whether or not there is a conductive condition and if the stapedius muscle reflex is present, the threshold levels may be used to predict residual hearing capacity (Sesterhenn and Brueninger, 1977). Absence of the reflex does not necessarily mean that there is abnormal hearing. Brain-stem evoked response (BSER) audiometry can without the aid of the patient assess auditorally stimulated neural activity up to and through the brain stem. Unfortunately it only gives a broad measure of high frequency hearing as a result of its use of click stimuli. While BSER is a non-invasive technique, it may prove necessary to sedate or apply a general anaesthetic prior to the measurement. Electrocochleography (E.Coch.G) is a surgical procedure for a multiply handicapped child in that it would need to be carried out under general anaesthetic. It assesses the neural activity close to the cochlea, when a needle electrode is put either in the ear canal or through the ear drum and on to the promontary near the cochlea itself. The E.Coch.G. test uses click stimuli or brief pure tones above 1 k Hz, so it is not possible to get accurate information about low frequency hearing. The E.Coch.G. test will not detect deafness if the site of the lesion is beyond the cochlea (retro-cochlea).

Given that the audiologist has access to the wide range of clinical facilities mentioned then it is possible to gain a picture of the child's hearing acuity however severely handicapped.

Educational Provision for Children with Multiple Handicaps

If we believe that children with deafness and no additional handicap are a heterogeneous group and require individualised educational programming then such is most certainly true of the additionally handicapped.

Additional impairments range from slight impairments with little overall additional effect on the deafness to the most severe neurological and physical handicaps which make any learning a great feat for the child and a wonderful testimony to the teacher's skill. The former child may need little additional programming, the latter will almost certainly require full-time special educational treatment in a school specialising in educating multiply-handicapped children. In the United Kingdom until fairly recently there were no such specialist schools and such children were either given no educational opportunity at all or were placed with non-deaf, severely subnormal children. Now there are several schools catering for severely multiply handicapped deaf children. This has been partly due to a growing expression of the view that such children were educable and partly to declines in the 'ordinary' deaf population which has put pressures on school numbers (Tucker, 1978). Some special schools have set up units/departments for severely/profoundly multi-handicapped sensory-impaired children.

Educational audiologists in co-operation with other educational colleagues are likely to be at least in part responsible for the decision making process for placement of multiply-handicapped deaf children and it is therefore important that, whatever their location, they are fully aware of both the child's needs for education and the availability and suitability of provision. Comprehensive diagnostic investigation of the child is an essential precursor to decisions on his educational management. Ives and Morris (1978) outlined a diagnostic advisory service at the Royal School for the Deaf in Manchester where the educational audiologist joined the specialist psychologist to provide information about placement, audiological management, and educational programming needs of multiply-handicapped hearing-impaired children. They also stress the need for manual assistance in communication methodology. This type of service, providing it is objective, is of great benefit to small authorities, particularly those without specialised staff. Both Ives and Morris (1978) and Bond (1982) have stressed the need for regional resource schools.

It is very difficult to group the additionally and multiply handicapped for comment on specific educational need, but it is worth highlighting three possible groupings outlined by Murphy (1977):

(a) The child with a primary severe or greater hearing loss who, on initial examination, appears to have no additional major physical intellectual or sensory handicap.

(b) The child with a primary severe hearing loss together with a severe additional handicap (for example, blindness), with severe physical or severe intellectual handicap.

(c) The child with a mild, moderate or profound hearing loss who has additional handicaps due to exogenous factors such as late diagnosis, bilingual background, socially deprived or emotionally disturbed home.

Bond (1982) developing the ideas of Murphy considered that on the face of it difficulties such as those in group (a) would be the most difficult to identify. Many workers consider that aetiological factors have been ignored or, at least, not treated seriously enough. This, when it is quite clear that such deafness-causing agents as rubella, anoxia and meningitis are frequently linked with specific psycho-neurological damage. Murphy (1977) noted discrepancies of function in several areas in group (a) children. He suggested certain mild central nervous system dysfunctions which seemed to be associated with deafness by trauma, genetic deafness, as a rule, being free from this additional handicap. Bond (1979, 1982, 1983) has outlined areas of difficulty commonly found in group (a) children. These specific difficulties adversely affecting learning include problems in all, some, or combinations of the following areas:

1. Various disorders of short-term visual memory (which might include memory for digits, colours, bead patterns, designs, pictorial information, sequence of movement, rhythmical sequence, etc.
2. Visual attention span.
3. Visual/motor sequencing.
4. Visual spatial planning and organisation.
5. Visual motor learning and visual perceptual skills.
6. Difficulties in simple imitation (for example, of gesture), both gross and fine.

He also suggested that such children have difficulties in temporal encoding and decoding (for example, speech-reading, finger-spelling) and appear to require a high degree of structure in their learning environment with plenty of opportunity for success. Bond has also added more factors which may apply to group (a) children. These are as follows:

1. Attention seeking or demanding and poor on-task and attention to task behaviours.
2. Distractability and impulsivity.
3. Difficulties in interpersonal relationships.
4. Failure in aural/oral approaches.
5. Underachievement in language and reading.
6. Educational records which contain a minimum of medical, aetiological, audiological and psychological information.
7. Involuntary motor behaviours.
8. Muscular rigidity/tension.
9. Clumsiness.
10. Anxiety about failure in reading, maths, written work, etc.
11. Function in verbal educational learning and communication at a much lower level than practical skills and abilities.
12. Occasional flashes of 'brilliance' at a much higher level than the child's assumed level of ability.

There is a great need to improve the methodology for detecting the children who will not make the progress that their hearing problem might indicate them capable of. Teaching methodology for the severely multiply handicapped hearing-impaired child also requires further research and development. The fact that learning is often very slow and depends on an achievement of one stage before another is attempted has led workers to propose objectives-based curricula where it is necessary to clearly define teaching objectives, assess current pupil performance, implement teaching procedures and follow up with evaluation of effectiveness of the teaching. This in a much more 'fine grain' way than with ordinary children. Techniques of behaviour analysis and behaviour and/or environmental management have been widely used with mentally handicapped children and are incorporated, with some children, in programmes for the multiply handicapped hearing-impaired. They attempt to change the child's responses in certain situations either by removing or reducing undesirable responses through consistent reinforcement or introduction of more appropriate activities. Specialist psychologists, in conjunction with teachers of the deaf, have to define how far teaching procedures can be based on 'enrichment' methods and how much needs to be done using 'task analysis' techniques where skills and experiences are identified, ordered into a hierarchy of difficulty, subdivided if necessary, taught, tested and the effectiveness of the teaching assessed.

What is certain is that special arrangements must be made for training teachers and psychologists and others involved in this very demanding work. Currently this training is sadly lacking in the United Kingdom.

Bond (1982) has been involved as a member of a team in setting up a department within a special school for hearing-impaired children and has highlighted some areas which are essential to the appropriate management and intervention with such children. The following list is adapted from his work.

1. Small units are important, with *all* staff sharing ideas on management and involved in the teaching strategies and follow-on assessment and re-evaluation of methods.
2. Adequate staffing ratios are important with one member of staff to two children not unusual.
3. Regular staff meetings which emphasise the learning role for all. These sessions can also act as in-service training sessions.
4. The unit must be well equipped and educational materials may need to be designed and made specially for one child according to needs. Appropriate well made equipment at particular stages in the development of multiply handicapped children is crucial.
5. A curriculum consisting of carefully structured developmental activities and experiences closely linked to skills, which have been analysed and organised in such a way that it is possible for children and their teachers to achieve realistic goals.
6. Improved liaison between home and school. The school might have a parent's flat, offer parent guidance and training and always be open for parent school interchange of ideas.
7. An attitude within the department which sets it out as a 'problem solving environment' always willing to try alternative strategies for encouraging learning in the child.

Dual or Multi-sensory Impaired Children

The primary cause of dual or multi-sensory impairment in children is rubella early in the mother's pregnancy. Others are retrolental fibroplasia, Usher's syndrome (retinitis pigmentosa), meningitis and a variety of unusual genetic syndromes. There are approximately 400 such children in Britain.

The National Association For Deaf-Blind and Rubella Handicapped which exists to serve the interests of this handicapped group is concerned that no official definition exists in this country. The present authors are concerned that definitions bring forth labels and labels do not necessarily say much about educational needs. On the other hand if there is no definition then there are no statistics and it is then difficult to assess the need for provision.

The American definition which might be adopted is

> a child who has auditory and visual handicaps regardless of the degree of impairment the combination of which causes such severe communication and other developmental and educational problems that he cannot be properly catered for in special education programmes either for the hearing handicapped child or for the visually handicapped child.

The pressure groups involved with deaf-blind children see 'definition' as one of the weapons for pressurising for more service. In the United Kingdom a substantial proportion of deaf-blind rubella handicapped children are receiving no formal education. There is no network of regional facilities and what we regard as most crucial is that there is no training for teachers which is based on the child as a multi-sensory deprived (MSD) child (McInnes and Treffry, 1982). Currently training is geared to blindness and/or deafness but not multi-sensory. A lack of all-round knowledge inevitably means that one of the senses, often the auditory sense, is neglected. In our view there are no grounds for depriving such children of auditory stimulation and there is no reason why aids should not be set and working efficiently. No reason, that is, other than the lack of knowledge and inefficiency of those who assess and manage them. We have seen MSD children with useful residual hearing with no aids or using aids not capable of providing them with useful auditory experience. These children almost always have useful residual hearing, very often more hearing than vision, and appropriate aids can at the least improve general awareness, reduce behaviour problems and increase their ability to receive other sensory stimuli. At most it can provide the child with an opportunity to hear and learn spoken language through hearing, an aim which must be high on anyone's list of goals.

All of the objective tests (described in Chapter 2) such as impedance, stapedius muscle reflexes, brain stem evoked response and electrocochleography along with behavioural and other free field tests are capable of giving very useful information about residual hearing.

There are some problems with the above measures, the child may reject the probe for impedance but the latest equipment operates so rapidly that measures can almost always be made satisfactorily. Electric responses can be affected by drugs used to sedate the child and by structural brain damage. BSER is very resistant to change from drugs. The Auditory Evoked Response (AER), which measures higher up the auditory pathway, is more affected by brain damage and by sedation and is not recommended for use with MSD children. Enormous strides are being made in the electric response area. The present authors have fitted aids to MSD children as young as three months on the basis of results on the above. We would obviously gear the amplification to factors such as severity of loss and physical manageability of the system, aiming for ear-level provision as early as practical, consistent with efficient amplification. Fitting would be binaural if both ears are affected. Radio transmission equipment would be used for certain situations but *selectively*. The use of a close microphone distance with such children is desirable because of their very limited 'environment'. This link helps to maintain the contact between parent and child.

Acceptance of aids is sometimes difficult, usually because of late diagnosis. All audiologists are aware of the ease of fitting children in the first year of life and the difficulty of fitting the mobile, dextrous and inquisitive two year old. They should be aware of the added difficulties of fitting the MSD child who, perhaps because of low functioning, may take longer to become aware of the beneficial effects of amplification, but that is no reason for not getting started. McInnes and Treffry (1982) have suggested useful steps in encouraging the child to accept the aid. These would include a gradual build-up of tactile awareness of the aid on the child. Parental observations are very important and the above-named authors have provided parents with a useful check-list related to the use of the auditory sense.

There is much controversy about the ability levels of MSD children stemming from the difficulties involved in testing them formally. However, many would agree that their abilities are underestimated. Formal intelligence tests cannot be reliably presented to hearing-impaired children using verbal instructions or to blind children using visual instructions, and to MSD children it is often only possible very gradually to build up a picture of the child's cognitive abilities by using parts of a variety of formal tests. Then of course the norms for these tests cannot be used, but a picture of the child's current level of functioning can be obtained. The testing, evaluation and programming of MSD children is heavily reliant on skill, experience and co-operation of a variety of professionals including the audiologist, ophthalmologist, psychologist, parent and educator. Stemquist (1968) from the Perkins School in the USA has outlined their use of formal tests such as the

Ontario School Ability Examination (OSAE) (Amos, 1936) and the Nebraska Test of Learning Aptitude (NTLA) (Hiskey, 1955). The OSAE yields a mental age and an intelligence quotient as well as mental levels of performance in various subject areas relating to visual perception, visual motor, attention and memory areas. In order to perform, the child requires useful vision. Since the OSAE only tests non-symbolic ability, items from the NTLA which use symbolic materials are used.

Evaluation of visual capacity in MSD children is also difficult in early childhood. Clinical examination and scores from visual efficiency tests tend not to provide a comprehensive enough picture to enable educators to prepare programmes. McInnes and Treffry (1982) reported a boy who was recorded as 'totally blind', 'light perception' or 'mobility vision' depending on who tested him, when and where. His mother, however, reported that he could locate a cookie on a table at three feet. She was correct and her observations provided the educators with a goal and also a starting point for programming.

Suggested Further Reading in the Area of Multi-sensory Impairment

The book *A Vision Guide for Teachers of Deaf-blind Children* by Efron and DuBoff (1976) is an excellent guide for teacher evaluation and for those involved in setting up programmes for deaf-blind children. *Understanding Deaf-Blind Children* by Freeman (1975), a parent of an MSD child, is well worth reading. Peggy Freeman is a leader, in the United Kingdom, in the battle for more and better services for MSD children. For those audiologists with a special interest in this area we would recommend McInnes and Treffry (1982) and Jurgens (1977).

References

Amos, H. (1936) *Ontario School Ability Examination*, the Ryerson Press, Toronto
Balkany, T.J., Berman, S.A., Simmons, M.A. and Jefek, B.W. (1978) 'Middle ear effusion in neonates', *Laryngoscope*, *88*, 398
Ballantyne, J.C. (1960) *Deafness*, (latest edn), J. & A. Churchill, London
Bond, D.E. (1979) 'Aspects of psycho-educational assessment hearing-impaired children with additional handicaps', *J. Brit. Assn. Teachers of the Deaf*, *3(3)*, 76-9
Bond, D.E. (1982) 'Management of hearing-impaired children who have additional learning and behavioural difficulties', *Report of the Proceedings of the Conference of Heads of Schools and Services for Hearing-Impaired Children*, University of Manchester, Manchester

Bond, D.E. (1983) Personal communication

Brill, R.G. (1961) 'Hereditary aspects of deafness', *Volta Review, 63*

Brooks, D.N., Woolley, H. and Kanjilal, G.C. (1972) 'Hearing loss and middle ear disorders in patients with Down's syndrome', *J. Ment. Defic. Res., 16*, 21-7

Cockburn, W.C. (1969) 'World aspects of the epidemiology of rubella', *Amer. J. of Diseases of Children, 118*, 112-22

Cunningham, C. and McArthur, K. (1979) 'Hearing loss and treatment in young Down's syndrome children', *Child: Care Health and Development, 7*, 357-74

Davies, B. and Penniceard, R.M. (1980) 'Auditory function and receptive vocabulary in Down's syndrome children' in I.G. Taylor and A. Markides (eds.), *Disorders of Auditory Function III*, Academic Press, London

De Graff, A.C. and Creger, W.P. (eds.) (1963) *Annual Review of Medicine*, George Banta, Palo Alto, California

De Souza, S.W., MaCartney, E., Nolan, M. and Taylor, I.G. (1981) 'Hearing, speech and language in survivors of severe perinatal asphyxia', *Archives of Disease in Childhood, 56(4)*, 245-52

De Souza, S.W. (1981) 'Outcome in survivors after severe birth asphyxia', *Proceedings of the Scientific Meeting of the British Association of Audiological Physicians and Community Paediatric Group*, Department of Audiology and Education of the Deaf, University of Manchester, Manchester

Dinnage, R. (1972) 'The handicapped child' in *Research Review* (vol. 2) – *Visual Impairment Hearing Impairment, Speech Disorders and Other Physical Handicaps*, Longman, London

Efron, M. and Duboff, B.R. (1976) *A Vision Guide for Teachers of Deaf Blind Children*, Dept. of Public Instruction, Raleigh NC

Fraser, G.R. (1976) *The Causes of Profound Deafness in Childhood*, John Hopkins, University Press, Baltimore

Freeman, P. (1975) *Understanding the Deaf-Blind Child*, Heinneman Health Books, London

Fulton, F.T. and Lloyd, L.L. (1968) 'Hearing-impairment in a population of children with Down's syndrome', *Amer. J. of Ment. Defic., 73*, 298-302

Glovsky, L. (1966) 'Audiological assessment of mongoloid population', *Training School Bulletin, 63*, 27-36

Hilson, D. (1966) 'The abnormally shaped ear', *Devel. Med. and Child. Neur., 8*, 210-12

Hiskey, M. (1955) *Nebraska Test of Learning Aptitudes*, University of Nebraska, Lincoln, Nebraska

Hope, P.L., Hazell, J.W.F. and Stewart, A.L. (1981) 'Sensorineural hearing loss in the very low birth weight survivor', *Proceedings of the Scientific Meeting of the British Association of Audiological Physicians and Community Paediatric Group*, Department of Audiology and Education of the Deaf, University of Manchester, Manchester

Ives, L.A. and Morris, T. (1978) 'The creation and subsequent development of a diagnostic and advisory centre for hearing-impaired pupils with particular reference to the multiply-handicapped', *J. Brit. Assn. Teachers of the Deaf, 2(2)*, 61-4

Jurgens, M.R. (1977) *Confrontation Between the Young Deaf-blind Child and the Outer World*, Swets and Zeitlinger BV

Kershman, S.M. and Napier, D. (1982) 'Systematic procedures for eliciting and recording responses to sound stimuli in deaf-blind multihandicapped children', *Volta Review, 84(4)*, 226-37

Lloyd, L.L. (1970) 'Audiological aspect of mental retardation' in N.R. Mills (ed.), *Research in Mental Retardation*, vol. 14, Academic Press, London

MacKay, R.P. (1964) *The Yearbook of Neurology, Psychiatry and Neurosurgery*,

Yearbook Medical Publishers, Chicago

McInnes, J.M. and Treffry, J.A. (1982) *Deaf-Blind Infants and Children: A Development Guide*, Open University Press, Milton Keynes/University of Toronto Press

McIntire, M.S., Menolasino, F.J. and Wiley, J.H. (1965) 'Mongolism – some clinical aspects', *Amer. J. of Ment. Defic.*, 69, 794-800

Michaels, R.H. and Mellin, G.W. (1960) 'Prospective experience with maternal rubella and the associated congenital malformations', *Pediatrics, 26*, 209-20

Miller, J.R. (1965) 'Pediatric disorders in communication IV. Some genetic counselling problems in families with congenital hearing defect', *Volta Review*, 67, 118-23

Murphy, L.J. (1977) 'The multi-handicapped deaf child' in *Proceedings of the N.Z. Conference of Teachers of the Deaf*, Kelston, New Zealand (January)

Nance, W.E. (1976) 'Studies of hereditary deafness: present, past and future', *Volta Review, 78*, 6-11 (monograph)

Nolan, M., MaCartney, E., McArthur, K. and Rowson, V.J. (1980) 'A study of the hearing and receptive vocabulary of the trainee of an adult training centre', *J. Ment. Defic. Res., 24*, 271-86

Rigrodsky, S., Prunty, F. and Glovsky, L. (1961) 'A study of incidence, types and associated etiologies of hearing loss in an institutionalised mentally retarded population', *Training School Bulletin, 58*, 30-44

Robbins, N. (1971) 'Educational assessment of deaf-blind and auditorially and visually-impaired children: a survey' in E. Lowell and C. Rovin (eds.), *State of the Art*, California State Department of Education, Sacramento, California

Sallomi, S.J. (1966) 'Rubella in pregnancy: a review of prospective studies from the literature', *Obstetrics and Gynecology*, 27, 252

Scott, H. (1976) 'Outcome of severe birth asphyxia', *Archives of Disease in Childhood, 51*, 712

Sesterham, G. and Brueninger, H. (1977) 'Determination of hearing threshold for single frequencies from the acoustic reflex', *Audiology, 16(3)*, 201

Steiner, H. and Neligan, G. (1975) 'Perinatal cardiac arrest. Quality of the survivors', *Archives of Disease in Childhood, 50*, 696

Stemquist, G.M. (1968) 'Some behavioural characteristics of Rubella: implications for educability' in *Proceedings of the International Conference on Education of Deaf-Blind Children*, St Michielsgestel, Netherlands

Taylor, I.G., Brasier, V.J., Hine, W.D., Morris, T. and Powell, C.A. (1973) 'Some aspects of the auditory of familial hearing loss' in W. Taylor (eds.), *Disorders of Auditory Function I*, Academic Press, London

Taylor, I.G., Brasier, V.J., Chiveralls, K. and Morris, T. (1975) 'A study of causes of hearing loss in a population of deaf children with special reference to genetic factors', *J. Laryng. and Otol.,* 87, 899-914

Taylor, I.G. (1981) 'Medicine and education', *J. Brit. Assn. Teachers of the Deaf*, 5(5), 134-43

Thompson, G., Wilson, W.R. and Moore, J.M. (1979) 'Application of visual reinforcement audiometry (VRA) to low functioning children', *J. Sp. Hearing Disorders, 44*, 80-90

Thomson, A.J., Searle, M. and Russell, G. (1977) 'Quality of survival in severe birth asphyxia', *Archives of Disease in Childhood, 52*, 620

Tucker, I.G. (1978) 'The incidence of hearing-impairment and trends in the hearing impaired school population', *J. Brit. Assn. Teachers of the Deaf*, 2(2), 43-7

Vernon, M. (1969) *Multiply Handicapped Deaf Children: Medical, Educational and Psychological Considerations*, Research Monograph, Council for Exceptional Children, Washington, DC

Yannet, H. (1964) 'Mental retardation' in W.E. Nelson (ed.), *Textbook in Paediatrics* (8th edn), W.B. Saunders, Philadelphia

INDEX

acoustic environment, educational 306
acoustic feedback 192-7
acoustic gain 215-16, 218, 220, 223, 289, 299-302
acoustic reflex testing 80-1
   see also electroacoustic impedance
adapting to having a hearing-impaired child 119-21
additional handicap
   aetiological factors 381-9
   educational provision 392-9
American National Standards Institute (ANSI) 220-2
amplification *see* hearing aids
amplification systems for education
   auditory training unit 131
   electromagnetic induction 244-6
   FM radio transmission: type 1 radio system 246-56; type 2 radio system 256-65
   group hearing aid 240-1
   infra-red system 241-4
asphyxia 388
audiogram 46-7
auropalpebral reflex (APR) 13
auxiliary aids to hearing
   radio set aids 282
   telephone 282-3
   television 277-82
   viewdata services 283-5

behavioural observation audiometry (BOA) 392
behavioural tests *see* tests of hearing
British Standards Institute (BSI) 218-20

communication methods
   acoupedic 316-17
   auditory-oral 316-17
   auditory-visual 316
   British Sign Language (BSL) 315
   child progress 321-2
   controversies about 318-20
   cued speech 315-16
   fingerspelling 315
   manual English 315

   Paget Gorman 316
   signed English 315
   signing exact English (SEE) 316
   signs supporting English 316
counselling *see* parent
couplers 207-15

deafness
   and mental retardation 389-92
deafness syndromes
   Jervell and Lange-Nielson's 384
   Klippel-Fiel 382
   Pendred's 384
   Treacher Collin 384
   Usher's 384
   Waardenburg's 384
deterioration of hearing 306-7
distortion 227-34
   see also harmonic distortion
dynamic range 302-3

ear
   cochlea 5-6
   middle 4
   pinna 4
earmould
   acoustics 187-9
   as part of the hearing-aid system 136-8
   damping 192
   horn effects 192
   management 186-7
   precision fitting 175-84
   recent developments in materials 197-200
   requirements of 172-3
   types of material: indirect 173-5; instant 173
   types of mould 184-6
   venting 190
earmould simulator 212-13
   see also Zwislocki coupler 213
educational audiologist 1-3, 109
educational management
   advising ordinary school teachers 368-9
   ongoing assessments 369-77

educational placement
    factors influencing mainstream
        placement: child 366-8; school
        364-5; teacher and teacher
        style 365-6
    legislation 359-60
    philosophy 361-4
educational provision
    children with multiple handicaps
        392-9
    legislation 359-60
    mainstream 355-8
    peripatetic teachers 357
    pre-schoolers 357-8
    special classes 356-7
    special schools 352-5
electric response audiometry
    brain stem electric response
        (BSER) 36-7, 101
    electrocochleography 36
    post-auricular muscle response
        17, 36
    slow vertex cortical potential
        36
electroacoustic impedance
    bridge 67-8
    compliance 66-7
    concept of 65-6
    gradient 78-80
    stapedial reflex 80-1; contra-
        lateral stimulation 81; ipsi-
        lateral stimulation 81; testing
        for 81-3
    tympanometry 68; eustachean
        tube dysfunction 75;
        grommets 78; middle ear
        fluid 75-6; neonate 74-5;
        normal 68-73; ossicular dis-
        continuity 76; otosclerosis
        76-7; perforation 77-8; scarred
        or flaccid membrane 76
electromagnetic induction 165-7,
    244-6, 261-2, 283

frequency specificity
    in behavioural testing, 27, 39-40
functional hearing loss
    causes and management 102
    counting test 100
    electric response audiometry 101;
        see also 36-7
    identification 94-8
    impedance and stapedial reflex
        thresholds 97

interview 94
pointing test 98
prevalence 93-4
pure-tone and speech audio-
    metry 95-8
say test 99
sex differential 94
sound localisation 97-8
Stenger test 101

harmonic distortion 219-20, 221-2,
    228-34
    see also distortion
hearing aid
    as a system 136; aid controls
        157-64, 165; amplifier 155-7;
        battery 138-46; earmould
        136-8 *see also under* earmould;
        earphone receiver 167-9;
        lead 164-5; microphone
        146-55; telecoil 165-7, 244-6,
        261-2, 283
    distortion 219-20, 221-2, 227-34
    effects of environment on 236-8
    fitting procedures: dynamic range
        302-3; loudness discomfort
        measures 291-3; prescriptive
        procedures 294, 298-302;
        relevance of speech signal
        295-8; selective procedures
        294; use of audiological infor-
        mation 290-1
    hand held test unit 204-6
    hearing aid test box 206-12,
        216-18
    influence of wearer on 225-7
    KEMAR 213
    management following fitting
        134, 200-4, 307-9
    output limitation: automatic gain
        control 160-4; peak clipping
        158-60; *see also* hearing aid as
        a system — aid controls
    performance: couplers 207-15;
        2cc coupler 211; ear simulator
        212-13; Zwislocki coupler 213
    real ear-v-coupler measurements
        214-15
    selection: acoustic environment
        306; binaural/monaural fitting
        305-6; body worn or post-
        aural 303-4; deterioration in
        hearing 306-7; electroacoustic
        properties 304-5

standard measures: American National Standards Institute (ANSI) 220-2; British Standards Institute (BSI) 218-20; definitions 215-16; Hearing Aid Industry Conference (HAIC) 222-3; International Electrotechnical Commission (IEC) 218-20
subjective assessment 202-4
Hearing Aid Industry Conference (HAIC) 222-3
hearing-impairment
  neonatal screening 13-17; auditory response cradle 14; crib-o-gram 14; electric response audiometry 17; high risk register 15; reflex responses 13
hearing loss
  conductive 48
  sensori-neural 49
heredity and deafness 382

initial reactions to hearing-impairment
  guilt 117-19
  relief 113-15
  shock 111-13
  stress 115-17
  why? 110-11
International Electrotechnical Commission (IEC) 218-20

Jervell and Lange-Neilson's Syndrome 384

Klippel-Fiel Syndrome 382

language development
  critical period for 10
  hearing-impaired children 325-32
  interaction measures 340-7
  lipreading 335-7
  normally hearing children 323-5
  parents' role 332-5
  play 337-40
late detection of deafness 9
lipreading 335-7

mainstreaming *see* educational placement
masking
  air conduction 52-6
  bone conduction 56

  examples of 59-65
  how to mask 56-9
  need for 51-2
  stimulus 54
  when to mask air conduction 54-5
  when to mask bone conduction 56
meningitis 384-5
mental handicap 92
multi-sensory impairment 396

neonatal screening 12-19

parent-child interaction 340-7
  see also language development
parent counselling
  client centred approach 122-3
  counsellor qualifications 124-5
  do's and don'ts 126-7
  interpersonal skills 127-9
  practice 124
  skill areas 125-6
  theory 121
  see also adapting, initial reactions
Pendred's Syndrome 384
prematurity 388-9
psychological tests 374

radio set aids 282
reading 371-4
reflex responses 13
reverberation 236-8
rhesus incompatibility 387-8
rubella 385-7

social adjustment 374-7
sound waves 6-8
speech
  characteristics of speech signal 295-7
  see also speech tests
speech tests of hearing
  AB lists 87
  Auditory Numbers Test 84
  Doll Vocabulary List 84
  5-sound Test 84
  Manchester Junior Word Lists 87
  masking for 89-90
  New Manchester Picture Test 85-6
  Word Intelligibility by Picture Identification Test 85

telephone aids 282-3
television aids 277-82
tests of hearing
    behavioural tests: co-operative
        31-3; distraction 19; perform-
        ance 33-4
    diagnostic procedures: aims 35;
        behavioural responses 37-9;
        brain stem electric response
        audiometry 36; electric
        response audiometry 36;
        narrow band noise 40; warble
        tones 40-3
    frequency specificity 24-7,
        39-40
    pitfalls of the distraction test
        26-31

pure tone audiometry 44-52;
    air conduction (diagnosis)
    46-8; air conduction
    (screening) 44; bone conduc-
    tion 48-52
Treacher Collins Syndrome 384

Usher's Syndrome 384

vibro-tactile thresholds 49
viewdata services 283-5
visual reinforcement audiometry
    (VRA) 391

Waardenburg's Syndrome 384

Zwislocki coupler 213